Handbook of
HEADACHE MANAGEMENT

A Practical Guide to Diagnosis and
Treatment of Head, Neck, and Facial Pain

Second Edition

Handbook of
HEADACHE MANAGEMENT

A Practical Guide to Diagnosis and
Treatment of Head, Neck, and Facial Pain
Second Edition

Joel R. Saper, M.D.

Stephen D. Silberstein, M.D.

C. David Gordon, M.D.

Robert L. Hamel, P.A.-C

with Sahar Swidan, Pharm.D.

LIPPINCOTT WILLIAMS & WILKINS
A **Wolters Kluwer** Company
Philadelphia · Baltimore · New York · London
Buenos Aires · Hong Kong · Sydney · Tokyo

Publisher: Kathleen Gaffney
Production Manager: Wendi L. Anderson-Neenan
Production Editor: Jeda Taylor
Copy Editors: Eileen Creeger and Eric Branger

Copyright © 1999
Lippincott Williams & Wilkins
351 West Camden Street
Baltimore, Maryland 21201-2436 USA

Copyright © by Lippincott Williams & Wilkins, Inc.: 1999

Accurate indications, adverse reactions, and dosage schedules for drugs are provided in this book, but it is possible that they may change. The reader is urged to review the package information data of the manufacturers of the medications mentioned.

Printed in the United States of America

First edition 1993
Second edition 1999

Library of Congress Cataloging-in-Publication Data

Handbook of headache management : a practical guide to diagnosis and treatment of
    head, neck, and facial pain.—2nd ed. / Joel R. Saper . . . [et al.]
        p.   cm.
    Includes bibliographical references and index.
    ISBN 0-781-72048-6
    1. Headache—Handbooks, manuals, etc. I. Saper, Joel R.
    [DNLM: 1. Facial Pain—diagnosis—handbooks.   2. Facial Pain—therapy—
handbooks.   3. Headache—diagnosis—handbooks.   4. Headache—therapy—
handbooks. WL 39 H236]
    RB128.H35 1999
    616.8'491—dc20
    DNLM/DLC
    for Library of Congress   92-23747
                                                                                          CIP

99 00
2 3 4 5 6 7 8 9 10

Preface to the Second Edition

This second edition of *Handbook of Headache Management,* like the first, represents a commitment to physicians and other health care professionals who treat headache disorders and require a practical, efficient manual that addresses the key features of diagnosis and management. This edition, like its predecessor, is not designed to provide an encyclopedic reference for all aspects of head and neck pain. Instead, it assumes some understanding of the problem and relies upon the more complete texts that are increasingly available to the student and practitioner. Some of the more authoritative texts are listed under the General Suggested Readings section. This edition of *Handbook of Headache Management* will provide the key and updated information necessary to diagnose and treat headache, hopefully offering it in a practical and highly usable manner.

Since the first edition of the book, major advances have occurred in both diagnosis and treatment of headache. The most important of these advances have been included in this edition. Though headache management is still not a "mainstream" discipline, a growing number of well-trained, dedicated, and scholarly professionals have chosen to pursue the field of headache management. This interest parallels the growing recognition that pain therapy has been a sadly ignored aspect of medical care, fraught with prejudice, mismanagement, and neglect. Pain and those who suffer from it have not historically benefited from the same scholarly vigor and therapeutic intensity that have been accorded far less pervasive and disabling conditions. Headache, as well as the other painful disorders, has traditionally been shrouded in myth, mistreatment, and neglect.

The patient with recurring or persisting headache is likely to encounter an assembly line of medical care and services and an array of explanations and treatments, many of which are narrowly focused along the lines of subspecialty care and training. From sinus disease to allergy, from mental duress to neck problems, from yeast purging to colon purging, the headache patient travels along a pathway of costly and sometimes damaging explanations and therapies that often aggravate the problem, delay the diagnosis, and complicate the eventual treatment. Everyone is frustrated, from the patient to the physician to the payor.

This book approaches the problem of headache from a neurobiological perspective, believing that most cases of headache reflect a biological disorder. The authors of this book fully recognize the importance and contribution of psychiatric, behavioral, and personality factors, many of which may share neuropsychiatric mechanisms with headache. However, we believe that the headache disorders, for the most part, arise as a result of biological factors. Contributing or coexisting psychological and behavioral issues are frequently found and must be treated. An overemphasis on these factors has traditionally ignored the likelihood that predisposing biology is the fundamental factor that determines who will have primary headaches and who will not.

In this edition, as in the first, the reader will note that major portions are presented in outline form, with an abundance of tables. It is hoped that this will facilitate the accessibility and usefulness of the material. The reader will encounter the word "selected" before various listings. The use of this word designates that an arbitrary selection of items has been made. The lists are not necessarily exhaustive and should be used only as a reference and a guide. When appropriate, additional information from various other authoritative sources and references must be obtained to supplement the information presented here.

Finally, on a philosophical note, recurring head pain, as we now know it, is most often a chronic illness. The wise clinician must avoid the cynicism and bias that have historically influenced illnesses that are not fully understood at the time treatment is required. The integrity of complaints must be trusted, unless compelling support forces an alternate attitude.

Patients suffering from headache and related painful disorders are often desperate and complex, frequently rejected by the health care system and often injured and compromised by a long list of failed and inappropriate treatments. Treating headache and pain is a far more challenging test of clinical skill and vigor than generally recognized. Taking the patient's symptoms to heart is at the core of prudent medical care. Ultimately, if skillful and compassionate physicians take up their cause, even those persons with illnesses and symptoms that are not fully understood can be treated effectively or at least benefit from care.

Joel R. Saper, M.D.
Stephen Silberstein, M.D.
C. David Gordon, M.D.
Robert L. Hamel, P.A.-C
Sahar Swidan, Pharm.D.

Acknowledgments

The authors wish to acknowledge the following individuals:

Debbie Johnston, who for over 12 years has served as my personal transcriptionist, for her diligent and skillful technical assistance, remarkable endurance, and most of all for her sustaining commitment, loyalty, talent, charm, and friendship;

Alvin E. Lake III, Ph.D., a founding member of the Michigan Head•Pain & Neurological Institute, with special thanks for the trust and friendship, and particularly for the knowledge, wisdom, long hours, and perspective that have been shared with colleagues, and without which the Institute and its work would never have been the same;

Grace Lobel, for tireless support and understanding beyond simple description, and for more than 18 years of friendship, help, devotion, and extraordinary patience;

Marjorie Winters, R.N., B.S.N., for her skillful and diligent help with this manuscript, for over 18 years of prudent advice, endurance, dedication, clinical judgment, and professional dignity, and

Our many other colleagues, friends, and our families for what they endure to allow such an effort to happen.

Joel R. Saper, M.D., F.A.C.P., F.A.A.N., 1998

About the Authors

Joel R. Saper, M.D., F.A.C.P., F.A.A.N., is the founder and Director of the Michigan Head•Pain & Neurological Institute in Ann Arbor, Michigan (1978), and its Head Pain Treatment Unit at Chelsea Community Hospital (1979), the nation's first comprehensive, accredited headache treatment program. A Clinical Professor of Medicine (Neurology) at Michigan State University, Dr. Saper is a past President of the American Association for the Study of Headache, a course director for the American Academy of Neurology, and a past or current member of the Board of numerous medical organizations, including the American Pain Society and the American Academy of Pain Medicine. Dr. Saper is the editor and primary author of "Topics in Pain Management," a national, monthly professional newsletter. He has authored or coauthored seven medical books, in addition to over 100 published medical chapters, medical articles, and abstracts. Dr. Saper is an invited speaker throughout the world and has presented his work internationally to medical and other professional forums. In 1995, Dr. Saper was appointed by the Michigan legislature as Chair of the Michigan Council on Pain and since 1993 has coordinated the congressional legislative efforts of the American Pain Society, the American Association for the Study of Headache, and the American Academy of Pain Medicine. Dr. Saper is the recipient of numerous clinical and teaching awards. He is a graduate of the University of Illinois School of Medicine and trained in neurology at the University of Michigan and received his board certification in neurology in 1975 and in pain medicine in 1996.

Stephen D. Silberstein, M.D., F.A.C.P., is the Director of the Comprehensive Headache Center at The Jefferson Headache Center at Thomas Jefferson University Hospital and Professor of Neurology at Thomas Jefferson University in Philadelphia, Pennsylvania. He received his M.D. degree from the University of Pennsylvania, where he also completed his medicine and neurology training. Dr. Silberstein received his board certification in neurology in 1975. He completed a Special Fellowship in Neurology at the National Hospital for Nervous Diseases at Queen Square, London, and was a research associate in the Toxicology Laboratory of Clinical Science at the National Institute of Mental Health in Bethesda, Maryland. Dr. Silberstein is a member of the Board and Scientific Program Chairman of the American Association for the Study of Headache. Dr. Silberstein is coeditor of the 6th edition of Wolff's *Headache*. He has presented his scientific work throughout the world and is a frequent invited lecturer at medical and professional gatherings and educational forums.

C. David Gordon, M.D., is a member of the medical faculty of the Michigan Head•Pain & Neurological Institute and is an attending physician to the Head•Pain Treatment Unit at Chelsea Community Hospital. Dr. Gordon is a graduate of Boston University School of Medicine and completed his residency training in internal medicine at Faulkner Hospital in Boston, Massachusetts. He spent two years in specialty practice at the John R. Graham Headache Centre in Boston, where he also completed a fellowship in headache management. He has written medical articles and contributed to chapters on migraine and its pathophysiology and recently coauthored several books, including one of Brazil's first textbooks on primary headache disorders. Dr. Gordon has particular interest and experience in the computer application of headache education and clinical care and serves as a primary clinical research and educational resource at the Institute on the integration of the principles of internal medicine to the treatment and evaluation of headache disorders.

Robert L. Hamel, P.A.-C, is currently a clinical associate at the Michigan Head•Pain & Neurological Institute in Ann Arbor and clinical liaison and member of the Management Team at the Head•Pain Treatment Unit at Chelsea Community Hospital. He has extensive experience in the evaluation, treatment, and clinical coordination of head-injured patients and is the Clinical Coordinator of the Head Injury Program at the Institute. Mr. Hamel received his Bachelor of Science degree and Physician's Assistant degree from Mercy College in Detroit, Michigan, and has a Bachelor of Arts degree in Psychology and a Master's degree in Management. Mr. Hamel's work has achieved national recognition, and he is frequently an invited guest lecturer on state and national levels, presenting educational seminars and lectures on headache and head injury topics.

Sahar Swidan, Pharm.D., R.Ph., obtained her Doctor of Pharmacy degree from the University of Michigan, where she also completed a two-year postdoctoral fellowship. She is currently the Director of Pharmaceutical Services at Chelsea Community Hospital, where she also serves as clinical pharmacist on the inpatient Head Pain Unit. Dr. Swidan is a Clinical Assistant Professor of Pharmacy at the University of Michigan, President of the Washtenaw County Pharmacists Association, and a chairperson and member of numerous other professional societies. She has published numerous articles in standard medical journals and is a frequently invited lecturer on the topic of pharmacotherapy in the areas of headache and pain, internal medicine, and neurology.

Contents

To Our Clinical Colleagues

At the heart of responsible and qualified medical care is the clinician who, armed with wisdom, compassion, and experience, applies the art of medicine to the care of patients. Though it is the scientist who must define objectively the biological markers of disease, it is the clinician who is called upon to give relief and guidance, even in the absence of a charted course.

Indeed, the distinction between objective and subjective disease may not be defined so much by the validity of the symptoms, but by the scientific sophistication during the era in which the disorder occurs. And when circumstances demand a thoughtful response in the absence of objective definition, it is the clinician who must rally to vigorously enlist the most creative of resources to bring comfort and direction to those who seek help.

What makes so difficult the task of the clinician who endeavors to manage pain is the need to master the diagnosis of hundreds of conditions that can produce it and then to treat this disruptive disorder in the absence of a full understanding of the process, sufficient tools to overcome it, and minimal knowledge of the complexities of human suffering.

Since our first edition in 1993, the influence of managed care has had a major impact on what has already been a difficult and at times impossible challenge. Economic forces have challenged and threatened, and at times clearly obstructed, the effort to reach out to this difficult and complex population of human beings and treat what is often their serious affliction. To my colleagues, I implore you to stand up and defend the principles of medicine and the culture of our profession, which has from its origins advocated on behalf of the patient and subjected the physician to severe risks in pursuit of that commitment. While sensitivity to the economic realities and cost is appropriate, physicians must confront the changes that are occurring in health care and resist those that compromise our ability to provide effective care to our patients. If managed care is to survive, then it must learn to influence costs through prudent practice innovations and long-term concepts regarding chronic illness. Short-term savings derived largely from devices to arbitrarily reduce utilization and deny care and access will not succeed and will ultimately prompt greater expenditures from a population of patients who often worsen when their condition is either treated improperly or neglected. Managed care may well have a very powerful and positive influence on the care of headache patients over time. But first, managed care must recognize that long-term savings can be achieved only if proper care is made available to patients with chronic and complex illnesses at a time and in a way to assure long-term clinical and cost-effectiveness and before the costs of mismanagement and neglect have taken their toll.

JRS, 1998

General Suggested Reading

Dalessio D, Silberstein SD (Eds). *Wolff's Headache and Other Head Pain*, 6th Edition. New York, Oxford University Press, 1993.

Goadsby PJ, Silberstein SD. *Headache (Blue Books of Practical Neurology)*. Boston, Butterworth-Heinemeann, 1997.

Headache and Facial Pain (continuum): A Program of the American Academy of Neurology. Silverstein SD, Lipton RB, Saper JR, Solomon S, Young WB (faculty), Volume 1, No. 5, November 1995.

Lance JW. *Mechanism and Management of Headache*, 5th Edition. London, Butterworth Heinemeann, 1993.

Markus DA. Migraine and tension-type headaches: The questionable validity of current classification systems. *Clin J Pain*, 8:28–36, 1992.

Mathew NT (Ed). *Neurologic Clinics: Advances in Headache*. Volume 15, No. 1. Philadelphia, WB Saunders, February 1997.

Olesen J. Classification and diagnostic criteria for headache disorders, cranial neuralgias, and headache pain. *Cephalalgia*, 8 (supp); 7:1–96, 1988.

Olesen J, Edvinson L (Eds). *Basic Mechanisms of Headache*. Amsterdam, Elsevier Science Publishers, 1988.

Olesen J, Tfelt-Hansen P, Welch KMA (Eds). *The Headaches*. New York, Raven Press, 1993.

Raskin NH. *Headache*, 2nd Edition. New York, Churchill Livingstone, 1988.

Rose FC (Ed). *Handbook of Clinical Neurology*, Volume 48. Amsterdam, Elsevier Science Publishers, 1986.

Saper JR. Changing perspectives on chronic headache. *Clin J Pain*, 2:19–28, 1986.

Saper JR. *Headache Disorders: Current Concepts and Treatment Strategies*, Littleton, Massachusetts, Wright-PSG Publishers, 1983.

Silberstein SD (Ed). *Intractable headache: Inpatient and outpatient treatment strategies. Neurology* (supp 2), March 1992.

Welch KMA. Drug therapy of migraine. *N Engl J Med*, 329:1476–1483, 1993.

1

Epidemiology, Cost Implications, and Classification of Headache

I. Epidemiology

Headache is a widespread and costly public health problem. In men, the lifetime prevalence for headache of any kind is 93%, and for women it is up to 99% (Rasmussen, 1991). Headache prevalence in children increases from 39% at age 6 to 70% by age 15. In a recent report from the Centers for Disease Control (1990), a 60% increase in the prevalence of migraine during the years 1980–1989 was noted. Eight percent (8%) of sufferers are hospitalized at least once yearly, and 4% of men and 3% of women have a persistently impaired existence. Subsequent studies lend support to the view that the prevalence of migraine is increasing (Sillanpää, 1994; Stang, 1992).

Among migraine sufferers, 86% of women and 82% of men report some disability with each attack. Thirty-one percent (31%) of persons with headache have regular, periodic functional impairment. Moreover, it is estimated that 1 million days of missed school and over 150 million days of lost work per year are attributable to headache. Lost productivity estimates for the United States work force per year range from $6.5 to $17.2 billion. This compares to just $2.6 billion lost to diabetes (Lipton, 1994; Osterhaus, 1992). Migraine accounts for 5.7 million days of restricted activity per month. Thirty-one percent (31%) of women with headache and 70% of men lose six or more days of work per year. It is estimated that the annual cost of a migraine sufferer to an employer is from $5256 to $6864 for men and from $3168 to $3600 for women.

A recent study of headache in a large managed care organization (Clouse, 1994) demonstrated that headache patients submitted twice as many medical claims, twice as many psychiatric claims, four times as many emercency room (ER) visits, and 2.5 times the medication claims compared to the same health mainenance organization (HMO) patients without severe headache. These patients underwent five times more diagnostic procedures and incurred seven times more diagnostic procedure costs as did non-headache patients. A significant portion of these increased costs was attributable not only to migraine itself but to the comorbid conditions that accompany many headache patients. In just 18 months, this population of 1300 HMO patients cost the HMO $1.5 million more in health care costs than 1300 non-migraine HMO patients.

Despite the painful, costly, and disabling impact of headache, many patients with headache do not seek medical care. Sixty percent (60%) of females and 70% of males with typical migraine have never been properly diagnosed (Lipton, 1994).

II. Classification

The *primary headaches,* i.e., migraine and cluster headaches, are those in which no consistently identified organic cause can be determined. As far as we now know, they reflect intrinsic disturbances of the brain's pain system or perhaps an intrinsic heightened sensitivity to intrinsic and extrinsic stimuli. In other words, the primary headache disorders reflect inherited or acquired disturbances of the brain and its relationship to the rest of the body. *Secondary headaches* are headaches that arise as a symptom of another disorder. Over 300 possible organic causes of headache are known.

Until the late 1980s, the primary classification of headache was based upon the Ad Hoc Committee Report, published in 1962. However, following an international effort engineered by Professor Jes Olesen of Copenhagen, the International Headache Society (IHS) has proposed a new classification on headache, informally known as the International Classification. This comprehensive document attempts to reconcile the many and complex aspects of headache into a usable system. Its ultimate acceptance and usability remain to be defined, but it has, if nothing else, comprehensively organized headache for the first time (see Table 1.1).

The new classification of headache gives more precision to the diagnosis of headache in general, and migraine specifically. *Common migraine* is now called *migraine without aura* and is defined in terms of duration, quality, and associated findings accompanying each attack.

Classic migraine is now called *migraine with aura,* and the features of the aura are delineated in great detail.

Tension-type headache is the term for what has previously been called tension headache, muscle contraction headache, stress headache, and ordinary headache. The classification distinguishes between patients with episodic (acute) tension-type headaches and chronic tension-type headaches, with subclassifications based upon the presence or absence of increased tenderness of the pericranial muscles or increased electromyographic (EMG) activity.

Cluster headache and chronic paroxysmal hemicrania are also classified, as are a variety of miscellaneous conditions and headache phenomena. Thirteen categories of headache are subdivided into 129 different subtypes.

TABLE 1.1. **NEW INTERNATIONAL HEADACHE SOCIETY CLASSIFICATION OF HEADACHE**

1. Migraine
1.1 Migraine without aura
1.2 Migraine with aura
1.3 Ophthalmoplegic migraine
1.4 Retinal migraine
1.5 Childhood periodic syndromes that may not be precursors to or associated with migraine
1.6 Complications of migraine
1.7 Migrainous disorder not fulfilling above criteria

2. Tension-type headache
2.1 Episodic tension-type headache
2.2 Chronic tension-type headache
2.3 Headache of the tension-type not fulfilling above criteria

3. Cluster headache and chronic paroxysmal hemicrania
3.1 Cluster headache
3.2 Chronic paroxysmal hemicrania
3.3 Cluster headache-like disorder not fulfilling above criteria

4. Miscellaneous headaches unassociated with structural lesion
4.1 Idiopathic stabbing headache
4.2 External compression headache
4.3 Cold stimulus headache
4.4 Benign cough headache
4.5 Benign exertional headache
4.6 Headache associated with sexual activity

5. Headache associated with head trauma
5.1 Acute post-traumatic headache
5.2 Chronic post-traumatic headache

6. Headache associated with vascular disorders
6.1 Acute ischemic cerebrovascular disease
6.2 Intracranial hematoma
6.3 Subarachnoid hemorrhage
6.4 Unruptured vascular malformation
6.5 Arteritis
6.6 Carotid or vertebral artery pain
6.7 Venous thrombosis
6.8 Arterial hypertension
6.9 Headache associated with other vascular disorder

7. Headache associated with nonvascular intracranial disorder

7.1 High cerebrospinal fluid pressure
7.2 Low cerebrospinal fluid pressure
7.3 Intracranial infection
7.4 Intracranial sarcoidosis and other noninfectious inflammatory diseases
7.5 Headache related to intrathecal injections
7.6 Intracranial neoplasm
7.7 Headache associated with other intracranial disorder

8. Headache associated with substances or their withdrawal
8.1 Headache induced by acute substance use or exposure
8.2 Headache induced by chronic substance use or exposure
8.3 Headache from substance withdrawal (acute use)
8.4 Headache from substance withdrawal (chronic use)
8.5 Headache associated with substances but with uncertain mechanism

9. Headache associated with noncephalic infection
9.1 Viral infection
9.2 Bacterial infection
9.3 Headache related to other infection

10. Headache associated with metabolic disorder
10.1 Hypoxia
10.2 Hypoercapnia
10.3 Mixed hypoxia and hypercapnia
10.4 Hypoglycemia
10.5 Dialysis
10.6 Headache related to other metabolic abnormality

11. Headache or facial pain associated with disorder of cranium, neck, eyes, ears, nose, sinuses, teeth, mouth, or other facial or cranial structures
11.1 Cranial bone
11.2 Neck
11.3 Eyes
11.4 Ears
11.5 Nose and sinuses
11.6 Teeth, jaws, and related structures
11.7 Temporomandibular joint disease

continued

TABLE 1.1.   **NEW INTERNATIONAL HEADACHE SOCIETY CLASSIFICATION OF HEADACHE**

12. Cranial neuralgias, nerve trunk pain, and deafferentation pain	12.5 Superior laryngeal neuralgia
12.1 Persistent (in contrast to tic-like) pain of cranial nerve origin	12.6 Occipital neuralgia
12.2 Trigeminal neuralgia	12.7 Central causes of head and facial pain other than tic douloureux
12.3 Glossopharyngeal neuralgia	12.8 Facial pain not fulfilling criteria in groups 11 or 12
12.4 Nervus intermedius neuralgia	**13. Headache not classifiable**

References

Clouse JS, Osterhaus JH. Health care resource use and costs associated with migraine in a managed care setting. *Ann Pharmacother,* 28:659–664, 1994.

Linet MS, Stewart WF, Celentano DE, et al. An epidemiological study of headache among adolescents and young adults. *JAMA,* 261:2211–2216, 1989.

Lipton RB, Stewart WF: Epidemiology and comorbidity of migraine. (In) *Headache: The Blue Book of Practical Neurology.* PJ Goadsby and SD Silberstein (Eds). Boston, Butterworth-Heinemeann, 1997.

Lipton RB, Stewart WF. Prevalence and impact of migraine. (In) *Neurologic Clinics,* NT Mathew (Ed). Pgs 1–13, Philadelphia, WB Saunders, February, 1997.

Lipton RB, Stewart WF, Vonkorff M. The burden of migraine: A review of costs to society. *Pharmacoeconomics,* 6:215–221, 1994.

Olesen J. The classification and diagnosis of headache disorders. (In) *Neurologic Clinics,* NT Mathew (Ed). Pgs 793–799, Philadelphia, WB Saunders, November, 1990.

Rasmussen BK, Jensen R, Olesen JA. A population-based analysis of the diagnostic criteria of the International Headache Society. *Cephalalgia,* 11:129, 1991.

Sillanpaa M. Headache in children. (In) *Headache Classification and Epidemiology.* J Olesen (Ed). Pg 273, New York, Raven, 1994.

Stang PE, Yanagihara T, Swanson JW, et al. Incidence of migraine headaches: A population-based study of Olmstead County, Minnesota. *Neurology,* 42:1657, 1992.

Ziegler DK. Headache: Public health problem. (In) *Neurologic Clinics.* NT Mathew (Ed). Pgs 781–792, Philadelphia, WB Saunders, November, 1990.

2

Stratification of Headache Care and Outcome Results

I. Introduction

The quality of headache care is often inconsistent and variable and it is frequently devoid of state-of-the-art strategies and interventions[1]. As in other chronic illnesses, delay of proper diagnosis and treatment increases costs through greater utilization, development of iatrogenic sequelae, and illness progression. To control costs related to headache disorders, it will be necessary to establish a concept of care which assures that complex cases of headache are promptly triaged to the clinical setting that can provide the most effective and timely treatment for the complexity and severity of the case at hand. It will be mandatory as well to apply evidenced-based interventions.

II. Background
A. Training Deficiency

Medical school and standard postgraduate training programs provide less than adequate training for the wide range of headache disorders, a circumstance which lends itself to inappropriate and ineffective treatments for headache patients, particularly those with complex disorders. Most practicing physicians possess only rudimentary pain care skills, sufficient to treat perhaps the most straightforward, uncomplicated cases, but not the more complex ones. Continuing medical education (CME) courses on headache care offer the most effective means available to advance the skills of interested professionals, but clearly these do not reach the majority of those who treat chronic headache cases in the United States.

B. Failure to View Chronic Headache as a Complex Disorder

Adding to this problem is the underrecognition that chronic headache disorders are often complex, multifactorial conditions that affect individuals in whom pain is deeply integrated into a fabric of other important coexisting phenomena, which include psychological and behavioral, addictive, socioeconomic, and others (Breslau, 1991, 1994, 1995; Lipton, 1997; Merikangas, 1993, 1997). Advanced and complicated headache cases (as distinct from straightforward, periodic headache cases) frequently affect

---

[1]*Excerpted from* Strategic Stratification of Headache Care: A Managed Care Concept for Cost-Effective Headache Treatment, *Joel R. Saper (in preparation).*

emotionally and physiologically complex individuals, many of whom suffer from comorbid contributing factors which influence the primary headache illness and confound treatment strategies. Moreover, as in other complex, chronic disorders, headache conditions are often progressive, worsening over time, either naturally or as a result of poor treatment or the failure to impose secondary preventive measures at critical times in the clinical course.

Indeed, this is the very heart of the problem: *headache disorders often span well beyond a simple physiological symptom but instead reflect the intermingling of numerous confounding variables and clinical phenomena.* Failure to address these in a timely and appropriate manner often constitutes the basis of treatment failure, progressivity, and high cost.

C. Severe Pain Cannot Be Ignored

Because severe pain has such a compelling influence over behavior and well being, it cannot and will not be ignored. This prompts painful patients and families to seek service after service, treatment after treatment, and professional after professional in pursuit of relief. Even when patients reach the so-called specialist level, they may encounter professionals who have but a single "tool" (monotherapy) to treat *all* (or most) headache patients that seek their help. Each "specialist" interprets and treats head-ache through the sometimes narrow window and perspective of his/her own discipline and specialty training. The otolaryngologist performs nasal and sinus surgery or sphenopalatine blockade; the psychologist addresses stress and conflict; the allergist treats allergies; the anesthesiologist offers nerve blocks; and the neurologist prescribes pills. The services are frequently inappropriate, misdirected, and disconnected from each other. Some are harmful. Commingling psychological and physiological factors are not addressed in a manner which effectively confronts the complexity and severity of the case with the necessary coordinated and integrated services.

D. Timing Is Everything

Such a pattern of care reflects clinical chaos rather than clinical orderliness. *Complex patients often fail to receive the services they require at a time when the services can be most effectively delivered, and when well conceived and appropriate strategies can influence long-term cost and quality-of-life measures.*

III. Solutions

Finding an effective solution to this problem begins with a rethinking and restructuring of our approach to headache and pain care, as well as an increasing reliance on evidence-based service.

A. Stratified Care (Levels of Care)

A critical element is the development of an organized system of care that strategically and promptly assigns patients to the appropriate level of care based upon the identified complexity of the case being confronted. *Promptly distinguishing between the straightforward case and that which is not ordinary is a fundamental requirement.*

Headache care can be stratified into three levels.

1. Level 1 (primary care)

Level 1, primary care, should be the entry point for patients with headache disorders. The primary care physician can effectively diagnose and treat most patients with headache, offering first-line diagnostic and treatment services, consistent with his/her training and experience. At the primary care level, diagnostic assessments and treatment of uncomplicated primary and secondary headache disorders would be undertaken. When necessary, the primary care physician would triage a patient (depending upon case severity, complexity, and/or treatment responsiveness) to secondary or tertiary level care. Triaging of patients beyond primary care would be prompted by the details of the case and its clinical complexity (see Staging section).

2. Level 2 (secondary care)

Secondary care is comprised of two levels. Level 2a consists of medical specialists and subspecialists and other professionals who are trained in various disciplines which have relevance to the overall headache diagnostic or management perspective. The care provided at this level would be through either consultation or selected therapeutic/procedural intervention, the need for which should be determined in conjunction with the primary care physician who would remain in overall charge of the case.

Professionals at level 2a would include general neurologists, psychiatrists/psychologists, dental professionals, anesthesiologists, physiatrists, and others. These professionals would treat cases in which their particular discipline would be of specific value, such as headache cases requiring certain procedures, complex pharmacotherapy, or treatment of a particular comorbid illness.

Level 2b is comprised of small-sized headache clinics. In general, these are currently staffed by a physician(s), often with added experience and knowledge in headache, together with a psychologist and/or physician extenders (P.A., nurse specialists, and others). These systems contribute an added dimension of clinical experience, service coordination, and interdisciplinary service than that which is provided at a primary or consultant level.

3. Level 3 (tertiary care)

Level 3 is composed of tertiary (? quanternary) systems of care, which are comprehensive, accredited systems that provide a full and coordinated range of services for patients with complex head-ache disorders. These systems would have credentialed and experienced staffs, advanced diagnostic and treatment services within the system, and services that are coordinated and administered by recognized headache experts who oversee and manage the care. Inpatient and outpatient services are available and provided as needed.

Patients most appropriate for tertiary care include those who are treatment-resistant or refractory to standard therapies, those who require hospital-level care, those whose conditions are confounded by important comorbid and accompanying illness or behavioral disturbances, and those whose outcomes likely require rehabilitation and/or advanced, multidisciplinary interventions. Triage to this level could occur directly from primary care or from secondary levels of care, depending upon case complexity and treatment responsiveness.

IV. Triage and Staging

In order for such a system to work, it will be necessary to develop generally accepted triage guidelines. These guidelines would be developed to assist in the assignment of care to a primary, secondary, or tertiary level. This process will be simplified and measurably enhanced by the use of a staging or severity rating system to determine the complexity of a case. The operating principle of such triage guidelines would be that case complexity, as reflected by the clinical stage or rating, would be strategically matched to the level of care to which the patient is referred.

A. A Staging Tool

Staging is a severity rating. It is a means by which individual cases can be rated (staged) on the basis of their complexity, severity, and/or degree of progression. Generally, chronic illnesses can be staged using both objective and subjective markers, which indicate disease progression or the presence of advanced pathological variables and markers. The task is more challenging for headache and pain disorders because they are largely subjective conditions.

Staging offers at least three distinct advantages toward solving the current headache care dilemmas. First, staging offers a "tool" to assist the primary care physician to better assess the case and to prompt and guide the triage decision. Second, staging provides a dynamic, somewhat objectifiable measure of clinical worsening or improvement. Third, staging could establish a sound basis for determining treatment fees and projection of costs.

Various severity rating systems are possible. I (J.R.S.) propose a staging system that is based upon four key clinical parameters: frequency of significant attacks, treatment and utilization pattern, the presence or absence of comorbidity, and the presence or absence of disability. The Michigan Headache Staging System (MHSS), a system based upon these parameters, has been under development and study for several years. This concept, now in its most usable form, provides the foundation for identifying case complexity, progression, and improvement by utilizing the same key clinical variables that influence treatment decisions for headache patients. This offers an important advantage, since it assists the primary physician in identifying those clinical variables which must be considered to effectively treat patients with headache.

Triage guidelines can be based upon the staging level (as well as other markers), so that various clinical stages would prompt referral to the appropriate level of care, just as staging levels for other chronic illnesses prompt specific treatment interventions and strategies. Lower stages would ordinarily remain at a primary level, whereas higher stages would more likely be triaged to a secondary or tertiary level. (Each managed care system could determine for itself which stages are to be treated at which level in their system, although standardization would be desirable.)

Staging might also afford a rational basis for realistic and responsible fee schedules and cost determinations. The cost of treating the headache patient is clearly a reflection of the time, staffing, training, overhead, and services required. These, in turn, are determined by the complexity and severity of the case (frequency of attacks, comorbidities, addictive disease, disability, etc.). An effective staging tool must accurately reflect cost-sensitive clinical variables.

An added advantage of an effective staging system is that it is likely to provide a dynamic measure of progression and improvement so that *upstaging* and *downstaging* reflect clinical worsening or improvement, respectively. Other advantages include those for research, outcome studies, and more.

B. Guidelines of Care at Each Level

Based upon the above model, appropriate care guidelines can be established for each of the three levels of care. The interdisciplinary disagreements that now plague any attempt to develop broadly accepted guidelines of care for headache might be less significant, since it will be easier to determine guidelines for care *at each level of care,* rather than across the entire spectrum of the multidisciplinary care system. Consensus should be more easily achieved.

V. Cost Implications, Opportunities, and Evidenced-Based Treatment

The cost to treat cases along the broad range of complexity and service needs varies considerably. In a well functioning and ideal system, service costs and fees should directly reflect the complexity of the case. More advanced cases require more time-intensive intervention, more experienced professionals, and often multidisciplinary services to confront the more numerous and severe clinical variables and comorbidities. Since expenditures should directly reflect the complexity and severity of the case, an effective staging tool would provide a basis for projecting service costs and establishing fees. The cost of care and fees could be estimated and negotiated based upon the stage, thus providing a reasonable and objective parameter for these calculations.

Dr. Dennis C. Turk, Ph.D., the John and Emma Bonica professor of anesthesiology and pain research at the University of Washington School of Medicine, has summarized data from meta-analyses reflecting research data on the effectiveness of tertiary treatment of patients with chronic pain (not specifically headache) (Turk, 1996). Based on over 65 published studies (3089 patients), 45–65% of patients treated at tertiary care settings returned to work following treatment, compared to only 20% of patients without tertiary care. Patients receiving tertiary care required one-third the number of surgical interventions and hospitalizations, compared to patients treated with conventional medical and surgical care. Those who were referred to tertiary systems of care had a much longer history of pain (averaging more than seven years) and were thus the most difficult and complex cases. Such patients utilize the health care system heavily, having spent an average of over $13,000 on health care in the year prior to referral.

Although Dr. Turk's data does not specifically reflect headache care, available data illustrating the immense direct and indirect costs related to headache provide the basis for suggesting that here, too, major savings might occur. Clouse and Osterhaus (Clouse, 1994) measured comparative costs between migraine patients and nonmigraine patients in a managed care system. They evaluated approximately 1300 Health Maintenance Organization (HMO) headache cases and compared these to the same number of HMO nonheadache patients during an 18-month period. In just a year and a half, the headache patients' utilization costs were $1.5 million more than the nonheadache patients' costs. A major contributing element to these added costs was the presence of comorbidity, found in many headache patients, and which required comprehensive, multidisciplinary intervention. The direct costs reflected clinic visits, prescription drugs, hospitalization, diagnostic tests, alternate practitioner visits, etc. Overall, the headache patients' health care costs were increased 64% over the nonheadache patients' costs, with a minority of the migraine group (those with the most complex cases) accounting for the greatest utilization and costs.

Indirect costs are even more dramatic, with annual lost productivity due to headache estimated to lie between $6.5 to $17.2 billion. This compares to just $2.6 billion lost to diabetes (Lipton, 1994; Osterhaus, 1992). Current estimates include 150 million workdays lost per year, with annual costs to employers estimated at $3600 per woman and $6800 per man. Migraine accounts for 5.7 million days of restricted activity per month (Stang, 1993). In a more recent study, 51% of women and 38% of male migraineurs missed the equivalent of six or more work days per year, based upon reduced efficiency and days lost as a result of headache (Stewart, 1996). Moreover, the prevalence of migraine appears to be on the increase, based upon at least two studies published in the past several years (Centers for Disease Control, 1991; Sillanpaa, 1994).

Even if the indirect costs (disability/impairment/work absences) are ignored, just extrapolating the direct costs to the lifetime trajectory of all headache sufferers, the direct costs for headache patients, compared to those without headaches, would be astronomical. Thus, it is particularly important to consider both the data of Turk, demonstrating cost savings for outcomes in general pain patients treated in tertiary centers, along with data from headache care outcome studies (Baumgartner, 1989; Herring, 1991; Lake, 1993; Rapoport, 1986; Saper, in press; Schnider, 1996; Silberstein, 1992). With some exceptions, because of study detail and design, outcome data from headache studies do not allow reliable projections on potential cost reduction, compared with the data from Turk. However, a review of the available data does provide a basis to suggest that advanced levels of care might have an important impact on long-term costs.

In a specific assessment of outcome and cost-sensitive variables, Saper and Lake (in press) evaluated 218 patients at 6 months following outpatient only treatment (84%) and/or inpatient and outpatient treatment (16%). The majority suffered from transformed migraine with daily headache. Emergent care visits dropped from 4.39 to 1.67 ($p<0.0001$). Headache-related work impaired days declined from 2.04 to 0.67 days/week ($p<0.0001$). A net annualized reduction of 71.24 impaired workdays/year per patient was noted. For full-time workers, missed workdays in 6 months dropped from 5.46 to 2.68 ($p<0.00261$). Total days of incapacitation per week dropped from 1.72 to 0.89 ($p<0.0001$), a mean improvement of 67%. Treatment satisfaction was reported by 89% of patients. Sixty-seven percent (67%) of patients had at least 50% reduction in headaches after a mean of 3.5 visits. Forty-three percent (43%) met with a psychologist. Seventy-two percent (72%) of patients met goal attainment scores on pain control, functioning, work performance, reliance on emergency care, depression, and overall satisfaction.

These data were remarkably similar to an earlier prospective outcome study assessing hospitalized patients with intractable headache (Lake, 1993). Taken together, these studies of a stratified tertiary population of patients referred to a tertiary referral program suggest that not only can complex cases be significantly helped, but that even within the tertiary group, the most complex of these cases (those requiring hospitalization) can achieve similar results if the intensity of service is properly matched to the level of complexity. Projected cost savings from both indirect and direct costs could be astronomical. Saper and Lake (1998) have suggested that given the mean age of 39 years of their patients, and assuming 26 more years in the work force until age 65, the projected cost *savings* for total work-related disability alone (LWDE) climbs well beyond the $100,000 level per patient. This number does not address the possible reduction of direct care costs or the beneficial economic impact of return to work for the 53% of patients who were on extended medical leave or disabled prior to treatment.

VI. A Word to Managed Care

Managed care must look beyond immediate cost savings and focus upon innovative and creative solutions for long-term, high-cost, chronic medical problems. Businesses already recognize this and have begun to establish innovative arrangements with creative professional groups. The concept delineated here would allow for stratification of care to enhance outcome and efficiency, for the development of realistic reimbursement for the services required at each level of care, and for a more reliable projection of costs than is currently possible. Lower costs should be expected for more straightforward cases, which stage at lower levels, whereas higher costs and fees are required for more complex (higher staged) cases. Stratification of care should improve outcome results (the data support this), resulting in significant long-term direct and indirect cost savings, not to mention the patient benefits. Moreover, risk sharing with professional systems is more likely if fees are realistic and stratified according to case severity.

VII. Conclusion

Cost-effective care requires that a headache case be treated at the appropriate time, by the appropriate professionals, and in the appropriate setting. *Severity of illness must match intensity of service* in order for savings to be achieved. This requires prompt triage to the appropriate system of care at a time before unnecessary expenditures are incurred and before treatable cases become more intractable because of inappropriate care, delay, or neglect.

References

Baumgartner C, Wessley P, Bingol C, et al. Long-term prognosis and analgesic withdrawal in patients with drug-induced headaches. *Headache,* 29:510–514, 1989.

Breslau N, Andreski P. Migraine: personality and psychiatric comorbidity. *Headache,* 35:382–386, 1995.

Breslau N, Davis GC, Andreski P. Migraine, psychiatric disorders, and suicide attempts: An epidemiological study of young adults. *Psychiatry Res,* 37:11–23, 1991.

Breslau N, Merikangas KR, Bowen CL. Comorbidity of migraine and major affective disorders. *Neurology,* 44(supp 7):S17–S22, 1994.

Centers for Disease Control (CDC). Prevalence of chronic migraine headaches — United States — 1980–1989. *MMWR,* 40:331–338, 1991.

Clouse JC, Osterhaus JT. Health care resource use and costs associated with migraine in a managed health care setting. *Ann Pharmacother,* 28:659–664, 1994.

Cull RE, Wells NEJ, Miocevich ML. The economic cost of migraine. *Br J Med Econ,* 2:103–115, 1992.

Cutler RB, Fishbain DA, Rosomoff HL. Does nonsurgical pain center treatment of chronic pain return patients to work? A review and meta-analysis of the literature. (In) Abstracts: *7th World Congress on Pain.* Seattle, IASP Publications, Pgs 601–602, 1993.

Diener HC, Tfelt-Hansen P. Headache associated with chronic use of substances. (In) *The Headaches.* J Olesen, P Tfelt-Hansen, KMA Welch (Eds). Pg 721, New York, Raven Press, 1993.

Fishbain DA, Rosomoff HL, Goldberg M, et al. The prediction of return to the workplace after multidisciplinary pain center treatment. *Clin J Pain,* 9:3–15, 1993.

Flor H, Fydrich T, Turk DC. Efficacy of multidisciplinary pain treatment centers: A meta-analytic review. *Pain,* 49:221–230, 1992.

Hering R, Steiner TJ. Abrupt outpatient withdrawal from medication in analgesic-abusing migraineurs. *Lancet,* 337:1442, 1991.

Kaa KA, Carlson JA, Osterhaus JT. Emergency department resource use by patients with migraine and asthma in health maintenance organizations. *Ann Pharmacother,* 29:251–256, 1995.

Lake AE, Saper JR, Madden SF, et al. Comprehensive inpatient treatment for intractable migraine: A prospective long-term study. *Headache,* 33:255–262, 1993.

Lipton RB, Stewart WF, Vonkorff M. The burden of migraine. A review of costs to society. *Pharmacoeconomics,* 6:215–221, 1994.

Mathew NT, Stubbits E, Nigam MR. Transformation of episodic migraine into daily headache: Analysis of factors. *Headache,* 22:66, 1982.

Merikangas KR, Merikangas JR, Angst J. Headache syndromes and psychiatric disorders: Association and familial transmission. *J Psychiatr Res,* 27:197–210, 1993.

Merikangas KR, Stevens DE. Comorbidity of migraine and psychiatric disorders. *Neurol Clin,* 15:1–13, 1997.

Osterhaus JT, Gutterman DL, Plachetka JR. Health care resources and lost labor cost of migraine headaches in the United States. *Pharmacoeconomics,* 2:67, 1992.

Osterhaus JT, Stang PE, Wanagihara T. Use of diagnostic procedures associated with the incidence of migraine headaches among Olmstead County, Minnesota residents, 1979–1981. Poster presentation.

Rapoport AM, Weeks RE, Sheftell FD, et al. The "analgesic washout period": A critical variability in the evaluation of headache treatment efficacy. *Neurology,* 36(supp 1):100, 1986.

Saper JR, Wake AE, Madden SF, et al. Comprehensive/tertiary care for headache: A six-month outcome study. In press.

Schnider P, Aull S, Baumgartner C, et al. Long-term outcome of patients with headache and drug abuse after inpatient withdrawal: Five-year follow-up. *Cephalalgia,* 16:481–485, 1996.

Silberstein SD, Silberstein JR. Chronic daily headache prognosis following inpatient treatment with repetitive IV DHE. *Headache,* 32:439, 1992.

Sillanpaa M. Headache in children. (In) *Headache Classification and Epidemiology,* J Olesen (Ed). Pg 273, New York, Raven, 1994.

Simmons JW, Avant WS, Demski J, et al. Determining successful pain clinic treatment through validation of cost effectiveness. *Spine,* 13:24–34, 1988.

Stang PE, Osterhaus JT. Impact of migraine in the United States: Data from the national health interview survey. *Headache,* 33:29–35, 1993.

Stewart WF, Lipton RB, Simon D. Work-related disability: Results from the American migraine studies. *Cephalalgia,* 16:231–238, 1996.

Turk DC. Efficacy of multidisciplinary pain centers in the treatment of chronic pain. (In) *Pain Treatment Centers at a Crossroads: A Practical and Conceptual Reappraisal,* MJM Kohn, JN Campbell (Eds). Pgs 257–273, Seattle, IASP Press, 1996.

3

Diagnostic Evaluation of the Patient

*"Patients have illnesses and symptoms long before doctors
understand them or have the means to diagnose or treat them."*
—Saper, 1992

I. The History

A detailed, comprehensive history is undeniably the most important aspect of establishing the diagnosis of a headache condition.

A. Important Variables

Patients must be specifically asked how many headache patterns they experience. The following features must be delineated for each type, where appropriate:

- Date, circumstances, and suddenness (rate) of onset and buildup;
- Intensity/character of pain;
- Duration of individual attack(s);
- Location(s);
- Frequency of attacks;
- Preceding and accompanying neurological or other physical symptoms;
- Seasonal variations;
- Evolution (progression) in symptoms and/or frequency;
- Provoking/aggravating factors;
- Relief measures;
- Current and past treatments, both failed and effective;
- Family history;
- Sleep patterns;
- Occupation;
- Emotional profile; and
- Impairment impact.

The distinction between benign (primary) headaches and those of more serious origin can sometimes be made by a determination of the rate/speed of buildup. Severe headache, escalating in intensity over a minute or two, is of significant concern (see Table 3.1).

B. Provoking Factors ("Triggers")

Primary headaches, such as migraine, are sometimes provoked by certain factors, such as menstruation, alcohol, weather changes, or missing meals. The recognition of this provocation can often help to establish the diagnosis.

TABLE 3.1.   **SELECTED FACTORS THAT HELP DISTINGUISH PHYSIOLOGICAL (PRIMARY) FROM SECONDARY (ORGANIC) HEADACHE**

1. Abruptness of onset (rate of buildup of headache)
2. Progression of headache pattern
3. Presence or absence of abnormal neurological or other physical findings or symptoms
4. Presence or absence of migraine-typical provoking factors
5. Treatability or refractoriness to appropriate interventions

Many patients have more than one pattern of pain, and each requires separate delineation. Failure to do so results in an inability to distinguish coexisting entities.

Most patients with *chronic recurring* headache have their affliction because of genetic or acquired biological predisposition. However, various external and internal events can provoke an individual or series of attacks. It is possible, nonetheless, that intrinsic factors, more than extrinsic ones, ultimately explain why and when an attack occurs and the frequency of attacks.

Table 3.2 lists the most commonly cited headache-provoking factors. Table 3.3 lists foods that are frequently identified as provoking headaches.

Modest and moderate caffeine intake (up to 300–400 mg/day) (see Table 6.2, Chapter 6) has no adverse effect on most patients. If taken as part of headache treatment and in a patient who is not on high daily amounts, caffeine enhances gastrointestinal absorption of medicines, acts as a cerebral stimulant, and has primary analgesic influences. However, continuous, excessive caffeine intake can aggravate and induce headaches. Toxicity from caffeine can produce a headache as one of its symptoms. Moreover, high daily chronic intake greater than 500 mg/day can produce dependency, leading to "withdrawal" headaches 8–16 hours after the last dose. This is a major cause of morning headaches in people with high caffeine intake. Table 6.2 in Chapter 6 lists the caffeine content of various foods and drugs. The total daily caffeine intake should be calculated, or at least carefully estimated, since caffeine overuse can be an important contributing factor in some cases.

II. The Physical Examination

The physical examination, particularly of the head and neck, is an essential element in a comprehensive evaluation for headache. It may be critical in the identification of alternate conditions that may mimic or coexist with a primary headache syndrome and that would otherwise not be identified were not a careful evaluation carried out.

In patients with primary headache disorders, except for the occasional presence of "soft neurological signs," the neurological and

TABLE 3.2.   **POSSIBLE/TYPICAL PROVOKING FACTORS FOR MIGRAINE***

Hormonal changes
    Oral contraceptives
    Menstruation
    Hormonal replacement
    Pregnancy
Certain medicines
Weather changes
Lack of or excessive sleep (i.e., more than customary, such as on weekends)
Certain foods/ingredients (see Table 3.3)
Missed meals
Stress, exhilaration, or "letdown"
Fluorescent lights
Smoke

*The reliability of any of these factors to provoke a headache consistently or at all remains arguable. Overemphasizing their importance is unwise. Hormonal factors, excessive sleep, missed meals, alcohol, and weather changes represent the most reliable provoking factors. Patients themselves often identify stress, but studies which identify the presence of stress and absence of headache are not available. Even the most disciplined patient cannot prevent many of his/her attacks, even with compulsive discipline, since factors out of his/her control are operative.

TABLE 3.3.   **COMMON FOODS THAT MAY PROVOKE HEADACHE**

Food Type	Examples
Aged cheeses	Cheddar, brick, mozzarella, Gruyère, Stilton, Brie, Camembert, Boursault
Alcohol	Beer, wine (especially red), liquor
Caffeine (excessive)/withdrawal	Coffee, tea, cola, certain over-the-counter, analgesics and other medications (see Table 6.2, Chapter 6 for caffeine content of selected foods and analgesics)
Chocolate	Sweets, foods, drinks
Concentrated sugar	Sweets, cookies, cake
Dairy products	Milk, ice cream, yogurt, cream, cheeses (aged)
Fermented, pickled foods	Herring, sour cream, yogurt, vinegar, marinated meats (cold cuts)
Fruits	Bananas, plantain, avocado, figs, passion fruit, raisins, pineapple, oranges, and most citrus
Meats with nitrites	Bologna, hot dogs, pepperoni, salami, pastrami, bacon, sausages, canned ham, corned beef, smoked fish
Monosodium glutamate (MSG)	Chinese food, Accent, Lawry's Seasoned Salt, instant foods such as canned soup, TV dinners, processed meats, roasted nuts, potato chips
Nutrasweet/saccharin	Soft drinks, diet foods
Sulfites	Salad bars, shrimp, soft drinks, certain wines
Vegetables	Onions, pods of broad beans (lima, navy), pea pods, nuts, peanuts
Yeast products	Yeast extract, fresh breads, raised coffee cakes, doughnuts

general examinations are usually normal, as is the neurodiagnostic evaluation. Exceptions occur. For example, neurological findings can be present during *migraine with aura*, and drooping eyelid (ptosis) and pupillary changes are characteristically seen during cluster headache. Occipitocervical tenderness is common in migraine and its variants, and the electroencephalogram (EEG) may be mildly abnormal in up to 30–40% of patients with migraine.

A neurological examination should be completed in detail. Particular attention should be paid to the cranial nerves, the carotid and temporal arteries, and the cervical region. Cardiac and peripheral vascular status, as well as mental status, should be evaluated. Palpation, auscultation, and careful observation are components of a detailed exam.

The following aspects of the clinical examination are emphasized:

- Palpation/percussion
    cranium
    jaw (temporomandibular joint and musculature)
    neck (range of motion, pain on movement, etc.)
    oral cavity
    ears
    sinuses;
- Vital signs;
- Mental status;
- Funduscopic exam;
- Visual acuity;
- Signs of trauma; and
- Cardiac and pulmonary status.

Pathological processes in and about the head or neck can provoke secondary headaches and also activate primary headaches, such as migraine. *Thus, even if the diagnosis is likely to be migraine, a careful search for accompanying or inciting illness is necessary.*

Nuchal rigidity is an important sign of infectious, structural, or hemorrhagic events. In the case of subarachnoid hemorrhage, nuchal rigidity may not be initially present. It may take as many as *six hours* for subarachnoid blood, e.g., from an aneurysm, to migrate to the cervical region and induce the irritational and inflammatory changes that provoke nuchal rigidity (which must be distinguished from muscle tenderness and guarding). *Thus, the absence of neck stiffness does not exclude recent hemorrhage.* Other headache-related causes of neck movement limitation include primary cervical disease, Arnold Chiari malformation Type I, meningitis, and others.

III. Laboratory Testing

Over 300 causes of secondary headache are known. (See Table 5.1, Chapter 5.) Causes or aggravating factors must be considered efficiently and thoroughly, particularly in patients with frequent, atypical, and progressive headache patterns. Table 3.4 is a suggested list of laboratory studies. A complete chemistry profile, complete blood count (CBC), endocrinological tests, and urinalysis should be obtained in those cases in which headache is increasingly frequent and progressive, does not conform to typical patterns of the primary headache disorders, are associated with abnormalities on examination, or in which there exists a reasonable suspicion that such testing

TABLE 3.4. **SELECTED LABORATORY EVALUATION**

BUN[a]
Creatinine
SGOT[a]
SGPT[a]
Alkaline phosphatase
Total bilirubin
Total protein
Albumin
Calcium
Phosphorus
Sodium
Potassium
Glucose
Triglycerides
Cholesterol
HDL[a] cholesterol
CBC[a] and differential
ESR[a]
Serum B_{12}
Folate
Serum estrogen (females)
Free T_4
TSH
Urinalysis
Urine drug screen
PT, PTT_a
EKG_a
Lyme titre
HIV_a
VDRL
ANA
Lupus anticoagulant
Anticardiolipin antibodies (see Levine, 1997, and Iniguez, 1991 in Chapter 8)

[a]BUN, blood urea nitrogen; SGOT, serum glutamic oxaloacetic transaminase; SGPT, serum glutamic pyruvic transaminase; HDL, high-density lipoprotein; CBC, complete blood count; TSH, thyroid stimulating hormone; erythrocyte sedimentation rate; EKG, electrocardiogram; PT, prothrombin time; PTT, partial thromboplastin time; HIV, human immunodeficiency virus.

may identify an important disturbance. (Several of these studies also assist in determining the baseline values to allow future monitoring and enhance safe administration of medications for headache.)

Urine and blood drug evaluations can be used for detecting the presence of unsuspected medication/drugs. *Patients may intentionally or inadvertently fail to report their use (or excessive use) of over-the-counter or prescribed analgesics, tranquilizers, or other medications or drugs that are relevant to both the origin of headache and to the safety of planned pharmacotherapy.* (In the authors' personal experience, urine drug studies have revealed many unexpected substances, including barbiturates, cocaine, alcohol, opioids, marijuana, and others in individuals who had failed to acknowledge the use of these substances. Recognition of these is important in both safety and diagnostic perspectives.)

In some individuals, including those being considered for treatment with the "triptans" and other potent vasoconstrictors, performance of an electrocardiogram and other tests for cardiovascular disease is appropriate on a case-by-cases basis.

IV. Standard Neurodiagnostic Studies

In general, we believe that most patients with recurring, frequent headache will require some neurodiagnostic testing. An exception may be those patients with occasional, stereotypical, and infrequent headaches and those headaches which are specifically and exclusively associated with key and well known migraine provoking factors, such as menstrual periods, red wine, weather changes, etc. However, those headaches that have atypical or variant forms, are associated with neurological abnormalities on examination, are of sudden or acute onset, or are associated with fever, stiff neck, or other findings suggestive of organic disease must be tested thoroughly. Similarly, those associated with troubling provocative factors, such as postural change or increased with coughing or straining, must be pursued diagnostically.

A. Computerized Tomographic (CT) Scanning
1. Neuroimaging

Neuroimaging is indicated to rule out structural disease, such as, but not limited to, tumor, abscess, hydrocephalus, stroke, acute sphenoid sinusitis (see later and Chapter 5), and hemorrhage. It is particularly important whenever there are neurological or mental symptoms or findings and in the presence of persistent, recurring, or progressive headache, whether effectively managed by treatment or not.

Even when the headache is well managed, a CT scan (or magnetic resonance imaging [MRI]) may nonetheless be prudent. Many analgesics and preventive medications can relieve or mask headache associated with organic disease. The headache of subarachnoid hemorrhage, for example, may respond to dihydroergotamine (DHE) or the "triptans," as well as analgesic treatment. Subdural hematomas, obstructive syndromes, and A-V malformations, among others, which can mimic the primary headache conditions or activate migraine (a point deserving repetition), can at least initially respond to standard headache treatment.

Acute sphenoid sinusitis (see Chapter 5) may initially present with neuralgic symptoms as well as severe headache, sometimes not unlike that of an acute migraine. Headaches associated with an aneurysm or cerebral vein thrombosis may not be associated with features that reveal or are characteristic of the underlying pathology.

Moreover, patients with preexisting headache, such as migraine, may develop a superimposed disorder that causes headache and which can be easily overlooked or discounted. It may be assumed that it is a variation of the migraine or cannot be distinguished from it clinically.

Thus, the question of testing is clearly a controversial one, both from a neurological as well as a cost-effective point of view. In a series of 373 consecutive patients with chronic headache, Dumas (1994) found that the detection rate on CT scanning was similar to that expected in the general population, provided the neurological findings are normal. However, testing can not be ignored when patients present with new onset or atypical or progressive symptoms, variant patterns, or those that for other reasons raise concern in the mind of the clinician.

The American Academy of Neurology (1994) guidelines on CT and MRI assert that the routine use of neuroimaging is not warranted in adult patients with recurring headaches that have been defined as migraine with no recent change in pattern, no history of seizures, and no focal neurological signs or symptoms. In patients with atypical headache patterns, a history of seizures, or focal neurological signs or symptoms, CT or MRI may be indicated, and the role of CT and MRI in evaluation of patients with headaches that are not consistent with migraine cannot be determined at this time because of insufficient evidence.

Thus, neuroimaging is recommended in the following circumstances:

- The first or worst headache;
- A change in frequency, severity, or clinical features;
- An abnormal neurological examination, including the presence of bruits;

- Progressive, atypical, or variant forms of headache or a persistent unremitting pattern;
- Neurological symptoms that do not meet the criteria of migraine with typical aura;
- Persisting neurological deficits;
- Definite EEG evidence of a focal cerebral lesion;
- Headaches that are refractory to aggressive and appropriate treatment interventions;
- Comorbid seizures;
- A severely anxious patient who cannot be assured that the condition is benign until testing is undertaken; and
- Unilateral headache that is consistently unilateral, is not typical of a primary disorder, and does not easily respond to treatment.

2. MRI and Magnetic Resonance Angiography (MRA)

An MRI of the head, and perhaps of the cervical spine and neck, is indicated for many of the same reasons as the CT scan, and that is to rule out secondary causes of headache. Diagnostic testing is based on the same principles as above. The MRI should be ordered *instead of* or in addition to the CT scan in order to:

a. Identify lesions in the brainstem and occipital-cervical junction that are not well visualized by CT scanning; such as Arnold-Chiari Type I malformation, cervical disc disease, and spondylosis. (Cine phase-contrast MRI may be of particular value in assessing cerebrospinal fluid [CSF] flow in the occipital/cervical junction [Pujol, 1995].)
b. Visualize the pituitary region better than can be achieved with CT scanning;
c. Avoid contrast material, as in a contrast-enhanced CT scan. However, a noncontrast MRI may not visualize tumors, as well as other conditions, but may nonetheless offer important diagnostic data (see below);
d. Rule out demyelinating, ischemic, or inflammatory disease;
e. Evaluate carotid and anterior neck soft tissue (carotodynia, suspected carotid dissection, etc.)—(see MR angiogram);
f. Evaluate facial and retropharyngeal regions;
g. When evaluating subtle findings only identifiable on MRI, such as small foci of high signal intensity on T2 weighted images (found in up to 40% of migraine patients compared to 11% of matched controls);

h. Evaluate for cerebrospinal fluid leak (slow flow and diffusion weighted MRI [flow-sensitive MRI] may be particularly helpful in assessing CSF leakage) (Kabuto, 1996; Levy, 1995; Vakharia, 1997);

i. Evaluate cerebral vein thrombosis;

j. Evaluate the presence of meningeal enhancement, as in cases of CSF hypotension (Mokri, 1997); and

k. For evaluation of the sphenoid sinuses, both MR and CT imaging can demonstrate sphenoid sinus regions. The CT scan is better for evaluation of bone structures. The MRI may demonstrate subtle pattern changes in the sphenoids that suggest distinctions between bacterial and fungal infection.[1]

The cost of MR imaging is considerably more than that of the CT scan. However, the CT scan is not an adequate study in some circumstances and can lead to a false sense of normalcy. *Clinical judgment must prevail, and cost considerations should not compromise prudent clinical judgment.*

Gadolinium enhancement increases signal intensity and may be particularly valuable in visualizing suspected tumors, for example.

MRA is rapidly improving and becoming increasingly reliable, but it has not yet entirely replaced arteriography in the evaluation of aneurysm and vasculitis. However, MRA does provide a means by which vascular anatomy can be evaluated without significant risk or discomfort. It is of particular value in evaluating cervical vascular disease, including dissection of the carotid artery, and allows for the detection of aneurysms as small as 4–5 mm (perhaps 3 mm) in the vicinity of the circle of Willis. However, there are limitations as well as both technical and interpretive variations in reliability and consistency from center to center. However, MRA is a safe tool and is increasingly important in evaluating vascular disease.

Because of its availability and value, many clinicians, including these authors, believe that MRA may be fast becoming an appropriate test in the initial assessment of "thunderclap" headache.

Although MR imaging is currently considered a safe procedure, pregnant women, particularly during the first and second trimester,

---

[1]*When sphenoid sinusitis is suspected, and a CT scan is ordered, it is essential that views of the sphenoid region be specifically requested, since standard views may not reveal the sphenoid region, and a report of "normal" may not have reflected visualization of the sphenoid area. In general, an MRI visualizes the sphenoids routinely, but certainty must be established on a case-by-case basis.*

should not undergo MRI. Concern exists that magnetic fields and radio waves may impose an adverse influence on the unborn fetus.

B. The Lumbar Puncture (LP)

The conditions that can be identified only or most conclusively by performance of an LP are:

1. Elevation or reduction in cerebral spinal fluid pressure;
2. Bleeding and/or infection, inflammation, or cellular infiltration (lymphoma, etc.) in the central nervous system; and
3. Disturbances of protein, protein ratios, sugar, or other biochemical or neurohumoral changes associated with central nervous system pathology.

The indications for an LP and CSF evaluation are listed in Table 3.5.

The LP should be performed after CT or MR imaging have ruled out the presence of space occupying intracranial structural disease, which could induce unforeseeable risk were an LP to be undertaken. One exception is the urgent need to evaluate the CSF when there is a suspicion of an intracranial infectious disorder and neither a CT scan nor MRI is available. (This is very rare today in the United States, but not in other locations worldwide.)

In the presence of acute sudden-onset headache, sufficient to raise concern regarding the possible presence of intracranial hemorrhage, a CT scan (first with and then without contrast) should be performed, followed by an LP within the first 48 hours to rule out subarachnoid hemorrhage. (After the first 24 hours, an MRI may be preferable to the CT scan in evaluating subarachnoid hemorrhage.) *The absence of blood in CSF does not in and of itself eliminate the possibility of subarachnoid hemorrhage, since blood may not enter the spinal canal for several hours after hemorrhage.* Delaying the LP for days or longer allows the blood to be resorbed, sometimes without a trace, although xanthochromic

---

TABLE 3.5.   **INDICATIONS FOR LP AND CSF EVALUATION**

1. Abrupt and sudden onset of headache;
2. Headache accompanied by signs or symptoms of infection (fever, stiff neck, etc.);
3. Suspicion of bleeding or infiltrative/inflammatory processes;
4. Suspicion of elevated or reduced pressure, the latter often indicated by a postural component to the headache;
5. Headache attacks associated with cranial nerve deficits that could result from infiltrative, tumor, or infectious involvement of the brainstem;
6. Headaches which are intractable, subacute or acute, and daily or almost daily; and
7. Suspicion of CNS degenerative disease, such as MS.

CSF fluid is generally evident for at least a week, and often longer, following the hemorrhage.

The CSF must be handled properly. At least two tubes must be evaluated for cellular components, thereby providing a comparative measurement. We suggest a cell count for tubes 2 and 4. CSF must be analyzed soon after it is obtained. The CSF should be centrifuged immediately in order to assess for the presence of xanthochromia. If neither centrifuged nor evaluated quickly, lysis of cells may occur, and the fluid may become xanthochromic from the cellular material, thereby confounding the interpretation of xanthochromic discoloration.

Accurate opening and closing pressures must be documented. An excessive, relative drop in pressure following routine-volume fluid collection may indicate vulnerability to CSF hypotension. Opening and closing pressures are also of importance in evaluating idiopathic intracranial hypertension (pseudotumor cerebri). If the opening pressure is elevated (see Chapter 18), the degree of drop at closing should be correlated with the amount of fluid removed. Changes in headache status following lowering of pressure should be recorded. However, some patients with chronic elevations of CSF pressure will not report improvement in headache even with significant transient reduction in CSF pressure following an LP.

C. Electroencephalography

The EEG assists in evaluating paroxysmal electrical activity (indicating a predisposition to seizures) and neuronal disturbances resulting from drug or metabolic illness and primary neurological disease. While a variety of EEG abnormalities have been reported in patients with migraine, and while noninvasive and relatively inexpensive, the EEG lacks both specificity and sensitivity and should not be considered a "routine" test for patients with typical forms of headache. However, the EEG may have value in certain clinical circumstances. These include alteration or loss of consciousness or level of alertness (including following head trauma); recent sudden change in clinical characteristics or severity of headache attacks; transient neurological symptoms with or without ensuing head-ache; suspected encephalopathy (metabolic, toxic, infectious, etc.); and residual and persisting neurological deficits. It is particularly important in the presence of periodic or continuous mental changes, such as confusion, memory impairment, amnesia, and personality change. Some clinicians recommend the EEG to determine seizure vulnerability prior to the use of high dosages of drugs, such as the antidepressants, which lower seizure threshold.

D. Electrocardiography (ECG)

Most medications used in the pharmacological treatment of headache can affect heart function, coronary flow, cardiac rhythm and rate, or blood pressure. These include the "triptans," ergot derivatives, antidepressants, beta blockers, calcium channel blockers, and others. Establishing a baseline ECG prior to the implementation of these treatments, particularly vasoconstrictive medication and those likely to produce cardiac arrhythmia, is often wise and medically protective. Sumatriptan and the other "triptans," as well as DHE nasal spray, carry warnings that recommend cardiac evaluation and screening before administration to patients who are at risk for cardiac disease.

It is possible that primary cardiac disease, such as periodic arrhythmias, coronary artery disease, or spasm, results in cardiac ischemia and related headache (Lance, 1998; Lipton, 1997).

E. Routine X-rays

Cervical spine and skull x-rays may rarely be indicated in specific circumstances, such as in suspected fracture or bone disease.

F. Arteriography/MR Angiography

These studies are generally not routinely required in the evaluation of head pain syndromes. They are indicated, however, when there is a strong suspicion of aneurysm, vasculitis, stroke, or other condition that can be evaluated only by the study of cervical and cerebral circulation. (MR angiography is not yet established as an entirely reliable test for these circumstances but is rapidly becoming more reliable, particularly in centers with advanced experience and technique.)

G. Ultrasound Testing

Ultrasound evaluation of the carotid vascular system and heart may be indicated to:

1. Evaluate the carotid arteries and the heart in cases of headache accompanied by periodic neurological events associated with headache; and
2. Evaluate carotid artery flow dynamics and to rule out carotid dissection.

The value of transcranial Doppler evaluation in the diagnosis of cerebral flow patterns remains uncertain in the routine evaluation of patients with headache.

H. Evoked Response Testing

Sensory, auditory, or visual evoked response testing has been employed in a variety of neurological conditions associated with headache. These include *post-concussion syndrome* (brainstem auditory evoked response), headache in the presence of significant visual disturbances (visual evoked response), and headache associated with various sensory symptoms (somatosensory evoked response). Its value remains uncertain.

V. Other Evaluations
A. Temporomandibular Disorders (TMD, TMJ, etc.) and Dental Evaluations

The jaw and dental structures, including the surrounding musculature, may be important in headache and face pain conditions. Migraine may be exacerbated, or a new headache can develop as a direct result of dental disease or procedures, such as root canal or extractions, and in the presence of significant jaw dysfunction. TMD can generally be identified by aggravation of pain upon chewing, jaw opening, and related motions (see Chapter 16).

Microabscesses subsequent to tooth extraction or neuromas secondary to root canal may produce chronic head or facial pain. Surgical procedures that interrupt the dental nerves (branches of the trigeminal nerve) may result in neuronal disturbances within the *nucleus caudalis* of the *trigeminal nerve* in the brainstem. Disruption in the trigeminal system, so closely related to the important pain modulating systems of the brainstem (see Chapters 4 and 16), may explain the unexpected onset of head and facial pain following dental procedures, including provocation of migraine.

Temporomandibular disorders can accompany chronic headache and in some instances provoke headache. Nonetheless, this set of disorders seems overstated and overtreated as a cause of primary headaches and facial pain. Nonetheless, disorders of the jaw and related musculature may be important in some instances and critical in others. The pain can arise from the joint itself, gum structures, and surrounding soft tissue and musculature. Perhaps in ways that are not fully delineated, neural impulses via the trigeminal system activate or alter threshold phenomena related to migraine in the brainstem, thereby accounting for the coexistence of both primary headache and pain from TMD. Inappropriate/overtreatment of TMD and TM joint disease often makes the head pain syndrome worse, not better. Most often conservative intervention is more appropriate.

MRI of the temporomandibular joints is primarily useful in assessing degenerative disease or displacement within the joint itself and is indicated in selected circumstances. We recommend referral to a qualified dental professional who understands headache and face pain and shares a conservative and prudent view toward the treatment of jaw disorders.

B. Selected Tests to Evaluate for Suspected Stroke or Vasculitis

Increased attention has focused on the possible risk of stroke in certain patients with headache who experience periodic neurological events. The presence of anticardiolipin antibodies, lupus anticoagulant, and other clotting abnormalities might predispose to stroke. Migraine itself is a modest risk factor for stroke in young women (Carolei, 1996) (also see Chapter 8). Table 3.6 provides a recommended (selected) laboratory diagnostic battery for assessing stroke risk in patients with significant periodic neurological events and headache and that should be employed in conjunction with standard neurodiagnostic testing. (Further discussion of stroke and headache can be found in Chapter 8.)

Inherited deficiencies of antithrombin III, protein C, and protein S are associated with arterial and venous occlusive brain infarction. These studies, in conjunction with a careful neurological examination and diagnostic assessment, including carotid ultrasound, MR studies of the brain and vasculature, transesophageal echocardiogram (to rule out valvular disease or right-to-left shunts through a patent foramen ovale, for example), and Holter cardiac monitoring, are among the tests indicated when significant periodic neurological events (other than simple visual auras) are present in patients with headache and who are suspected of having ischemic phenomena. They are indicated in the presence of *migraine with prolonged aura* (*complicated migraine*). Migraine with prolonged aura is defined as migraine with one or more aura symptoms lasting more than 60 minutes, but with full recovery within three weeks and a normal late CT scan or MRI. If the CT scan or MRI is abnormal after 21 days, an infarction (migrainous infarction) is likely.

TABLE 3.6.   **SELECTED LABORATORY EVALUATION FOR ASSESSING STROKE RISK IN HEADACHE PATIENTS**

Hemoglobin, hematocrit, platelet count, prothrombin time, partial thromboplastin time
Anticardiolipin antibodies (see Levine, 1997; Iniguez, 1991 in Chapter 7)
Lupus anticoagulant
Antinuclear antibody (ANA)
Double and single-stranded anti-DNA antibodies (if ANA-positive)
Protein C, S
Antithrombin III
Sedimentation rate
Fasting lipid profile, glucose
Others

C. Diagnostic Blocks

Diagnostic blocking of structures such as the occipital nerve, C2–C3 facet joints and nerves, supraorbital nerve, sphenopalatine ganglia, the styloid process, stylomandibular ligament, as well as trigger point injections may provide clues to diagnosis and/or offer a specific treatment intervention as well. Recent interest has been drawn to the C2-C3 roots, nerves, and facet joints in traumatic, as well as nontraumatic, headache. Facet joint and related neuroblockade may provide substantial relief to some otherwise refractory patients, particularly those with chronic whiplash injury (Lord, 1996; Wallis, 1997) (see Chapter 19).

Establishing a definitive diagnosis based solely upon the value of any of the blocking procedures, however, is tenuous, as these procedures can relieve pain by blocking nerves and tissues not directly related to the pathological process. The blocked nerves or ganglia are perhaps involved in the transmission of pain impulses from a number of sources, and therapeutically effective blocking may not of itself constitute the basis for reliable localization or diagnosis.

Summary

Recurring head, neck, and face pain must be evaluated with the same intensity, completeness, and objectivity as that accorded to other important clinical conditions. The diagnosis of migraine or other primary headache disorder cannot be made without consideration and perhaps exclusion of certain conditions that can mimic, ac-

---

TABLE 3.7. **SELECTED INVESTIGATIONS FOR HEAD, NECK, AND FACE PAIN**

History and physical examination (including neurological exam)
Laboratory evaluation (see text)
CT scan, including special views of the sphenoid*
MRI and MRA
Electroencephalography
Lumbar puncture/CSF evaluation
Ultrasound studies (carotid, vertebral, transcranial, cardiac)
Cardiac evaluation
Dental/jaw evaluation
Diagnostic blockade
EMG of cervical musculature
Myelogram
Arteriography
Evoked response tests
Otolaryngological evaluation
Ophthalmological evaluation

*When sphenoid sinusitis is suspected and a CT scan is ordered, it is essential that views of the sphenoid region be requested specifically, since standard views may not reveal the sphenoid region. The report may indicate normal findings, and the physician may assume, inappropriately, that the sphenoid region has been visualized.

company, or activate primary headache syndromes. Invasive testing can usually be avoided, but the occasional need for it cannot be overlooked. Table 3.7 lists selected investigations for head, neck, and face pain evaluation.

Diagnostic testing should not replace a comprehensive history and physical examination, but a history and physical examination cannot substitute for adequate laboratory and diagnostic testing.

References

Carolei A, Marini C, DeMatteis G. History of migraine and risk of cerebral ischemia in young adults. *Lancet,* 347:1503–1506, 1996.

Dumas MD, Pexman JHW. Computed tomography evaluation of patients with chronic headache. *Canadian Medical Association Journal,* 151:1447, 1994.

Headache and facial pain. Continuum, Life-long learning in neurology. A program of the American Academy of Neurology. Volume 1. No. 5. November, 1995.

Kabuto M, Kabuta T, Kobayashi H. MRI imaging of cerebrospinal fluid rhinorrhea following the suboccipital approach to the cerebral pontine angle and the internal auditory canal: Report of two cases. *Surg Neurol,* 45:336–340, 1996.

Lance JW, Lambros J. Unilateral exertional headache as a symptom of cardio ischemia. *Headache,* 38:315–316, 1998.

Levine SR, Salowich-Palm L, Sawaya KL, et al. IgG anticardiolipin antibody titre > 40 GPL and the risk of subsequent thrombo-occlusive events and death. *Stroke,* 28:1660–1665, 1997.

Levy LM, Gulya AJ, Davis SW. Flow-sensitive magnetic resonance imaging in the evaluation of cerebrospinal fluid leaks. *Am J Otol,* 16:591–596, 1995

Lipton RB, Lowenkopf T, Bajwa ZH, et al. Cardiac cephalgia: A treatable form of exertional headache. *Neurology,* 49:813–816, 1997.

Lord SM, Barnsley L, Wallis BJ, et al. A randomized, double-blind, controlled trial of percutaneous radiofrequency neurotomy for the treatment of chronic cervical zygoapophyseal joint. *N Engl J Med,* 335:1721–1726, 1996.

Mokri B, Pipgras DG, Miller GM. Syndrome of orthostatic headaches in diffuse pachymeningeal gadolinium enhancement. *Mayo Clin Proc,* 72:400–413, 1997.

Obuchowski N, Modic MT, Magdinec M, et al. Current implications for the efficacy of noninvasive screening for occult intracranial aneurysms in patients with family history of aneurysms. *J Neurosurg,* 83:42–49, 1995.

Pujol J, Roig C, Capdevila A, et al. Motion of the cerebellar tonsils in Chiari Type I malformation studied by cine phase-contrast MRI. *Neurology,* 45:1746–1757, 1995.

Quality Standards Subcommittee. American Academy of Neurology. Practice parameter. The utility of neuroimaging in evaluation of headache in patients with normal neurological examinations (summary statement). *Neurology,* 44:1353–1354, 1994.

Quality Standards Subcommittee. American Academy of Neurology. Practice parameter summary. The electroencephalogram and headache. *Neurology,* 45:1411–1413, 1995.

Vakharia SB, Thomas S, Rosenbaum AE, et al. Magnetic resonance imaging of cerebrospinal fluid leak and tamponade effect of blood patch in postural puncture headache. *Anesth Analg,* 84:585–590, 1997.

vanDusseldorp M, Katan MB. Headache caused by caffeine withdrawal among moderate coffee drinkers switched from ordinary to decaffeinated coffee: A 12-week, double-blind study. *BMJ,* 300:1558–1559, 1990.

Wallis BJ, Lord SM, Bogduk N. Resolution of psychological distress of whiplash patients following treatment of radiofrequency neurotomy. A randomized, double-blind, placebo-controlled trial. *Pain,* 73:15–22, 1997.

4

Mechanisms and Theories of Head Pain

I. Introduction

The precise etiology of recurring, benign (chronic) head pain has not yet been established, but important advances have been made in the past decade. There is increasing support for the concept that benign recurring head pain originates in the structures of the brain. Disturbances of neurotransmitter/receptor function and neurovascular control and inflammation are the focus of much current research.

We present a brief and selected review of current thinking regarding the mechanisms of headache, particularly migraine. It is not intended to be an all-encompassing study of the topic. The reader is directed to more extensive reviews (see References) for further discussion.

II. Anatomical Considerations

A. Pain-Sensitive Structures

Pain-sensitive intracranial structures include the skin and blood vessels of the scalp; the head and neck muscles; the venous sinuses; the arteries of the meninges; the larger cerebral arteries; the pain-carrying fibers of the fifth, ninth, and tenth cranial nerves; and parts of the dura mater at the base of the brain. The brain itself is insensitive to pain.

B. Pain Pathways

In general, pain is transmitted from the periphery by *small myelinated (α-Δ) fibers (sharp pain) and* unmyelinated c-fibers *(aching, burning pain) that terminate in the dorsal horn of the spinal cord and the trigeminal nucleus caudalis. Secondary neurons from the dorsal horn reach the thalamus via the spinal thalamic pathways.*

Substance P, a neuropeptide, may be a pain neurotransmitter for the primary sensory neurons. Interneurons in the dorsal horn use *enkephalins* and perhaps *γ-aminobutyric acid (GABA)* as inhibitory neurotransmitters to block pain transmission.

Figure 4.1 illustrates the pain fiber pathways transmitting pain from the face, head, and neck regions. The upper cervical spinal cord contains pain fiber systems for the entire head and neck region. (See Chapter 19 for a more extensive discussion of neck structures and frontal and occipital neural pathways.)

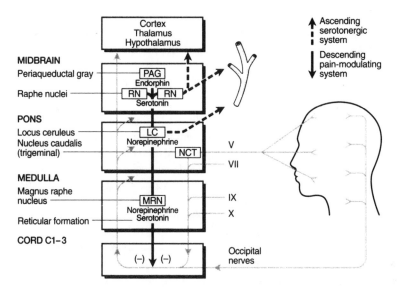

Figure 4.1. Pain pathways.

1. Ascending pain pathways

The neothalamic pathway (quality of pain) terminates in the ventrobasal nucleus of the thalamus, which projects to the somatosensory cortex. The paleothalamic pathway (emotional content of pain) sends projections to the reticular formation of the brainstem, the periaqueductal gray (PAG), the hypothalamic, and the medial and intralaminar thalamic nuclei.

Within the brainstem is an *ascending serotonergic system* that originates in the midbrain raphe region, innervates the cerebral blood vessels, and is distributed to the thalamus, hypothalamus, and cortex. The neurons of this system appear to be involved in cerebral blood flow, sleep, and neuroendocrine control, among other influences.

2. Descending pain-modulating system

The *descending pain-modulating system* originates in the *PAG* in the midbrain and synapses in the raphe magnus in the medulla, and from there connects to the spinal tract of the trigeminal nerve and the dorsal horn of the first, second, and third cervical roots in the spinal cord. Norepinephrine, serotonin, and opiates mediate this important system that modulates (inhibits) pain transmission from most regions of the head and neck.

Thus, within this brainstem and spinal cord there exists a system to carry pain to the thalamus and cortex and a system to modulate pain or inhibit it (the descending pain-modulating system).

III. Physiological Considerations
A. Pain Mechanisms

Head pain is mediated by the trigeminal system and the upper cervical nerves, as well as cranial nerves VII, IX, and X. Pain fibers descend in the brainstem and converge on cells in the posterior horn of the upper cervical spinal cord, which also receive input from the upper cervical sensory roots, as well as other sources. *This convergence is likely to be the basis of pain referral from the neck to the forehead and supraorbital area.* Head pain arising from organic causes can be the result of traction, displacement, inflammation, or pressure on nociceptors in pain-sensitive structures. Nociceptor information is then relayed to the brainstem and spinal cord. Peripheral activation of nociceptors alone, however, is not likely to be the primary cause of migraine or muscle-type headaches. Quite possibly, pain can be generated by *a primary dysfunction within the central ascending and/or descending pain-related systems and involve input from supraspinal, vascular, and myogenic sources* (see Olesen, 1991).

B. Neurogenic Inflammation

Neural connections exist between the trigeminal nerve and intracranial blood vessels. Substance P, calcitonin gene-related peptide (CGRP), and neurokinin A (NKA) are located in the trigeminal sensory neurons, which innervate the cephalic blood vessels.

According to the model of Moskowitz (1984), trigeminal activation results in the release of these neuropeptides, producing neurogenic inflammation with increased vascular permeability, dilation of blood vessels, plasma extravasation, and platelet injury. These changes may be blocked by specific antimigraine drugs, such as DHE and the "triptans."

Migraine and cluster headache have traditionally been called "vascular headaches" because of the suspected involvement of blood vessels. Initially, constrictive or vasodilatory changes were considered to be the primary mechanism by which pain or neurological symptoms occurred. It is now believed that constriction or dilation are epiphenomena, and are not the cause of neurological symptoms or pain, respectively.

It is not currently known whether the neurogenic inflammation is the primary or only mechanism of head pain. The intracranial release of substance P and CGRP may explain why dilation of intracranial vessels during migraine may be accompanied by pain but not under normal physiological circumstances such as physical exertion or a hot bath. CGRP is, in fact, released in the jugular venous blood during an attack of migraine.

The antimigraine drugs dihydroergotamine (DHE) and sumatriptan prevent neurogenic-induced inflammation in the rat dura mater by blocking neurotransmission in small myelinated C-fibers peripherally or within the brain itself. This action appears unrelated to constriction of the blood vessels, no longer thought to be a primary mechanism by which so-called vasoconstrictive antimigraine medications work. In addition, 5-HT_1 agonists relieve headache and normalize CGRP levels in venous jugular blood.

IV. Traditional Concepts in Headache Pathogenesis
A. The "Muscle Theory"

The muscular contraction (tension) concept of headache states that tension-type headaches are secondary to increased muscle contraction in the pericranial and cervical musculature. Studies, however, do not support this mechanism as a primary cause of pain. Muscles may be more tender in tension-type headache, but there is no correlation to increased muscle contraction. In fact, more muscle contraction may be present in migraineurs than in tension headache patients!

B. The "Vascular Theory"

It was once believed that migraine aura was due primarily to cerebral ischemia from vasoconstriction, and the headache itself the result of reactive vasodilation. Pain was thought to be enhanced by vasoactive polypeptides in the tissues surrounding the external carotid artery.

However, blood flow studies do not entirely support the traditional vascular theory. In migraine with aura, a wave of reduced blood flow (oligemia) spreads anteriorly from the occipital area and precedes the aura. It persists into the headache phase. Positron emission tomography (PET) scan technology has confirmed the presence of spreading oligemia in a migraineur who did not have typical aura, suggesting the possibility of "silent" spreading oligemia in some migraine with aura patients (Woods, 1994).

Historically important work by Leão (1944) demonstrated that electrically stimulated rabbit cortex exhibited a wave of *spreading electrical depression* that moved over the cortex at a rate of

2–3 mm/minute. This rate of *spreading depression* is similar to the spread of oligemia (reduced blood flow) in patients with *migraine with aura*.

Lashley (1941), a researcher who himself suffered migraine with aura, mapped out the rate of progression of his own scintillating scotoma across his visual field. He calculated that it corresponded to a rate over his occipital cortex of 2–3 mm/minute.

Thus, the rate of development of the scotomata, spreading oligemia, and spreading electrical depression are approximately the same. Many authorities now believe that the oligemia is secondary to a primary neurogenic event.

V. The Neurogenic Concepts

The neurogenic theory of migraine suggests that migraine is caused by a primary disturbance of brain function. Cerebral blood flow studies in migraine with aura are most consistent with a primary neuronal event producing secondary vascular changes. Magnetoencephalographic studies of the brain during a migraine attack support the concept of spreading depression in migraine, as described above.

In favor of the neurogenic concept of migraine are:

- The presence of premonitory (prodromal) symptoms suggestive of hypothalamic origin;
- The visual aura that crosses vascular territories (due to spreading depression?);
- Associated symptoms, such as nausea/vomiting, and hypersensitivity to sensory stimuli;
- Magnetoencephalographic findings confirming spreading depression; and
- Magnetic resonance spectroscopy showing increased high-energy phosphate consumption and low intracellular magnesium.

Researchers have shown that the brain of migraineurs is different than that of nonmigraineurs even between attacks (see Welch 1990, 1997). Visual information is processed more quickly, and there may be a relative deficiency of energy metabolism in some areas of their brains and muscles. PET scanning technology (see below) has shown brainstem activation in migraine during migraine attacks. The visual association cortex and auditory association cortex, as well as cingulate cortex, are activated, in addition to an area of the brainstem between the dorsal raphe nucleus and locus ceruleus, the region now thought to be the "migraine generator." Sumatriptan reverses the headache and cortical changes but not the activation in the "generator" region (see below). (Perhaps this is related to the phenomenon of recurrence.)

In 1995, researchers (Diener, 1996; Weiller, 1995) using PET scanning, found what is believed to be the migraine "generator" in the dorsal raphe nucleus and locus ceruleus area of the brainstem, a region referred to as the *Talairach space*. Dysfunction of these brainstem nuclei is likely to affect antinociception and intracerebral vascular control, findings with important implications for migraine, perhaps other primary headaches, and migraine comorbidities.

A. Serotonin Considerations

Serotonin, 5-hydroxytryptamine (5-HT), is widely distributed throughout the body. Major concentrations occur in the gastrointestinal tract (90%), the platelets (8%), and the brain. Blood serotonin, which is mainly in the platelets, falls at the time of a migraine attack but is normal between attacks. A low molecular weight platelet serotonin-releasing factor has been identified in the blood only during migraine attacks. Moreover, platelet serotonin content is low in patients with chronic tension-type headaches, which may support the concept that the tension-type headache is a variant of migraine.

A relationship between serotonin and migraine is further suggested by the observation that migraine can be precipitated by reserpine (a serotonin-depleting agent) and relieved by serotonin and serotonin agonists.

B. Serotonin Receptors (5-HT)

There are at least seven classes of 5-HT receptors: 5-HT_1, 5-HT_2, 5-HT_3, 5-HT_4, 5-HT_5, 5-HT_6, and 5-HT_7, with subtypes of each of these classes (Figure 4.2). All have been identified in the brain. The 5-HT_1 and 5-HT_2 receptors are influenced by estrogen. Aging results in a decrease in serotonin receptors. The 5-HT_1 receptors are most dense in the hippocampus, the dorsal raphe, and the substantia nigra, with lesser concentrations in the cortex. 5-HT_1 receptors are inhibitory, while the remainder are excitatory. 5-HT_2 is excitatory, and inhibition may provide migraine prophylaxis. 5-HT_3 is also excitatory and has a role in emesis. Blockade with the HT_3 blocker ondansetron (Zofran) is the basis of the drug's antiemetic action.

5-HT_1-inhibitory (acute migraine relief)
5-HT_2-excitatory (migraine prophylaxis)
5-HT_3-excitatory (antiemetic)
5-HT_4-excitatory
5-HT_5-excitatory
5-HT_6-excitatory
5-HT_7-excitatory

Figure 4.2. Mechanisms of Action of 5-HT (Serotonin) Receptors.

In humans, there are at least five 5-HT$_1$ receptor subtypes, including 5-HT$_{1a}$, 5-HT$_{1b}$, 5-HT$_{1c}$, 5-HT$_{1d}$, and 5-HT$_{1f}$. Stimulation of the 5-HT$_{1a}$ receptor is implicated in anxiety mechanisms.

5-HT$_{1d}$ may be preferentially neuronal (on nerve terminals) and is the most widespread serotonin receptor in the brain. It functions as an autoreceptor modulating neurotransmitter release. Receptor activation inhibits release of 5-HT, norepinephrine, and acetylcholine and substance P, among others.

The 5-HT$_{1b}$ receptor may be preferentially vascular and found on cerebral blood vessels and also on trigeminal ganglia, but not on nerve terminals. Stimulation results in closure of A-V shunts in dogs and cats and appears to produce vasoconstriction, bronchoconstriction, gastrointestinal smooth muscle contraction, and platelet aggregation.

There are three subtypes of the 5-HT$_2$ receptor (a, b, and c).

VI. Tentative Concepts on the Pharmacology of Antimigraine Drugs

Many of the drugs that are effective in migraine are believed to affect one or more of the various serotonin receptors. Methysergide, cyproheptadine, dihydroergotamine (DHE), tricyclic antidepressants, and verapamil interact with the 5-HT$_2$ receptor. β-propranolol, sumatriptan, and DHE interact at the 5-HT$_{1a}$ receptor, while sumatriptan and other triptans, as well as DHE, also work at the 5-HT$_{1b}$ and 5-HT$_{1d}$, and perhaps the 5-HT$_{1f}$ receptor as well.

DHE and the triptans block neurogenic inflammation, and both may help in the modulation of the central serotonin pain system.

DHE, sumatriptan (after disruption of the blood-brain barrier), and zolmitriptan either bind to and/or inhibit the firing of the trigeminal nucleus caudalis—the major relay nucleus for head pain—after stimulation of the superior sagittal sinus. Potentially, specific migraine drugs could work by vasoconstriction, blocking neurogenic inflammation, inhibiting brainstem pain transmission, deactivating the brainstem "generator," blocking spreading oligemia, enhancing pain modulation, or desensitizing neurons.

VII. An Integration of Current Theory on Migraine Pathogenesis

Reconciling and unifying the current concepts with respect to the aura, pain, and other symptoms of migraine has recently been attempted by Welch (1997).

A. The Aura and Spreading Depression

It is believed that spreading depression is the best explanation for the migraine aura, and two mechanisms are proposed. One is founded in the concept of potassium physiology and the other is upon the release of the excitatory amino acid glutamate. Magnesium ($Mg++$) is capable of blocking glutamate-induced spreading depression. Glutamate-induced spreading depression may also be blocked both competitively and noncompetitively by N-methyl-D-aspartate (NMDA) receptor antagonists. Both magnesium and NMDA receptor antagonists are the subject of studies in the treatment of general pain as well as migraine.

B. The Mechanism of Headache

The animal model of head pain, developed by Moskowitz (1984), suggests that the local release of peptides from sensory axones of the trigeminal nerve supplied to dural meningeal tissues, dural arteries, dural sinuses, and extracranial arteries clearly explain a pain-sensitive state (neurogenic inflammation) that promotes local vasodilation. CGRP is released into the venous blood during a migraine attack. Sumatriptan blocks this release, thus blocking the neuropeptide-mediated inflammatory response after trigeminal stimulation. Sumatriptan has selective agonist influence at the b and d subtype of $5-HT_1$ receptors in the peripheral trigeminal nerve terminals that supply pain-sensitive vascular and meningeal structures. (The $5-HT_{1d}$ may be preferentially neuronal, inhibiting $5-HT_1$, NE, acetylcholine, substance P, and CGRP release. The $5-HT_{1b}$ has similar properties of $5-HT_{1d}$ but may be preferentially vascular (located on blood vessels).

The trigeminal vascular model, extended by the work of Goadsby (1995) to involve the sagittal sinus/brainstem model, and the work of Diener (1996), Weiller (1995), and others reporting blood flow changes and brainstem activation (migraine generator) further focuses attention on brainstem, trigeminal, and blood flow interplay. Moreover, brain hyperexcitability exists in the interictal state, and this may be explained by a mitochondrial defect or brain magnesium deficiency. Moreover, an ion channel abnormality, as supported by the gene studies on hemiplegic migraine (chromosome 19) (see Chapter 8), may lend further to understanding the underlying pathophysiology and vulnerability related to migraine.

Thus, migraine sufferers appear to be at the end of a physiological spectrum determined in large measure by genetic factors. The threshold for migraine is lower in these individuals, and when external and internal conditions are right, the mechanisms for a migraine attack are activated. Disordered neurogenic control of the intrinsic and extrinsic circulation may be secondary to the primary process of the attack. As Goadsby (1997) suggests, central intrinsic biogenic amine neurotransmitter dysfunction, as well as that involving the sympathetic nervous system, may be at the heart of the process. Stress and a variety of other migraine "triggers" could result in a functional change within the intrinsic neurotransmitter systems, thus lowering the threshold for migraine activation through an enhancement of neuronal excitability.

Genetically, migraine patients may be predisposed to brain hyperexcitability. Magnesium deficiency, mitochondrial defects, ion channel abnormalities, and central intrinsic biogenic amine disturbances may play a role. Hyperexcitability leads to brainstem and visual cortex activation and trigeminal activation. The aura of migraine cannot be explained by ischemia alone, if at all, and may involve neuronal dysfunction, possibly related to a variety of phenomena, including potassium efflux, the excitatory amino acid glutamate, and calcium channel abnormalities. Magnesium and NMDA receptor antagonists appear to block glutamate-induced spreading depression. Pain may be in part provoked by trigeminal activation and subsequent neurogenic inflammation. At least this part of the process may be blocked by specific antimigraine drugs. The "migraine generator," located in the region between the dorsal raphe nucleus and locus ceruleus, appears to be involved in antinociception and intracerebral vascular control, as well as other important phenomena, and in some way yet to be determined, may play a central role in the entire migraine process.

References

Bogduk N. The clinical anatomy of the cervical dorsal rami. *Spine,* 7:319–330, 1982.

Buzzi MG, Moskowitz MA. The antimigraine drug sumatriptan (GR43175) selectively blocks neurogenic plasma extravasation from blood vessels in dura mater. *Br J Pharmacol,* 99:202–206, 1990.

Diener HC, May A. New aspects of migraine pathophysiology: Lessons learned from positron emission tomography. *Currt Opin Neurol,* 9:199–201, 1996.

Goadsby PJ. Central processing of trigeminal vascular inputs: Relationship to migraine. (In) the American Academy of Neurology: *Scientific Basis of Migraine.* Presented at the 49th Annual Meeting of the AAN, Boston, MA, 1997.

Goadsby PJ, Edvinsson L. Sumatriptan reverses the changes in calcitonin gene-related peptide seen in the headache phase of migraine. *Cephalalgia,* 11(supp 11):3, 1991.

Goadsby PJ, Keay KA, Hoskin KL. Distribution of pain process in trigeminal vascular neurons and the brainstem in high cervical spinal cord of the monkey. *Cephalalgia,* 15(supp 14):57, 1995.

Goadsby PJ, Zagami AS, Lambert GA. Neuroprocessing of craniovascular pain: A synthesis of the central structures involved in migraine. *Headache,* 31:365–371, 1991.

Lashley KS. Patterns of cerebral integration indicated by scotomatas of migraine. *Arch Neurol Psychiatry,* 46:331, 1941.

Lauritzen M. Links between cortical spreading depression and migraine: Clinical and experimental aspects. (In) *Migraine and Other Headaches: The Vascular Mechanism,* Volume 1. J Olesen (Ed), Pgs 143–151, New York, Raven Press, 1991.

Leão AAP. P1A1 circulation and spreading activity in the cerebral cortex. *J Neurophysiol,* 7:391, 1944.

Moskowitz MA. Basic mechanisms in vascular headache. (In) *Neurologic Clinics.* NT Mathew (Ed). Pgs 801–815, Philadelphia, WB Saunders, November, 1990.

Olesen J. Clinical and pathophysiological observations in migraine and tension-type headache explained by integration of vascular, supraspinal, and myofascial inputs. *Pain,* 46:125–133, 1991.

Ramadan NM, Halvorson H, Vande-Linde AMQ, et al. Low brain magnesium in migraine. *Headache,* 29:590–593, 1989.

Raskin NH. Serotonin receptors and headache. *N Engl J Med,* 325:353–354, 1991.

Raskin NH, Hosobuchi Y, Lamb S. Headache may arise from perturbation of brain. *Headache,* 27:416–420, 1987.

Saito K, Markowitz S, Moskowitz MA. Ergot alkaloids block neurogenic extravasation in dura mater: Proposed action in vascular headaches. *Ann Neurol,* 24:732–737, 1988.

Schoenen J, Sianard-Gain KO, Lenaerts M. Blood magnesium levels in migraine. *Cephalalgia,* 11:97–99, 1991.

Sessle BJ, Hu JW, Amano N, et al. The convergence of cutaneous, tooth pulp, visceral, neck, and muscle afferents onto nociceptive and non-nociceptive neurons in trigeminal subnucleus caudalis (medullary dorsal horn) and its implications for referred pain. *Pain,* 27:219–235, 1986.

Silberstein SD. Advances in understanding the pathophysiology of headache. *Neurology,* 42 (supp 2):6–10, 1992.

Silva JE, Brown JD, Watson BV, et al. Temporal arteritis presenting as bilateral brachioplexopathy (Abstract). *Neurology,* 1998.

Weiller C, May A, Limmroth V, et al. Brainstem activation in human migraine attacks. *Nat Med,* 1:858–860, 1995.

Welch KMA. Synthesis of mechanisms. (In) the American Academy of Neurology: *Scientific Basis of Migraine.* Presented at the 49th Annual Meeting of the AAN, Boston, MA, 1997.

Welch KMA, Andrea GD, Tepley N, et al. The concept of migraine as a state of central neuronal hyperexcitability. (In) *Neurologic Clinics: Headache.* NT Mathew (Ed). Pgs 817–828, Philadelphia, WB Saunders, 1990.

Welch KMA, Levine SR, D'Andrea G, et al.. Preliminary observations on brain energy metabolism and migraine, studied by in-vivo phosphorous 31 NMR spectroscopy. *Neurology,* 39:538–541, 1989.

Woods RP, Iacoboni M, Mazziotta JC. Bilateral spreading cerebral hypoperfusion during spontaneous migraine headache. *N Engl J Med,* 331:1689, 1994.

5

Differential Diagnosis of Headache

I. Introduction

Over 300 entities cause headache. The *primary headache disorders,* such as migraine, tension-type headache, and cluster headache, are those in which headache represents the primary symptom or at least one of the primary symptoms of a physiological disorder. These disorders generally do not have identifiable gross microscopic pathology, although actual or presumed physiological disturbances, such as the recently identified "migraine generator," are suspected (see Chapter 4). The primary headache conditions often have an inherited biological predisposition, and genetic disturbances are now being identified.

The *secondary headache conditions* are those in which the headache represents a symptom of a pathological, organic process. Table 5.1 lists selected categories of illness that can produce secondary headache and mimic benign disorders, such as migraine or cluster headache.

A headache differential diagnosis can be approached in several ways, though admittedly none is entirely satisfactory. We have chosen to approach the differential diagnosis of headache from a clinical temporal perspective, that is, certain conditions produce headache with a characteristic pattern of onset, buildup, and evolution. Some are explosive and sudden in onset. Others begin insidiously or subacutely and progress slowly or aggressively in intensity and frequency.

This chapter reviews the key differential diagnostic possibilities within the context of three temporal patterns of headache. Because many of the conditions demonstrate more than one temporal pattern, conditions may be listed in more than one category. Clearly, assignment to a category is arbitrary, and an awareness of the many differential diagnostic possibilities is required in all settings.

The three temporal categories include:

1. Sudden, abrupt-onset headache (acute buildup);
2. Subacute onset with persistent or intermittent pattern; and
3. Insidious onset with slow buildup (persistent or episodic).

All cases of "new onset" headache must be evaluated carefully. The term "new onset" headache refers to headaches that have never been present before or in which the pattern or accompanying symptoms are new. Such headaches often have significant clinical importance. Moreover, new onset headache may be superimposed upon an existing and continuing headache pattern.

TABLE 5.1. **SELECTED CATEGORIES OF ILLNESSES THAT CAUSE HEADACHE**

Intracranial structural disease
Infectious disease (including AIDS, Lyme disease, sinusitis, etc.)
Cerebrovascular ischemia
Cerebral vein thrombosis
Metabolic/toxic disturbances
CNS disturbances of intracranial pressure (high or low)
Vasculitis and connective tissue disease
Hemorrhage (parenchymal and subarachnoid)
Head trauma
Withdrawal syndromes
Severe hypertension
Dental, cranial vault, temporomandibular disorders, and myofascial disease
Cervical spine and occipitocervical jjunction disease (Arnold Chiari Type I
    malformation, facet joint syndromes, etc.)
AV malformations/aneurysms
Intraocular disease (glaucoma, etc.)

II. Sudden-Onset, Rapidly Worsening, Severe Headache ("Acute Buildup, 'First or Worst,' etc.")
A. Description

A sudden-onset, "first or worst" headache must always be assumed to be the result of an acute neurological event, although it may reflect nothing more than a severe migraine or cluster attack. Migraine can be associated with a "thunderclap" pattern, also referred to as "crash migraine." Changes in awareness or cognition, or the presence of neurological signs or symptoms suggest, but do not in themselves establish with certainty, the presence of an intracranial or systemic process. On the other hand, the absence of these disturbances does not rule out organic disease.

Central nervous system (CNS) organic disease can provoke what would otherwise appear to be typical migraine attacks. A rapid-onset, severe migraine may be difficult to differentiate from the symptoms of a subarachnoid hemorrhage (SAH), cerebral venous thrombosis, or headache associated with stroke.

Among the key and worrisome features are:

1. Abrupt-onset headache (unexpected event) that rapidly progresses in seconds to minutes;
2. Accompaniments, which may include nausea and vomiting, fever, stiff neck, focal neurological findings, papilledema, changes in mental function or level of consciousness, or other neurological events; and
3. A continuing, persistent, or progressive pattern. In some serious conditions, acute-onset headache may be associated with temporary reduction or cessation of the pain, as with a *sentinel*

headache associated with aneurysm (see below). However, in most instances a persistent headache is present. Table 5.2 lists selected diagnostic possibilities characterized by sudden-onset severe headache.

B. Selected Conditions
1. Subarachnoid hemorrhage (SAH)

SAH from a ruptured aneurysm occurs in 28,000 people per year in North America. It typically presents as an acute, sudden-onset, bilateral severe headache (often called "thunderclap headache") associated with nuchal rigidity (within 24 hours), photophobia, nausea, vomiting, and perhaps obtundation or coma. A *sentinel headache* is a severe sudden-onset headache that often abates temporarily, and usually represents a warning of impending catastrophic hemorrhage. (The now well-known case described by Day and Raskin (1986) is a good example of this condition. Three acute headache events occurred prior to the arteriographic demonstration of an aneurysm.) The *sentinel headache* may manifest as a severe headache alone or in association with nausea, vomiting, and, occasionally, stiff neck. It is not easily distinguished from an acute migraine, and in a person

---

TABLE 5.2. **CONDITIONS ASSOCIATED WITH SUDDEN-ONSET HEADACHE (ACUTE BUILDUP)**

Intracranial hemorrhage
   SAH
   Intracerebral hemorrhage
   Subdural or epidural hematoma
   Pituitary hemorrhage
Acute severe hypertension
   Pressor response
   Pheochromocytoma
   Malignant hypertension
Acute glaucoma
Internal carotid or vertebral dissection or other acute carotid syndromes
Acute obstructive hydrocephalus (from tumor, etc.)
Head trauma (hemorrhage, cavernous sinus thrombosis, etc.)
Spontaneous or traumatic low pressure syndrome (may also be subacute in onset)
"Crash" migraine (thunderclap migraine)

The following conditions may cause sudden-onset attacks but are more likely to be
   subacute in presentation and have rapid but not sudden buildup.
Encephalitis/meningitis
Sinusitis/periorbital cellulitis
Cerebral vein thrombosis (may present with "thunderclap" headache)
Optic neuritis
Migraine
Ischemic cerebrovascular disease
Cerebral vasculitis

with a history of migraine, it may not be distinguishable at all by history alone.

Subarachnoid hemorrhage from an arteriovenous (A-V) malformation may be less dramatic than from an aneurysm.

If frank subarachnoid hemorrhage or impending hemorrhage is suspected, an extensive neurological evaluation is necessary, including a computed tomography (CT) scan (with and without contrast) and lumbar puncture (LP). The importance of magnetic resonance imaging (MRI) and/or MR angiography (MRA) to rule out an aneurysm is gaining support, and most authorities now believe that MRA can rule out aneurysms of 5 mm in size or larger (perhaps even smaller). They are the most likely to be problematic. The need for arteriography in suspected cases must be determined on an individual basis. Up until now, it has been the prevailing view that if the CT scan (without contrast) and an LP are normal within 24 hours of the attack, further invasive studies, such as arteriography, are not necessary. However, cases such as that of Day and Raskin (1996) in which three acute-onset (sentinel) headaches were accompanied by a normal CT scan and lumbar puncture, and the availability of reliable MR angiography, lend support to the greater application of MRA in this clinical setting. MRA, when skillfully performed and rigorously interpreted, is approaching the accuracy of conventional arteriography in the diagnosis of intracranial aneurysms, according to some authorities. Although Wijdicks (1988) presented data suggesting that a CT scan and LP accurately evaluated the presence or absence of aneurysm in patients with sudden onset headache, the availability of a relatively safe and painless technology, along with its growing sophistication, appear to be shifting the attitude toward using these studies in the workup of patients with bona fide "thunderclap" events.

2. Spontaneous, acute brain (parenchymal) hemorrhage

Cerebral and cerebellar hemorrhage may cause sudden-onset headache, and have also been reported in patients with migraine, with and without previous hypertension. Whether migraine is itself a risk factor to hemorrhage remains uncertain. Unlike subarachnoid hemorrhage, acute parenchymal hemorrhage is more likely associated with acute neurological signs. Distinguishing the headache due to parenchymal hemorrhage from that of subarachnoid hemorrhage may be difficult if blood enters the ventricular system and if neurological events are present. Parenchymal hemorrhage can also result from bleeding into a brain tumor. Pituitary apoplexy can present with severe headache and be difficult to diagnose.

3. Acute, severe hypertension

Suddenly elevated hypertension (greater than 25% rise in diastolic pressure or a combined pressure of 180/130 mm Hg) can produce a severe, sudden-onset headache. More moderate elevations of systolic and/or diastolic pressure, though frequent accompaniments of migraine, generally do not cause headache. Stupor, seizures, or focal neurological signs are present in *hypertensive encephalopathy*. Pressor responses result from toxic or medication effects (e.g., monoamine oxidase inhibitor [MAOI] etc.). *Pheochromocytoma* is associated with diaphoresis, palpitations, and anxiety symptomatology and is diagnosed by chemical and imaging tests (see page 50).

4. Acute angle closure glaucoma

Glaucoma often presents with sudden-onset orbital and eye pain associated with headache, pupillary changes conjunctival injection, lens clouding, and sometimes nausea, vomiting, and other symptoms. The demonstration of elevated intraocular pressure is diagnostic. *Onset may occur following the use of anticholinergic drugs.* Tables 5.3 and 5.4 list the ocular and otolaryngological causes of headache. (Also see Chapter 16.)

5. Spontaneous internal carotid artery dissection

Spontaneous dissection of the carotid artery is an uncommon but important cause of sudden-onset headache and acute neurological symptoms. The headache is often unilateral and located in the orbital, periorbital, frontal, or neck regions. Stroke-related symptoms and pupillary changes (including a Horner's syndrome) can accompany or precede the headache. Internal carotid artery dissection should be considered in the presence of acute-onset headache or neck pain, pupillary disturbance or Horner's syndrome, tinnitus, and the presence of stroke-like symptoms. MRI/MRA of the neck can be diagnostic in most instances, although carotid arteriography may be required. Ultrasound studies, when expertly performed and interpreted, are also considered reliable.

Giant cell arteritis, atherosclerotic thrombosis, fibromuscular dysplasia, and carotid aneurysm, as well as parenchymal brain hemorrhage, may produce a similar clinical picture. (See Chapter 14 for further discussion of spontaneous internal carotid and vertebral artery dissection.)

TABLE 5.3. **SELECTED OCULAR CATEGORIES OF HEADACHE (SEE CHAPTER 16 FOR ADDITIONAL LISTINGS)**

Glaucoma
  Narrow angle (acute) glaucoma
  Neovascular glaucoma (from neovascularization secondary to disease, such as carotid
    stenosis, retinal vein or artery occlusion, diabetic retinopathy, etc.)
Corneal and conjunctival disease
Asthenopia
Retrobulbar neuritis
Ischemic ocular inflammation
Uveitis (intraocular inflammatory disease)
Diseases of the orbit
  Cellulitis
  Inflammatory or noninflammatory orbital pseudotumor
  Orbital myositis
  Lacrimal gland disease (tumors, cysts, infection)
  Posterior scleritis
Herpes zoster opthalmicus
Painful ophthalmoplegia (Tolosa-Hunt syndrome)
Cavernous sinus thrombosis, fistula, aneurysm

TABLE 5.4. **SELECTED OTOLARYNGOLOGICAL CATEGORIES OF HEADACHE (SEE CHAPTER 16 FOR ADDITIONAL LISTINGS)**

Cerumen impaction
External otitis
Herpes zoster oticus
Myringitis (tympanic membrane inflammation)
Otitis media
Mastoiditis
Gradenigo syndrome (CN VI palsy, eye pain, and sometimes discharge from the ear)
  from temporal bone infection (petrositis)
Eagle's syndrome (elongation of the styloid process)
Ernest syndrome (stylomandibular ligament syndrome)
Carotodynia
Temporomandibular joint syndrome
Cranial neuralgias (glossopharyngeal neuralgia, superior laryngeal neuralgia)
Malignancy (primary and metastatic), infiltrative nasopharyngeal cancer, etc.
Denture misfittings
Nasal disease/septum deformities
Sinus disease (sphenoid sinusitis is particularly virulent)
  Infectious (bacterial or fungal), granulomatous, abscess
  Occlusive/obstructive
Others

III. Subacute, Intermittent, or Persistent Headaches (Rapid But Not Sudden Buildup)
A. Description

The distinction between this pattern of buildup and the sudden, acute onset (thunderclap) pattern is the intensity and rapidity of the buildup period. Arbitrarily, buildup in the sudden, acute-onset (thunderclap) pattern occurs over seconds to a minute or so, whereas the buildup in the subacute form occurs over minutes, hours, or days. Overlap occurs, and benign disorders, such as migraine, cerebral vein thrombosis, and others, may present in either pattern. Moreover, awareness of the existence of previous similar headache attacks is helpful in placing subsequent attacks into the proper diagnostic perspective. Table 5.5 lists illnesses capable of producing a subacute-onset and recurring or persistent headache.

B. Selected Topics

1. A-V malformation

A-V malformation may present with either acute, sudden-onset subarachnoid hemorrhage (thunderclap) or with less dramatic, progressive, or episodic bouts of migraine-like headaches, sometimes preceded by neurological symptoms mimicking typical migraine with aura. Other patterns are possible.

2. Cerebral ischemia

Cerebral ischemia and stroke may result in persistent or episodic headaches that may precede, accompany, or follow the acute neurological event. Neurological symptomatology is usually evident within 48 hours of headache onset, but not always. Approximately 35% of patients with stroke initially present with headache, and 25% of patients with a transient ischemic attack (TIA) experience headache. The headache is nonspecific. Clinical differentiation between embolic, thrombotic, and hemorrhagic disease is often impossible on clinical grounds. Table 5.6 lists the cerebrovascular causes of headache. (See Chapter 8 for a discussion of stroke and migraine.)

3. Cerebral vein thrombosis

Thrombotic occlusion of the dural sinus and cerebral veins can produce acute, severe intermittent, or continuous headache. Sometimes it can present as a "thunderclap" headache (de Bruijn, 1996). Thrombosis of the cerebral sinuses or veins can result in headache, intracranial hypertension with papilledema, or focal neurological seizures, and if hemorrhagic infarction (with or without subarachnoid hemorrhage or intraparenchymal hemorrhage) occurs, the result can be major neurological events and progressive obtundation.

Cavernous sinus thrombosis, which can result from sphenoid sinusitis (see later in this Chapter and in Chapter 16), causes pain around the eye and over the forehead and progressive unilateral visual disturbances, together with conjunctival changes, proptosis, ophthalmoplegia, and occasionally edema of the face.

TABLE 5.5. **CONDITIONS ASSOCIATED WITH SUBACUTE-ONSET**

Cerebrovascular ischemia (TIA, embolic disease, etc.)
Cerebral vein thrombosis, including cavernous sinus thrombosis, fistula, etc.
Obstructive hydrocephalus, including Arnold-Chiari malformation type I
Pheochromocytoma
Neuralgic syndromes
Cluster headache, chronic paroxysmal hemicrania
Migraine
Cerebral vasculitis
Cerebral tumors (most commonly a progressive, worsening course, but can be
  intermittent initially)
Intracranial hypertension (pseudotumor cerebri)
Recurring hemorrhage from A-V malformation
Headache associated with substances or their withdrawal (ergotamine, caffeine, narcotics,
  etc.)
Subdural hematoma (usually progressive, but can be intermittent)
Occipitocervical junction disease
CSF hypotension (can be sudden onset; from spontaneous or traumatic cause)
Dental, cranial vault, TM joint disease
Cranial, paranasal sinusitis (see Druce, 1991; see Chapter 16)

TABLE 5.6. **CEREBROVASCULAR DISEASES CAUSING HEADACHE**

Occlusive vascular disease
  Emboli
  Transient ischemic attack (TIA)
  Internal carotid or vertebral artery occlusion or dissection
  Occlusion of middle cerebral artery
  Thrombosis of cerebral veins or dural sinus
  Fibromuscular hyperplasia
  Vasculitis (giant cell arteritis, etc.)
Severe hypertension
Hemorrhage
  Pituitary
  Subarachnoid hemorrhage
  Cerebellar/cerebral parenchymal hemorrhage
  Subdural and epidural hematoma

For venous thrombotic syndromes, contrast CT scanning, venous-phase MRI/MRA, and/or arteriography are important diagnostic interventions, as are appropriate laboratory studies to rule out coagulopathic illnesses, including antiphospholipid antibody syndrome.

Treatment of cerebral vein thrombosis includes reduction of intracranial pressure, anticoagulation, and treatment of seizures, if present. Thrombolytic treatment following catheter placement into the involved sinuses is also used. Headache may improve with resolution of the condition but may prove resistant to early treatment, other than with narcotic analgesics. Patients may present with features similar to those of pseudotumor cerebri (benign increased intracranial pressure; see later in this Chapter and Chapter 18), particularly when there is involvement of the lateral sinus (*otitic hydrocephalus*).

4. Obstructive hydrocephalus

Obstructive hydrocephalus may produce headache with gait disturbances, changes in cognition, or other neurological events. Postural abnormalities, worsened by exertion or neck posture, are noted frequently. Enlargement of the ventricular system, as seen by CT scanning or MRI, and increased intracranial pressure are diagnostic features. Headache is usually improved with reduction in pressure. Intermittent elevations result in periodic headaches. Headaches associated with Arnold Chiari Type I malformation typically produce headaches during straining or cough (increases intracranial pressure), and with neck movement. In addition, other forms of headache, including persistent headache, may be associated with Arnold Chiari malformation (Khurana, 1991; Stovner, 1993). The technique of cine-phase MRI assessment of Arnold Chiari Type I malformation may improve the diagnostic accuracy for the diagnosis of cervical occipital obstructions (see Chapters 15, 17, 19, and others, Arnold-Chiari Type I malformation).

5. Pheochromocytoma

Pheochromocytoma can produce episodic headache, often provoked by exertion or from certain medications such as β-adrenergic blocking agents. Periodic or sustained elevations of blood pressure, excessive perspiration, and palpitations and anxiety symptoms are usually present. A family history is noted in approximately 10% of cases. This disorder can be associated with *neurofibromatosis* and *cafe au lait spots*. The diagnosis of pheochromocytoma is based on biochemical evidence, including elevated urinary catecholamines and related metabolites (metanephrine, normetanephrine, and vanillylmandelic acid) from a 24-hour urine specimen and CT, ultrasound, or MRI evidence of a suprarenal mass.

IV. Insidious Onset Headache with Slow (Chronic) Buildup

A. Description

This category frequently includes those illnesses that have an insidious onset and a progressive course, although episodic pain may be present initially. Table 5.7 lists selected conditions characterized by insidious onset, persistent, and progressive headache patterns.

B. Selected Topics

1. Chronic subdural hematoma

Chronic subdural hematoma can produce severe or milder forms of progressive, bilateral, or unilateral headache, at times

TABLE 5.7. **CONDITIONS ASSOCIATED WITH SUBACUTE TO INSIDIOUS BUILDUP, PERSISTENT, AND/OR PROGRESSIVE HEADACHE (SLOW BUILDUP)**

Chronic subdural hematoma
Brain tumor
Brain abscess
Cerebral vein thrombosis, including cavernous sinus thrombosis (often rapid buildup)
Idiopathic intracranial hypertension (pseudotumor cerebri)
Central nervous system (CNS) infection (fungal, Lyme, viral meningitis, etc.)
Giant cell arteritis, etc.
Migraine and its variants
Hemicrania continua
Progressive metabolic abnormalities (hypoxia, renal or liver failure, hypercapnia, etc.)
Headache associated with substances or their withdrawal
Cerebrospinal fluid (CSF) hypotension (postural) (often rapid buildup)
Cervical spine, occipitocervical junction disease
Dental, cranial vault, temporomandibular (TM) joint disease
Cranial, paranasal sinusitis

with an insidious onset and fluctuating intensity. Changes in cognition, personality, and neurological signs are common accompaniments. Less than half of the patients give a prior history of head trauma. Thus, a high index of suspicion is necessary to make the diagnosis. Cranial percussion tenderness may occur over the site of hematoma.

2. Brain tumor

Headache occurs as the presenting symptom of *brain tumor* in approximately 40% of patients. But, by some estimates, headaches are present in less than 50% of patients with brain tumor, and this data may reflect the now earlier detection because of CT scanning and MRI (Forsyth, 1993). Increased intracranial pressure, tumor size, and the amount of midline shift seem to be factors associated with brain-tumor-related headache. A prior history of headache is more likely to be associated with the development of headaches with brain tumor.

Differentiating headache due to brain tumors from migraine and tension-type headache is difficult. The "classic" headache associated with brain tumor, i.e., severe, worse in the morning, and associated with nausea and vomiting, occurs in less than 20% of patients, and most of these patients have increased intracranial pressure. The headache is usually generalized but can overlie the tumor. The headaches may be mild to moderate in severity, and commonly are accompanied by nausea and vomiting (seen in about 40% of patients). If an intermittent and throbbing pattern is present, differentiation from migraine is difficult. Altered position, coughing, or exertion may aggravate the headache in approximately 32% of patients. The most common headache is described as a dull ache or pressure. It is usually bifrontal but frequently worse on the ipsilateral side. It is most commonly seen with supratentorial tumors or increased pressure. Twenty-five percent of patients have unilateral headaches, and these are generally on the side of the tumor. In those patients with headache associated with increased intracranial pressure, the distinctive features included severity, nausea and vomiting, and resistance to common analgesics. Many patients describe "the worst pain they had experienced." A progressive pattern eventually occurs. Brain tumors may undergo spontaneous, parenchymal hemorrhage.

Overall, the "classic" brain tumor description is relatively uncommon, and the headache associated with the tumor is more likely to be nonspecific and may even be mild. It is frequently intermittent. It is not the quality of the headache but the accompanying symptoms and signs that suggest a brain tumor. Headaches associated with a brain tumor are similar to tension-type headache in 77%, migraine in 9%, and other types in 14% (Forsyth, 1993).

3. Brain abscess

The headache of *brain abscess* is similar to that of brain tumor. However, the course is usually more rapid. Associated meningitis and/or other signs of infection may be evident.

4. Idiopathic intracranial hypertension (pseudotumor cerebri)

Pseudotumor cerebri, also called *idiopathic* or *benign intracranial hypertension,* is associated with headache that sometimes correlates with pressure elevation, but which may have features more reminiscent of migraine variants including daily, persistent headache. Visual obscuration and papilledema are noted in most but not all cases. The condition is most common, though not exclusively, in obese women, often with hormonal or endocrine disturbances. It has been reported following administration of antibiotics and danocrine, as well as other agents. It may be associated with postconcussional syndrome and with cases that appear otherwise typical of daily chronic, persistent headache (Mathew, 1997). Diagnosis must be established by lumbar puncture that demonstrates elevation of cerebral spinal fluid pressure.

Headaches characteristically, but not always, improve following a lumbar puncture. Pain can become persistent, despite the reduction of increased pressure. *Moreover, approximately 5–15% of patients do not demonstrate papilledema, either be-*

cause of anatomical variation in the sheath or in chronic cases, due to atrophic changes in the optic disc. (See Chapter 18 for a more complete discussion.)

5. Giant cell arteritis (temporal arteritis)

Temporal arteritis, giant cell arteritis (GCA), is a painful inflammation of the cranial arteries. It is more properly considered a vasculitis of the aortic arch and its branches. Thus, it can be associated with a wide spectrum of vascular disturbances, including anterior ischemic optic neuropathy and sudden visual loss. Cerebral infarction, myocardial infarction, and aortic rupture are the most serious complications of GCA. Headache is an important symptom and occurs in approximately 70% of patients. It is the initial symptom in approximately one-third of patients. GCA is frequently associated with systemic signs and symptoms, including general malaise, myalgias, arthralgias, and anemia. Headache, the most consistent complaint, may localize anywhere about the scalp but is most often in the temples (half of cases). The condition often begins insidiously and may persist for weeks, months, or years. Orbital pain, anorexia, weight loss, and diaphoresis may be accompaniments.

Other important symptoms of GCA are ischemia (and claudication) of jaw and tongue muscles, cranial neuropathic syndromes, carotodynia, optic neuropathy, ocular motility disorders, brachioplexopathy (Silva, 1998), and other neurologic events, including encephalopathy. Polymyalgia rheumatica (PMR) occurs in approximately 50% of patients and may represent the initial symptom in up to one-fourth of patients with GCA.

Sudden visual loss or stroke-like symptoms are the most serious complications of GCA. The diagnosis is suspected by clinical history, the presence of a tender, nonpulsatile temporal artery, and an elevation of erythrocyte sedimentation rate (range 60–120 mm Westergren). *A normal or only modestly elevated sedimentation rate is seen in 3–25% of patients.* Other acute-phase reactant proteins may also be increased. A complete blood (cell) count (CBC) may reveal normochromic, microcytic anemia. Mild elevation of the serum transaminases and alkaline phosphatase occurs in a small percentage of people, and elevation of plasma alpha-2 globulins occurs in 72% of patients. Temporal artery biopsy and/or arteriography are generally required to confirm the diagnosis.

The damage due to the vasculature by GCA is the result of activation of CD4+T helper cells that respond to an antigen presented by macrophages. Thus, the condition represents a disease of cellular immune mechanisms. The inflammatory response occurs around the internal elastic lamina.

Most cases of GCA occur in persons after the age of 50, but the condition has been reported in younger patients.

Steroid therapy is the treatment of choice. Other immunosuppressant drugs may also be required (see Goadsby and Silberstein, 1997).

Other vasculitides must also be considered. Idiopathic granulomatis angiitis of the CNS presents with headache, altered neural function, and focal neurological deficits. It may resemble neoplastic, demyelinating, and vascular disorders. Arteriography and brain biopsy are generally required to establish the diagnosis (Finelli, 1997; Younger, 1997).

6. Systemic or intracranial infection

Systemic or intracranial infection can produce severe headache. Alternately, severe migraine or migraine-like headaches may be activated by systemic or CNS infection. The presence of fever or signs of infection accompanying headache mandates a complete evaluation. A stiff neck may or may not be present. Photophobia is common. In most instances, infection produces a progressive or persistent headache pattern, but it may be intermittent initially.

a. Benign viral meningitis

Benign viral meningitis may present with subacute severe headache associated with mild nuchal rigidity and significant photophobia. The cerebrospinal fluid (CSF) usually demonstrates the presence of mild to moderate leukocytosis. The condition is generally self-limited, but the headache requires treatment. Short-term analgesic administration seems most appropriate.

b. Lyme Disease

Lyme borreliosis is a multisystem infection resulting from infection by the spirochete Borrelia bugdorfi. In the early phases, patients may have a characteristic cutaneous infection called erythema migrans. Some patients develop disseminated and chronic infections with prominent rheumatological, cardiac, and neurological manifestations. During the erythema migrans phase, headache occurs in 38–54% of patients. Most problematic are the patients who present with headache as an isolated manifestation of Lyme disease. Four causally related forms of neurologic disease or dysfunction occur: lymphocytic meningitis with or without cranial neuritis or painful radiculoneuritis or both; encephalomyelitis; peripheral neuropathy; and encephalopathy.

Only rare reports point to headache as the most prominent neurological manifestation of CNS Lyme disease. Halperin et al. (1989) reported the case of a woman with chronic headache and a positive CSF Lyme Antibody Index; headaches completely resolved after treatment with ceftriaxone. Other cases have also been reported in which the CSF Lyme Antibody Index was positive and the headaches resolved after intravenous antibiotic therapy.

The appropriate workup for patients with headache and suspected Lyme disease is problematic. Recommended testing includes serologic testing (enzyme-linked immunosorbent assay [ELISA]), the Western Blot test, demonstration of intrathecal antibody production, and culture and polymerase chain reaction studies.

Selsa et al. (1995) offer the following recommendations:

- Testing for Lyme is not recommended as a matter of routine in patients presenting with typical headaches alone (false-positive tests would lead to inappropriate evaluation or treatment).
- If headache is accompanied by clinically apparent systemic or neurological manifestations of Lyme disease, serum antibody testing by ELISA is suggested.
- In patients with atypical headaches, ELISA testing for Lyme should be considered.
- Suspected false-positive ELISAs should be confirmed by Western Blot for Borrelia-specific antigens.
- Patients with headache as the only neurological manifestation and a positive ELISA and Western Blot should be treated with oral doxycycline 100 mg. p.o. b.i.d. for 3–4 weeks.
- In patients with headache and evidence of other suspected Lyme-related neurological disorder/dysfunction (encephalopathy, cognitive deficits, focal deficits, etc.), neuroimaging or lumbar puncture for cell count, protein, glucose, and Lyme Antibody Index is recommended. If CNS disease is present, intravenous therapy should be considered.

c. Acquired Immune Deficiency Syndrome (AIDS)

AIDS is a disturbance of cell-mediated immunity resulting in opportunistic infections and demyelinating disorders. Headache may be the presenting symptom in persons with CNS involvement and is most likely caused by cryptococcal meningitis and other HIV-related meningitides. The headache is generalized and diffuse and is most prominent in the frontal and occipital regions. Nausea and vomiting are common.

d. Other Infections

Systemic viruses may either spread directly to the CNS or impart "remote effects," in which direct spread is not apparent. Persistent headache, mood and mental disturbances, sleep abnormalities, and fatigue, among other phenomena, are common. Current speculation suggests that neurotransmitter/receptor disturbances result from either direct viral involvement or remote influence on CNS mechanisms. The *chronic fatigue syndrome* may be the most apparent example.

(For other meningitides or encephalitis, including those caused by herpes simplex and others, consult standard neurological textbooks.)

7. Sinusitis

Acute sinusitis of the paranasal sinuses is a cause of headache. *Subacute sinusitis* may well cause headache itself or activate preexistent headache conditions, such as migraine. *Chronic sinusitis* of the paranasal sinuses may potentiate existing migraine tendencies as well.

Acute sphenoid sinusitis must be distinguished from other forms of paranasal sinusitis. The sphenoid sinuses lie within the middle cranial fossa, inferior to the pituitary region and medial to the cavernous sinuses. Acute sphenoid sinusitis represents a neurological emergency. Headache, neuralgic pain in the distribution of trigeminal V1 or V2 branches, progressive monocular visual loss, and impairment of ocular motility may accompany progressively severe headache. The headache is often located at the vertex but may occur anywhere throughout the cranium. Progressive symptoms, inability to sleep, and failure to respond to pain therapy are noteworthy characteristics. Acute sphenoid sinusitis may result from bacterial infection or fungal involvement. Progression may lead to rupture into the cavernous sinus which lies laterally. Catastrophic neurological implications result. Fatality has resulted from spread into the leptomeninges, and rapidly evolving permanent visual impairment from involvement of the ipsilateral optic nerve make the aggressive pursuit of symptoms mandatory. Acute sphenoid sinusitis does not generally respond to oral antibiotics but requires intravenous antibiotics and/or surgical drainage in up to 50% of cases. A CT scan, with specific views of the sphenoid sinuses, and/or MRI imaging are required to establish the initial diagnosis. Endoscopic assessment and treatment are likewise required in some instances.

V. Summary

The clinician must have a broad perspective when considering the differential diagnosis of headache. The clinical overlapping of symptoms and signs that is apparent in the various presentations listed in this chapter reflects the difficulty in approaching this challenge within the limits of any one perspective. Diagnostic studies must be determined by the presence of specific signs or symptoms or headache patterns that raise reasonable concerns regarding the possible presence of organic pathology. The following phenomena should alert the clinician to this possibility:

1. New onset headache, particularly persistent headache;
2. A variation from a preexisting pattern;
3. The presence of medical or neurological signs or symptoms;
4. Atypical headache features, varying from typical episodic primary headache patterns;
5. Progressive headache;
6. Acute-onset (rapid or sudden buildup) headaches; and
7. Resistance or refractoriness to standard treatment

While none of the above may in and of itself indicate the presence of pathology, they might! Similarly, headaches of significant pathological origin may present with what initially appears to be a benign, and at times ordinary, headache. *Reappraisal and retesting is required in chronic headache disorders.* The superimposition of a new disorder on a preexisting primary headache condition is all too familiar. From time to time the clinician must reappraise and challenge the diagnosis. All too often, the long-term presence of a benign headache syndrome has resulted in failure to take a new headache pattern seriously, by either the patient or the clinician.

References

Antiphospholipid Antibodies and Stroke Study Group (APASS). Anticardiolipin antibodies are an independent risk factor for first ischemic stroke. *Neurology,* 43:2069–2073, 1993.

Bindoff LA, Hezeltine D. Unilateral facial pain in patients with lung cancer: Referred pain via the vagus? *Lancet*, 1:812–825, 1988.

Brinck T, Hansen K, Olesen J. Headache resembling tension-type headache as the single manifestation of lyme borreliosis. *Cephalalgia*, 13:207–209, 1993.

Brook I, Overturf GD, Steinberg EA, et al. Acute sphenoid sinusitis presenting as aseptic meningitis: A pachymeningitis syndrome. *Intl J Pediatr Otorhinolaryngol*, 4:79–81, 1982.

Cant RS, Daniel FI. Glossopharyngeal neuralgia in a child. *Arch Neurol*, 43:301–302, 1986.

Caplan L. Intracerebral hemorrhage revisited. *Neurology*, 38:624–627, 1988.

Cole AJ, Aube M. Migraine with vasospasm and delayed intracerebral hemorrhage. *Arch Neurol*, 47:53–56, 1990.

Cox LK, Bertorini T, Lassiter RE. Headaches due to spontaneous internal carotid artery dissection: Magnetic resonance imaging evaluation follow-up. *Headache*, 31:12–16, 1991.

D'Angelejan-Chatillon J, Ribeiro V, Mas JL, et al. Migraine—a risk factor for dissection of cervical arteries. *Headache*, 29:560–561, 1989.

de Bruijn SF, Stam J, Kappelle LJ. Thunderclap headache as first symptom of cerebral venous thrombosis. *Lancet*, 348:1623–1625, 1996.

Day JW, Raskin NH. Thunderclap headache: Symptom of unruptured cerebral aneurysm. *Lancet*, 2:1247–1248, 1986.

DeAngelis LM, Payne R. Lymphomatous meningitis presenting as atypical cluster headache. *Pain*, 30:211–216, 1987.

de Bruijn SF, Stom J, Kappelle LJ. Thunderclap headache as first symptom of cerebral venous thrombosis. *Lancet*, 348:1623–1625, 1996.

Druce HM, Slavin RG. Sinusitis: Critical need for further study. *J Allergy Clin Immunol*, 88:675–677, 1991.

Dwyer A, Aprill C, Bogduk N. Cervical zygapophyseal joint pain patterns I: A study in normal volunteers. *Spine*, 15:453–457, 1990.

Finelli PF, Onyiuke HC, Uphoff DF. Idiopathic granulamatous angiitis of the CNS manifesting as diffuse white matter disease. *Neurology*, 49:1696–1699, 1997.

Fisher CM. The headache and pain of spontaneous carotid dissection. *Headache*, 22:660–665, 1982.

Forsyth PA, Posner JB. Headaches in patients with brain tumors: A study of 111 patients. *Neurology*, 43:1678–1683, 1993.

Goldstein J. Headache and acquired immunodeficiency disorder. (In) *Neurologic Clinics*. NT Mathew (Ed). Pgs 947–960, Philadelphia, WB Saunders, November, 1990.

Halperin JJ, Volkman DJ, Wu P. Central nervous system abnormalities and Lyme neuroborreliosis. *Neurology*, 41:1571–1582, 1991.

Hannerz J. A case of parasellar meningioma mimicking cluster headache. *Cephalalgia*, 9:265–269, 1989.

Hannerz J. Recurrent Tolosa-Hunt syndrome. *Cephalalgia*, 12:45–51, 1992.

Harling DW, Peatfield RC, Van Hille PTE, et al. Thunderclap headache: Is it migraine? *Cephalalgia*, 9:87–90, 1989.

Khurana RK. Headache spectrum and Arnold-Chiari malformation. *Headache*, 31:151–155, 1991.

Levine SR, Salowich-Palm L, Sawaya KL, et al. IgG anticardiolipin antibody titre > 40 GPL and the risk of subsequent thrombo-occlusive events and death: A perspective cohort study. *Stroke*, 28:1660–1665, 1997.

Lew D, Southwick FS, Montgomery WW, et al. Sphenoid sinusitis: Review of 30 cases. *N Engl J Med*, 309:1149–1155, 1983.

Marcelis J, Silberstein SD. Spontaneous low cerebral spinal fluid pressure headache. *Headache,* 30:192–196, 1990.

Mathew NT, Ravishkar K, Sanin LC. Coexistence of migraine in idiopathic intracranial hypertension without papilledema. *Neurology,* 46:1226–1230, 1996.

Metzer WS. Trigeminal neuralgia secondary to tumor with normal exam, responsive to carbamazepine. *Headache,* 31:164–166, 1991.

Nelson DA, Halloway WJ, Kara-Eneff SC, et al. Neurologic syndromes produced by sphenoid sinus abscess. *Neurology,* 17:981–987, 1967.

Nightingale S, Williams B. Hind brain hernia headache. *Lancet,* 1:731–734, 1987.

Nordeman L, Lucid EJ. Sphenoid sinusitis, a cause of debilitating headache. *J Emerg Med,* 8:557–559, 1990.

Obuchowski N, Modic MT, Magdinec M. Current implications for the efficacy of noninvasive screening for occult intracranial aneurysms in patients with family history of aneurysms. *J Neurosurg,* 83:42–49, 1995.

Ramadan NM. Headache caused by raised intracranial pressure and intracranial hypotension. *Curr Opin Neurol,* 9:214–218, 1996.

Raskin NH, Howard MW, Aaronfield WK. Headache as the leading symptom of thoracic outlet syndrome. *Headache,* 25:208–210, 1985.

Reik L, Steere AC, Bartenagen NH, et al. Neurologic abnormalities of Lyme disease. *Medicine,* 58:281–294, 1979.

Rond R, Keane JR. The minor symptoms of increased intracranial pressure: 101 patients with benign intracranial hypertension. *Neurology,* 38:1461–1464, 1988.

Rothrock JF, Lim V, Press G, Gosink B. Serial magnetic resonance and carotid duplex examinations in the management of carotid dissection. *Neurology,* 38:686–692, 1989.

Ruggieri PM, Poulos N, Nasaryk TJ, et al. Occult intracranial aneurysms in polycystic kidney disease: Screening with MR angiography. *Radiology,* 191(1): 33–39, 1994.

Selsa NN, Lipton RB, Sander H, et al. Headache characteristics in hospitalized patients with Lyme. *Headache,* 35:125–130, 1995.

Shankland WE II. Ernest syndrome (insertion tendonosis of the stylomandibular ligament) as a cause for craniomandibular pain: Diagnosis, treatment, and report of two patients. *J Neurol & Orthopedic Med & Surg,* 8:253–257, 1987.

Sicuteri F, Nicolodi M, Fusco BM, et al. Idiopathic headache as a possible risk factor for phantom tooth pain. *Headache,* 31:577–581, 1991.

Silberstein SB. Intractable headache: Aseptic meningitis and sphenoidal sinusitis. *Cephalalgia,* 14:376–378, 1994.

Silberstein SB. Migraine in pregnancy: A review. *Neurol Clin of North America,* (15:1), 1997.

Silva JE, Brown JD, Watson BV, et al. Temporal arteritis presenting as bilateral brachioplexopathy (Abstract presented to AAN April 1998).

Silvestrini M, Cupini LM, Calabresi P, et al. Migraine with aura-like syndrome due to arteriovenous malformation. The clinical value of transcranial Doppler in early diagnosis. *Cephalalgia,* 12:115–119, 1992.

Smith RG, Cherry JE. Traumatic Eagle's syndrome: Report of a case and review of the literature. *J Oral Maxillofac Surg,* 46:606–609, 1988.

Stovner LJ. Headache associated with chiari type I malformation. *Headache,* 33:175–181, 1993.

Teitjen GE, Day M, Norris L, et al. The role of anticardiolipin antibodies in young persons with migraine and transient focal neurological events: A prospective frequency-matched study. *Neurology* (in press).

Vakharia SB, Sebastian Thomas P, Rosenbaum AE, et al. Magnetic resonance imaging of cerebral spinal fluid leak and tamponade effect of blood patch in post-dural puncture. *Anesth Analog,* 84:585–590, 1997.

Wijdicks EF, Kerkhoff H, van Gijn J. Long-term follow-up of 71 patients with thunderclap headache mimicking subarachnoid hemorrhage. *Lancet,* 2:68–70, 1988.

Winston AR. Whiplash and its relationship to migraine. *Headache,* 27:452–457, 1987.

Younger DS, Calabrese LH, Hays AP. Granulomatous angiitis of the nervous system. *Neurol Clin,* 15:821–834, 1997.

6

Medications Used in the Pharmacotherapy of Headache

Introduction

This chapter contains a comprehensive review of the pharmacological agents used to treat various types of head, face, and neck pain. Also included are tables, charts, and other listings to provide the reader with a detailed reference of agents used in the treatment of head and face pain.

This chapter should be used in conjunction with subsequent chapters in which treatment recommendations are provided for specific clinical entities.

Special Warning

Many of the agents recommended in this text have not been approved for such usage by the Food and Drug Administration (FDA). Moreover, many of the drugs that are listed, while widely administered, have not been subjected to well-controlled studies to determine efficacy. Evidence-based data exist for only some of the many agents used in the treatment of migraine and other headaches and pain syndromes. This text, because of its design, will not review the evidence-based efficacy data, nor will it list only those drugs for which FDA approval for the treatment of headache has been received, except to note in Table 6.21 those agents that have received FDA approval for migraine, as of the date of this publication. The reader, however, must recognize the importance of these issues. It is recommended that, at least initially, preference be given to those therapies for which evidence-based data supporting efficacy have been established and that have received approval by the FDA.

Also, as mentioned in the Preface, various listings in this chapter will contain the word "selected." Its use designates that an arbitrary choice of items was made, based upon the authors' judgement. Particularly in the case of side effects and contraindications, the reader must take full responsibility to obtain complete and comprehensive prescribing and safety information. This book is intended to serve as a guide only.

Finally, many of the drugs noted in this chapter are not recommended for standard treatment. Their inclusion is to inform the reader of available treatments for resistant, severe cases. Many of these agents should be administered only by experienced physicians with advanced knowledge of headache and prescribing information about these agents. Moreover, many of these drugs should be given only to resistant cases of severe headache, in settings where careful monitoring and frequent visits, patient education, and safety procedures can be provided. Before administering any of the medications recommended in this text, the physician must consider the clinical circumstances individually and carefully. Keep in mind that pharmacotherapeutic needs vary widely between patients. Also, while every effort was made to ensure accuracy in this book, printing errors may have occurred. It is always best to verify dosages.

I. Symptomatic (Abortive) Treatment vs. Preventive (Prophylactic) Treatment

The reader should note that throughout this text we will use the terms "symptomatic" and "abortive" interchangeably. The literature is confusing on the use of these terms. The term "abortive" is sometimes used to designate only those agents that have a specific effect on the headache mechanism, such as sumatriptan or dihydroergotamine, whereas the term "symptomatic" is often used to describe agents that treat the pain in a general way (such as analgesics) or address the accompaniments to headache, such as nausea. In this text, however, we will use the term "symptomatic" to refer to agents that treat both the pain and its accompaniments.

A. Symptomatic Treatment

The *symptomatic treatment* of head pain involves the use of agents that reverse, abort, or reduce pain once it has begun, or the symptoms accompanying headache. The objective of symptomatic treatment is the reduction of the intensity and duration of pain, as well as its attending features. The choice of medication often depends upon such factors as:

- frequency;
- the severity of the attack;
- the presence or absence of accompaniments, such as vomiting;
- the time to peak; onset of action of the medication;
- the bioavailability of the drug;
- the drug's route of administration;
- comorbid medical conditions;
- the adverse effect profile of the drug; and
- a patient's previous medicine-use history.

Generally (exceptions exist), the use of symptomatic medications (particularly those that can cause rebound) should not exceed two, and at most three days per week. Symptomatic medications are frequently used along with preventive medications to treat breakthrough attacks. Symptomatic treatments are generally administered alone (without preventive therapies) when:

- Attacks are infrequent (two or less per week);
- Preventive medication is contraindicated;
- When effective use of preventive medication is not achievable or is inappropriate; and
- When symptomatic treatment is satisfactory.

For frequent attacks, a combination of preventive and symptomatic treatment is often necessary.

The route of administration can be critical. Gastric emptying delay (gastroparesis) is common during acute attacks of migraine and related headaches. Rectal, nasal, or parenteral forms of medication are of particular value in such instances. Reduction or reversal of gastroparesis can be achieved by pretreatment with metoclopramide.

B. Preventive Treatment

Preventive (prophylactic) treatment is used to prevent attacks and reduce the frequency and severity of headache events. Preventive treatment should be considered when:

- Attacks of significant acute pain occur more than four times per month, particularly if treatment with symptomatic medications is not satisfactory;
- The severity or duration of attacks justifies the use of preventive treatment, even if attacks occur less often;
- When the use of symptomatic medications is excessive in frequency or dose;
- Symptomatic treatment cannot be used because of medical contraindication; and
- To enhance the efficacy of symptomatic medication.

In most instances in which preventive treatment is employed, symptomatic medication must also be used for the treatment of acute attacks that escape preventive measures.

II. Symptomatic Drugs Used to Treat Headache and Face Pain

(Note to readers: At the end of this chapter are various tables and summaries that might be of additional value when considering drug treatment of head and face pain.)

A. Analgesics and Analgesic Combinations (see Table 6.1)

1. General comments

Simple analgesics and analgesic combinations are appropriate for the treatment of periodic, mild to moderate headache. Simple analgesics or simple analgesic combinations may also be appropriate as adjunctive treatments with more specific, symptomatic or preventive therapies. Opioid analgesics are appropriate for very severe headaches unresponsive to other agents or when other therapies are contraindicated.

Analgesic agents are generally safe when used periodically. Overuse and the development of rebound headache are risks.

TABLE 6.1. **SELECTED ANALGESIC PREPARATIONS**

Simple analgesics and analgesic combinations	
Aspirin	100% aspirin
Tylenol	100% acetaminophen
Excedrin*	acetaminophen 250 mg, aspirin 250 mg, caffeine 65 mg per tablet
Other mixed over-the-counter preparations	
Combinations analgesics containing barbiturates	
Fiorinal	aspirin 325 mg, caffeine 40 mg, butalbital 50 mg
Fioricet, Esgic	acetaminophen 325 mg, caffeine 40 mg, butalbital 50 mg
Phrenilin	acetaminophen 325 mg, butalbital 50 mg
Combination analgesics containing codeine	
Fiorinal w/codeine	aspirin 325 mg, caffeine 40 mg, butalbital 50 mg, codeine 30 mg
Tylenol w/codeine III	acetaminophen 325 mg, codeine 30 mg
Phrenilin w/codeine	acetaminophen 325 mg, butalbital 50 mg, codeine 30 mg
Narcotic analgesics/analgesics containing opioids	
Darvon CPD-65	propoxyphene HCL 65 mg, aspirin 389 mg, caffeine 32.4 mg
Darvocet-N	propoxyphene napsylate 50/100 mg, acetaminophen 325 mg
Vicodin	hydrocodone 5 mg, acetaminophen 500 mg
Vicodin ES	hydrocodone 7.5 mg, acetaminophen 750 mg
Percocet	oxycodone 5 mg, acetaminophen 325 mg
Percodan	oxycodone 4.5 mg, aspirin 325 mg
Demerol	meperidine 50/100 mg tablet; injectable
Oxy Contin	oxycodone, long-acting form
Dilaudid	hydromorphone
	1/2/3/4 mg tablets
	3 mg suppository
	1, 2, 4 mg/ml injections
Stadol	butorphanol (IV, IM, or nasal spray)
Talwin NX	pentazocine 50 mg/naloxone 0.5 mg (oral)
Nubain	nalbuphine 10 mg/ml, 20 mg/ml
Dolophine	methadone 5 mg
Morphine Sulfate	short- and long-acting forms; oral formulations, injectable
Duragesic Patch	fentanyl; several dose preparations

*Excedrin Migrane has been shown to effectively treat mild to moderate (and sometimes severe) migraine in controlled studies (Lipton, 1997), using a population of patients which excluded the most severe cases of migraine (those requiring bedrest and/or experiencing vomiting with 20% or more of their attacks).

Monitoring is necessary for both over-the-counter (OTC) and prescribed medications.

Advocates of combination analgesics have traditionally justified their use with the following points:

- Enhanced analgesia from multiple mechanisms of action;
- Enhancement of gastrointestinal (GI) absorption (caffeine); and
- Enhanced control of anxiety via tranquilization and a primary effect on the pain mechanism from barbiturates, in those agents containing barbiturates.

Recently, the combination and dose of agents found in the popular OTC formulation Excedrin was found, in controlled studies (Lipton, 1997), to effectively treat migraineurs with moderate or severe headache pain who meet IHS diagnostic criteria for migraine with or without aura. The combination was also found to effectively treat the disability and associated symptoms of migraine. The most severely disabled segment of migraineurs, whose attacks usually required bedrest or who experienced vomiting with 20% or more of their attacks, were excluded from the study. On the basis of these studies, the combination of asprin, acetaminophen, and caffeine may have a role as a safe and cost-effective first-line agent for intermittent mild to moderate migraine or as an adjunctive agent, in addition to its historical use for tension-type headache. This formulation is also marketed as Excedrin Migraine per the mandate of the FDA to ensure appropriate distribution of migraine-specific information.

2. **Proposed mechanisms**
   a. **Aspirin**—prostaglandin and leukotriene synthesis inhibitor (prostaglandins may sensitize nociceptors and produce hyperalgesia); may affect neurogenically mediated inflammation; may influence 5-HT neurotransmission.
   b. **Acetaminophen**—prostaglandin synthesis inhibitor within the central nervous system; a proposed effect on endorphin/opioid system; inhibition of nociceptive activity via 5-HT receptors.
   c. **Opioids**—stimulation of endogenous opioid receptors
   d. **Caffeine**—stimulation of adenosine receptors; enhanced analgesia; increased GI absorption; may have a primary analgesic effect

3. **Recommended use**
   The analgesics and analgesic combination treatments may be used in all infrequently occurring head and face pain disorders (see below). Usage more than 2 days per week should be

restricted. The use of opioids for periodic treatment of severe headache is appropriate, particularly when other agents are contraindicated. The use of opioids in maintenance treatment is still subject to study, and while there is an increasingly enlightened attitude toward their usage for appropriate cases, the long-term outcome for headache has not been determined, although currently under study (Saper, 1997). (See later in this chapter for further discussion.)

Children should avoid aspirin for headache, since the headache event may be an early component of a viral syndrome that serves as a prelude to Reye's syndrome.

4. Principles of use (see Table 6.21)

In general, analgesics should not be regularly used more than two days per week, and ideally less often, due to "*rebound phenomenon.*" (See Chapters 8 and 9.) More frequent use may be justified during self-limited and defined episodes of pain, such as menstrual periods. It may also be acceptable in limited numbers of patients in whom frequent use of analgesics, including opioids, is considered justifiable because of health or intractable pain considerations (see later). The effectiveness of a simple analgesic has been enhanced by administration with agents such as metoclopramide, which promote gut motility and absorption. (Dopamine antagonists may also provide a primary effect on headache, as well as an antiemetic role.) Analgesics may also be used as adjunctive agents to enhance the efficacy of specific antimigraine medications, though unnecessary combining of medications is discouraged.

5. Drugs in this group (see Table 6.1)

Many other oral and parenteral agents, including agonist/antagonist agents, are available. See Table 6.2 for the caffeine content of analgesic preparations and foods. See Table 6.3 for opioid equivalency estimates.

The periodic, symptomatic use of opioids in the treatment of benign head pain is controversial. However, clinical circumstances exist in which the use of opioids is justified. Opioids can generally be considered in patients without a past profile of serious overuse or dependency/addiction, who have severe, debilitating pain, or do not respond to alternate choices safely or effectively. Patients with severe pain disorders, or patients with alcoholism who are no longer drinking, can occasionally use opioids safely, provided appropriate safeguards and careful monitoring are undertaken (Dunbar, 1996). (See page 127 for discussion of sustained opioid therapy.)

TABLE 6.2.   **CAFFEINE CONTENT OF COMMON FOODS AND DRUGS**

Product	Example	Caffeine Content (mg)
Cocoa and chocolate	Baking chocolate (1 oz)	35
	Chocolate candy bar	25
	Cocoa beverage (6 oz mixture)	10
	Milk chocolate (1 oz)	6
Coffee	Decaffeinated (5 oz)	2
	Drip (5 oz)	146
	Instant, regular (5 oz)	53
	Percolated (5 oz)	110
Over-the-counter drugs	Anacin	32
	Excedrin	65
	No-Doz tablets	100–200
	Vanquish	33
	Vivarin tablets	200
Prescription drugs	Esgic	40
	Fioricet	40
	Fiorinal	40
	Norgesic	30
	Norgesic Forte	60
	Supac	33
Soft drinks (12 oz)	7-Up/Diet 7-Up	0
	Coca Cola	34
	Diet Pepsi	34
	Dr. Pepper	38
	Fresca	0
	Ginger Ale	0
	Hires Root Beer	0
	Mountain Dew	52
	Pepsi-Cola	37
	Tab	44
Tea	1-minute brew (5 oz)	9–33
	3-minute brew (5 oz)	22–46
	5-minute brew (5 oz)	20–50
	Canned ice tea (12 oz)	22–36

Butorphanol nasal spray (Stadol NS) offers a transnasal formulation for the treatment of acute pain. Butorphanol is a synthetic agonist/antagonist opioid analgesic that exerts its effect on the mu, kappa, and sigma opioid receptors. Butorphanol's analgesic effect seems to be exerted through the agonist action on the kappa and sigma receptors and mixed agonist/antagonist activity on the mu receptors. Because of an antagonist action at the mu receptor, butorphanol is reported to cause less respiratory depression, euphoria, and physical dependence than pure opioid analgesics. After transnasal administration of butorphanol, onset of action occurs within 15 minutes, with peak blood levels occurring in 30–60 minutes. Medication half-life is 4.7 hours in younger patients but more prolonged in older patients. The drug has adverse effects that are generally similar to those of other opioids.

TABLE 6.3. **SELECTED OPIOID (OR ANTAGONIST/AGONIST) EQUIVALENCY ESTIMATES COMPARED WITH 10 MG INTRAMUSCULAR MORPHINE SULFATE**[a]

Drug	Trade Name	Equivalent Parenteral Dose (mg)	Equivalent PO Dose (mg)
Anileridine	Leritine	25	75
Buprenorphine[b]	Buprenex	0.3	—
Butorphanol[b]	Stadol	2.0	
Codeine phosphate	Codeine	120	200
Diphenoxylate	Lomotil	—	300
Fentanyl	Sublimaze/Innovar	0.1	—
Hydrocodone	Hycodan, Vicodin		10–15
Hydromorphone	Dilaudid	2	4
Levorphanol tartrate	Levo-Dromoran	2	4
Meperidine	Demerol	75	300
Methadone	Dolophine	10	20
Morphine		10	20–30
Immediate-release	Roxanol	10	20–60
Controlled-release	MS Contin	—	20–60
Nalbuphine[b]	Nubain	10–15	—
Naloxone[c]	Narcan		
Naltrexone[c]	Trexan		
Oxycodone w/ASA	Percodan	—	10–15
Oxycodone w/ACET	Percocet	—	10–15
Oxymorphone	Numorphan	1	—
Pentazocine[b]	Talwin	60	180
Propoxyphene	Darvon	—	120

[a]Modified from the Analgesic Study Section, Sloan-Kettering Institute for Cancer Research, New York, and Purdue Frederick, Inc., Toronto.
[b]Agonist/antagonist.
[c]Pure antagonist.

The use of butorphanol nasal spray in treating acute headaches is controversial. Excessive administration, improper selection, and use for frequent headaches have led to numerous cases of physical and psychological dependence, many of which required prolonged hospital treatment for withdrawal symptomatology (personal observations). Usage patterns exceeding a bottle of butorphanol a day are not uncommon. Patients describe increasing headaches and drug use (rebound), euphoria (or perhaps dysphoria), and an irresistible desire for more medication. Recent work suggests that withdrawal from butorphanol results in focal increases in extracellular levels of glutamate within the locus ceruleus which may act through the N-methyl-D-aspartate glutamate receptor (Hoshi, 1996).

When used properly and administered with appropriate restrictions and proper patient selection, butorphanol nasal spray may provide an important rescue medication for patients who either cannot take alternate treatments or have failed to respond to them. Reduced dosing may also minimize the sedation and other untoward effects reported with current dosing schedules. Recently the FDA scheduled butorphanol as a Schedule IV analgesic.

Symptomatic use of opioids may provide effective pain control in those who would otherwise not achieve it. Moreover, there is growing sentiment that physicians have the unavoidable obligation to provide effective pain relief when possible. The risks of opioid therapy are at times minimal compared to the impact upon patient, family, and society when severe pain is not effectively treated or when large (toxic) amounts of more "acceptable" agents are required.

The following are guidelines for the administration of opioids in patients with intermittent headache:

- Use the lowest dose and least potent agent available, when possible;
- Administer via the most appropriate and efficient route (oral, rectal, nasal spray, or parenteral) for the specific clinical circumstances;
- Carefully review other concurrently used medications to avoid enhanced sedation, respiratory suppression, or other untoward reactions;
- Calculate and prescribe the appropriate number of pills to be used between visits, based on frequency of attacks and attack requirements (refills are discouraged, as are call-in requests for additional medication);
- Carefully delineate, preferably in writing, the guidelines for usage, including for which type of headache, how many times per day the drug can be used, and how frequently per week it can be used;
- Establish a visit pattern that is consistent with the frequency of headaches and the amount and type of medications prescribed;
- Consider past history for patterns of noncompliance, excessive use, obsessive drug-taking behaviors, etc.;
- Continue to seek alternative options if possible; and
- Insist upon one prescribing physician and, if possible, one dispensing pharmacy.

6. Selected major untoward reactions and contraindications:

- Aspirin—asthma, rash, gastrointestinal irritation and ulceration, effects on coagulation, liver toxicity, and renal disease;
- Acetaminophen—liver toxicity and high dose may potenti-

ate oral anticoagulants; chronic use may contribute to renal disturbances;

- Opioids—nausea, vomiting, respiratory depression, sedation, constipation, physical and/or emotional dependence, or addictive disease[1]; and
- Barbiturates—drowsiness, physical and emotional dependency, and effects on coagulation.

All drugs in this group can potentially produce "rebounding" when used frequently. Barbiturates and low-dose aspirin may be exceptions.

See standard references for additional untoward reactions, guidelines, contraindications, and warnings.

B. Nonsteroidal Anti-Inflammatory Drugs

1. General comments

Numerous nonsteroidal anti-inflammatory drugs (NSAIDs) are available. Though similar in many ways, the analgesic effect may differ between agents. They are potentially useful in both symptomatic and preventive regimens, but it is advisable to avoid prolonged, frequent use whenever possible for reasons of safety. GI changes may be preventable with the simultaneous administration of misoprostol and perhaps proton pump inhibitors (Koch, 1996). Renal changes remain a risk with long-term use.

2. Proposed mechanisms

The proposed mechanisms of agents in this group include

a. Inhibition of cyclooxygenase (inhibits prostaglandin synthesis);
b. Inhibition of lipoxygenase (inhibits leukotriene synthesis);
c. Prostaglandin receptor antagonism; and
d. Interference with cell-membrane processes.

3. Recommended use (selected)

a. Mild to moderate migraine and tension-type headache;
b. Exertional and menstrual headache;
c. Benign orgasmic cephalgia;

---

[1] *Addictive disease, as distinct from physical dependency, implies the* inappropriate *use of medications that cause dependence and includes antisocial, surreptitious behavior, drug hoarding, illegal acquisition, multisourcing, etc. While physical dependency can occur with many agents, addictive disease is a more profound problem and requires more aggressive and specific "drug abuse" treatment strategies. Obsessive drug-taking or simple overuse/excessive use patterns in patients with difficult-to-control pain disorders should not in and of itself be considered addictive disease. See Chapter 11 for further discussion on terminology for drug overuse.*

    d. Chronic paroxysmal hemicrania (indomethacin);

    e. Hemicrania continua (indomethacin);

    f. "Icepick" syndromes (indomethacin); and

    g. Acute or intractable migraine requiring parenteral treatment (parenteral ketorolac).

4. Principles of use (see Table 6.21)

These agents should be taken at the first sign of a headache. Ordinarily, administration should not exceed three usage days per week, but more frequent, continuous use for defined, self-limited periods of time may be acceptable, such as around a menstrual period.

5. Selected drugs in this group (see Table 6.4)

6. Selected major untoward reactions and contraindications

Risks associated with nonsteroidal anti-inflammatory agents appear to increase with age and in those with predisposing risk

TABLE 6.4. **SELECTED NONSTEROIDAL ANTI-INFLAMMATORY DRUGS**

Type	Available Size (mg)
Carboxylic acids	
Acetylated	
Aspirin	
Nonacetylated	
Choline magnesium trisalicylate (Trilisate)	500/750/1000
Salsalate (Salflex, Disalcid)	500/750
Propionic acids	
Ibuprofen (Motrin, Advil)	200/400/600/800
Naproxen (Naprosyn)	250/375/500
Fenoprofen (Nalfon)	200/300/600
Naproxen sodium (Anaprox)	275/550
Ketoprofen (Orudis)	25/50/75
Oxaprozin (Daypro)	600
Aryl and heterocyclic acids	
Tolmetin (Tolectin)	200/400/600
Indomethacin (Indocin)	25/50/75
	50 rectal
Diclofenac (Voltaren)	25/50/75
Sulindac (Clinoril)	150/200
Fenamic acids	
Mefenamic acid (Ponstel)	250
Meclofenamate (Meclomen)	50/100
Enolic acids	
Piroxicam (Feldene)	10/20
Pyrrolo-pyrrole	
Ketorolac (Toradol) (PO, IM, IV)	Because of renal and GI risks, usage should be limited and avoided in those with renal risk factors and GI disease

factors for either GI or renal disease (Strom, 1996). Duration of use and dose are important as well.

a. **Major untoward reactions**

1) GI ulcers/bleeding
2) Oral ulcers
3) Colitis activation/aggravation
4) Headache, lightheadedness, and dizziness
5) Somnolence
6) Tinnitus
7) Fluid retention
8) Asthma activation/aggravation
9) Hypertension aggravation
10) Nephrotoxicity

b. **Contraindications/cautionary recommendations**

1) Active ulcer disease
2) Gastritis
3) Renal disease
4) Bleeding disorders
5) Aspirin-sensitive asthma
6) Severe hypertension
7) Colitis (active or in remission—a relative contraindication)
8) Severe dehydration, elderly patients, and those with renovascular disease and/or diabetes appear to be particularly at risk (most notably but not exclusively with ketorolac)

See standard references for additional untoward reactions, guidelines, contraindications, and warnings.

7. Special considerations

Ketorolac has been established as effective as opioids in the treatment of acute migraine (Davis, 1995; Duarte, 1992; Shrest, 1996). However, the risks are significant, even with short-term usage. Considering the availability of other agents with less risk for the acute treatment of headache, ketorolac should be reserved as a second- or third-line agent. Parenteral dosages of 30–60 mg IM or 7.5–10 mg administered intravenously should be reserved for those patients *without* significant renal risk, who are otherwise healthy, and in whom other more acceptable agents are ineffective or contraindicated. Risk factors include renovascular disease, GI disease, moderate to severe dehydration, significant diabetes, and older age.

Frequent use of oral or rectal NSAIDs requires monitoring of GI blood loss, renal function, and blood pressure. The therapeutic dose may vary from patient to patient. When failure to respond to one agent occurs, another agent can be tried.

Ibuprofen has been associated with a sterile meningitis (Horn, 1997) and leptomeningeal enhancement (Van Gerpen, 1998).

C. Isometheptene
1. General comments

The most well-known agent containing isometheptene is Midrin. Midrin is a combination of three active ingredients: isometheptene mucate, 65 mg; acetaminophen, 325 mg; and dichloralphenazone 100 mg. The combination is effective for symptomatic treatment of mild to moderate (and sometimes severe) headache (migraine, tension-type headache) and is usually safe and well tolerated. Many authorities consider the drug a major first-line agent for mild to moderate migraine because of its safety and long-standing prominence as an effective agent. It is additionally important because many patients cannot take ergot derivatives, NSAIDs, aspirin containing products, or the triptans but require an orally administered, generally safe drug for migraine and tension-type headache.

2. Proposed mechanisms

The mechanism of action reflects individual components. Isometheptene mucate is a sympathomimetic vasoactive agent, which probably impacts headaches centrally. Acetaminophen has analgesic properties, and dichloralphenazone, a tranquilizing agent, may affect central pain mechanisms.

3. Recommended use
a. Mild to moderate migraine
b. Tension-type headache (probably a migraine variant)
c. Menstrual migraine

4. Principles of use (see Table 6.21)

Isometheptene compounds should be used for symptomatic treatment and can be combined with nonsteroidal anti-inflammatory agents for greater efficacy. Short-term, self-limited, daily use around menstrual periods or for prolonged headache is sometimes acceptable. Concern for rebound should be maintained.

5. Drugs in this group
Midrin
Isocom

6. Selected major untoward reactions and contraindications

Drugs containing isometheptene are contraindicated in patients using monoamine oxidase inhibitors (MAOIs) and patients with partial spinal cord lesions. Sympathomimetic stimulation and severe hypertensive reactions have occurred in patients with partial spinal cord lesions. Because safety is uncertain, Midrin should not be used concurrently with the triptans.

a. Common untoward reactions

1) Transient dizziness
2) Sedation

b. Contraindications/cautionary warnings

1) Glaucoma
2) Severe renal disease
3) Severe hypertension
4) Severe heart or liver disease
5) MAOI therapy
6) Patients with spinal cord lesions

See standard references for additional untoward reactions, guidelines, contraindications, and warnings.

D. Ergot Derivatives

1. General comments

Prior to the availability of sumatriptan, the ergot derivatives (ergotamine tartrate and dihydroergotamine) were the only symptomatic treatments for moderate to severe migraine and related headaches and became the agents of first choice for severe migraine. Despite the increasing and appropriate attention now being given to the triptans, many, but not all, authorities still believe that parenteral dihydroergotamine (DHE) maintains its earned prominence because of its efficacy and overall safety record. Dihydroergotamine (DHE) is now available in both parenteral and nasal spray formulations (Migranal).

Ergot alkaloids are derived from the rye fungus (Claviceps purpurea) (see Table 6.5). Ergots have a high, irreversible affinity for a wide range of receptors (see below).

DHE is distinct from ergotamine tartrate (e.g. Cafergot) in several important ways. These include:

DHE

• Is a *weak* arterial constrictor (ergotamine tartrate is a more potent arterial constrictor);

TABLE 6.5.   **SELECTED SYMPTOMATIC DRUGS CONTAINING ERGOT DERIVATIVES**

Cafergot tablets
Wigraine tablets
Migrogot tablets
DHE-45 (parental DHE)
Migranal (DHE nasal spray)

- Has selective venoconstricting properties;
- Has substantially less emetic (nauseating) properties;
- Has less uterine effects; and
- Is less likely to cause rebound.

2. Proposed mechanisms

The ergot derivatives are considered pharmacologically nonselective, having a wide and complex influence. Both ergotamine tartrate and DHE have:

- High affinity for the 5-HT_{1b}, 5-HT_{1d}, 5-HT_{1f}, and 5-HT_2 receptors[2];
- Low to moderate affinity for 5-HT_{1c} and 5-HT_3 receptors;
- Affinity at alpha- and beta-adrenoreceptors and dopamine D_2 receptors;
- Vasoconstrictive effects via stimulation of arterial smooth muscle through 5-HT receptors;
- Venous capacitance vessel constriction;
- Reuptake inhibition of noradrenaline at sympathetic nerve endings; and
- Reduction of vasogenic/neurogenic inflammation (via influence on serotonin receptors).

Current belief is that the fundamental action of ergot derivatives on migraine may be via inhibition of neurogenic inflammation of the trigeminal vascular system, not necessarily via vasoconstriction. Other central neurotransmitter effects are also likely. DHE passes through the blood-brain barrier and localizes to nuclei in the brainstem and spinal cord involved in pain transmission and modulation. Its possible influence on the brainstem "migraine generator" is of significant

---

[2] *Currently, 5-HT_{1d} receptors (located on nerve terminals) appear to be of primary importance in migraine because of their role in inhibiting release of substances believed to cause perivascular inflammation, such as calcitonin gene-related peptide (CGRP), substance P, and others. 5-HT_{1b} receptors, localized on vessels, may result in vasoconstriction when activated (see Chapter 4).*

interest. A high density of DHE binding sites has been identified in the dorsal raphe nuclei (Goadsby, 1991), the location
of the generator (Weiller, 1995).

3. Recommended use

Ergot derivatives, particularly DHE, are appropriate in the
symptomatic treatment of the following conditions:

a. Moderate to severe migraine, including menstrual
    migraine
b. Cluster headache
c. Intractable migraine (status migrainosis) (parenteral DHE
    to interrupt)
d. Intractable, chronic daily headache (parenteral DHE to
    interrupt)

4. Principles of use (see Table 6.21)

a. **Ergotamine tartrate**—ergotamine tartrate (oral and
    rectal) has lost its historical prominence to DHE nasal
    spray (Migranal), sumatriptan (Imitrex), and the other
    triptans. Pharmacy compounded suppositories are still
    available and widely used. Because of concern for
    "rebound" and ergot dependency syndrome (see later), it
    is advisable to limit its use to 2 days per week, except
    perhaps for cluster headache or menstrual migraine,
    during which more extended but still limited usage is
    acceptable in patients not at risk for vascular disease.
b. **DHE**—DHE is available for administration via
    intravenous (IV), intramuscular (IM), subcutaneous (SC),
    and now intranasal routes. It is appropriate for:

    - Moderate to severe individual attacks of migraine or
      cluster headache (DHE-parenteral or nasal spray); and
    - Prolonged intractable attacks (the parenteral form).

    For prolonged intractable attacks, DHE should be used in
    a 3–5 day intravenous protocol (see Table 6.6, Figure 6.1, and
    Chapter 9). Personal experience with children and adoles-
    cents suggests a likelihood of headache intensification at stan-
    dard doses; reduced dosing or avoidance is often necessary.

    DHE is an important drug in the treatment of migraine
    and related headaches. It is a less potent arterial constric-
    tor than ergotamine tartrate, and although it causes nausea
    in some individuals, it has some antiemetic qualities. It is
    not associated (at this time) with rebound, as is ergotamine
    tartrate and possibly the triptans. Intravenous administra-
    tion can abort up to 90% of attacks (Saadah, 1992). Be-

TABLE 6.6. **INTRAVENOUS PROTOCOL FOR DIHYDROERGOTAMINE (DHE) ADMINISTRATION**

Protocol

- 0.25–0.5 mg IV "push" (test dose), over 2 minutes via heparin lock apparatus.
- If tolerated, DHE 0.5–1 mg IV "push" q 8 hours for 3–5 days.
- Administer 10 mg metoclopramide (IV[a] or IM) before DHE administration, if nausea occurs.
- Maintain for 3–5 days, if tolerated. May repeat program one time.

Guidelines for use

1. Administer metoclopramide before or at DHE administration if necessary to control nausea. Discontinue if not necessary.
2. DHE to be administered via 1–2 minute slow "push."
3. Most patients stabilize at end of day 3, but extension of program for 2–3 more days may be necessary.
4. Discontinue DHE via a 1–3 day gradual reduction program if patient is pain-free for 2 days or fails to respond after 3 days.
5. Hospitalization is most appropriate for therapy, during which careful monitoring for blood pressure elevation, chest pain, severe nausea, etc. can be carried out and necessary concurrent therapies can be administered, including establishment of an effective preventive program.
6. Discontinue or substantially reduce dose if severe nausea, chest pain, severe leg cramps, or other significant adverse reactions occur.

[a]10 mg slow "IV push" or in 50 cc 5% dextrose in water (D5W) over 20–30 minutes.

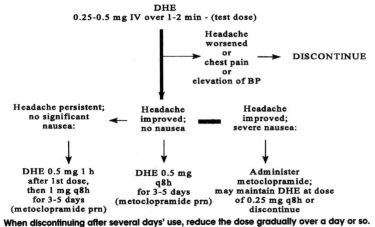

Figure 6.1. IV DHE Administration Algorithm

cause of its irreversible receptor binding, the biological half-life is considerably long (greater than 10 hours), and this may explain the lower likelihood of headache recurrence (see page 81), than with sumatriptan and perhaps the other short-acting triptans. Parenteral DHE has become the primary agent used to terminate prolonged and persistent migraine in the inpatient setting, as well as in many emergency departments.

The recent availability of DHE in nasal spray formulation (Gallagher, 1996) has provided an even greater dimension of use for this agent. Current studies estimate relief in 65% (at 4 hours) of patients using DHE nasal spray compared with placebo (Dihydroergotamine Nasal Spray Multicenter Investigators, 1995).

In a recent study comparing subcutaneous DHE and subcutaneous sumatriptan (Winner, 1996), approximately similar efficacy was demonstrated for both agents. Sumatriptan (Imitrex) demonstrated a more rapid rate of onset but was associated with a higher rate of headache recurrence. At 2 hours, 73% of patients receiving DHE and 85% of patients receiving sumatriptan had pain relief, whereas at 3 hours the rates were 86% (DHE) and 90% (sumatriptan). Headache recurrence within 24 hours occurred in 18% of DHE-treated patients but was higher in the sumatriptan-treated patients. (Because many DHE-treated patients required a second injection due to an inadequate initial response, it was not clear whether the rate of recurrence difference was due to the longer action of DHE or to the repeated dose protocol [Ferrari, 1997].) Chest symptoms were more frequent with sumatriptan, but nausea occurred more frequently after DHE administration.

DHE is effective in treating an individual attack of cluster headache or menstrual migraine and controlling headache during rebound and detoxification of patients with migraine who have excessively used ergotamine tartrate or analgesics for frequent headaches. Self-injected subcutaneous DHE is appropriate for reliable patients with occasional, severe headache who do not respond otherwise. DHE is relatively unstable and poorly soluble in other solutions. Parenteral DHE is best administered immediately after removing it from the ampule.

The warnings and contraindications accompanying DHE nasal spray and parenteral forms must be followed. However, DHE nasal formulation at current dosing range is generally not likely to cause cardiac symptoms in otherwise healthy individuals (see below). Thus, it is considered a front-line treatment of moderate to severe migraine when more modest treatments, such as Midrin, analgesics, and NSAIDs, are not effective.

5. Selected drugs in this group (see Table 6.5)
6. Selected major untoward reactions and contraindications

All ergotamine preparations are capable of producing nausea, vomiting, paresthesias, muscle cramps, and angina in sensitive individuals. Initially, low-dose administration may be helpful in reducing symptoms. Continued usage at symptom-producing doses should be avoided. These effects seem less likely with DHE. However, despite its reduced arterial constricting properties, the drug should be avoided and is considered contraindicated in patients with coronary artery disease, significant peripheral vascular disease, severe hypertension, and high risk for coronary or cerebral vascular disease. DHE should be used cautiously and only after appropriate screening in patients considered at mild to moderate risk or with an early family history of cardiac disease. The drug should be used cautiously in patients with impaired renal or hepatic function and pregnancy.

For other contraindications and cautionary warnings, see Table 6.7.

7. Special considerations

Ergotism, which is a rare but serious and at times life-threatening condition usually resulting from acute overdosage or chronic dependency on ergotamine, is accompanied by severe vasoconstriction. Discontinuation of the ergot preparation and attempts to reverse the vasospasm with direct-acting vasodilators are necessary. Frequent use of ergotamine tar-

TABLE 6.7.   **CONTRAINDICATIONS TO ERGOT DERIVATIVES**[a]

Age over 60 years (relative contraindication)
Concurrent use of a triptan
Pregnancy
Breast-feeding
Bradycardia (moderate to severe)
Cardiac valvular disease (moderate to severe)
Collagen vascular disease, vasculitis
Coronary artery disease
Hypertension (moderate to severe)
Impaired hepatic or renal function (moderate to severe)
Infection or fever/sepsis (enhances vasoconstriction)
Peripheral vascular disease
Cerebral vascular disease
Severe pruritus

[a]See standard references for additional untoward reactions, guidelines, contraindications, and warnings. Avoid ergot-containing agents in pregnancy, and encourage effective birth control methods in patients using these medications.

trate—more than 2 days per week—can result in ergot dependency (see Table 6.8). This condition will be discussed further in Chapters 8 and 9. Currently, the prevailing belief is that DHE does not induce the rebound phenomenon.

Table 6.9 provides a listing of the components of selected ergotamine preparations.

Bioavailability of ergotamine tartrate is dependent upon route of administration. Oral absorption is erratic, but rectal absorption provides a substantial increase and is generally considered 85–90% effective when taken appropriately for acute migraine.

When administering parenteral DHE or rectal ergotamine tartrate, treatment with antiemetic agents is advisable when nausea occurs as part of the migraine or is induced by the ergot derivative and cannot be avoided at therapeutic doses (see Table 6.21).

TABLE 6.8.   **SYNDROME OF ERGOTAMINE TARTRATE DEPENDENCE[a]**

Ergotamine tartrate dependence is characterized by:
1. The initial presence of intermittent migraine;
2. Insidious increase of headache frequency and ergotamine tartrate usage;
3. The dependable and irresistible use of ergotamine tartrate as the only effective agent; and
4. Attempts to discontinue the medication results in intensification of pain and accompaniments (withdrawal), thereby promoting continual usage.

[a]"Rebounding" is not currently believed to occur with dihydroergotamine usage.

TABLE 6.9.   **COMPONENTS OF SELECTED ERGOT DERIVATIVES**

Cafergot (oral tablet)	ergotamine tartrate 1 mg, caffeine 100 mg
Wigraine (oral tablet)	ergotamine tartrate 1 mg, caffeine 100 mg
Dihydroergotamine (DHE-45)	dihydroergotamine 1 mg/ml ampules (IM, SC, IV)
Migranal (DHE Nasal Spray)	0.5 mg/spray (up to 4 sprays/headache)

E. The Triptans
1. General comments

In the early 1990s, sumatriptan was introduced and has become the most extensively investigated pharmacological agent for acute migraine. Its introduction set the stage for development of numerous second generation agents that are now entering the market.

In general, the triptans are "receptor-specific" agonists to a growing list of serotonin receptors (see Chapter 4). The triptans now available or planned for marketing in 1998 and 1999 are purported to vary in onset of action, efficacy, response rate, recurrence rate, and side effect profile. In addition to sumatriptan, zolmitriptan, naratriptan, and rizatriptan are now marketed in the United States. Actual practical differences between these drugs and sumatriptan will require adequate post-marketing experience. All are likely to carry the same cardiovascular restrictions and warnings.

The triptans appear to have greatest affinity for the $5-HT_{1b}$, $5-HT_{1d}$, and $5-HT_{1f}$ subclass of receptors (see page 75), and it is suggested that some newer agents have a higher affinity than sumatriptan for some receptors. Naratriptan, rizatriptan, and zolmitriptan appear more lipophilic than sumatriptan (see Table 6.10) and may thus be more likely to penetrate the brain. Whether this matters remains to be determined.

Sumatriptan has the shortest half-life of the available compounds, and it is suggested (though not proven) that this reduced half-life is responsible in part for *recurrence*. *Recurrence* is the return of pain, after initially dissipating, within 12–24 hours after administration. Naratriptan, with a longer half-life, appears to have the lowest recurrence rate among the triptans.

Rizatriptan and zolmitriptan, with a more rapid T_{max}, may have relatively fast onset of action and greater early efficacy (see Table 6.10). The T_{max} of naratriptan is longer, suggesting a slower onset of action. Moreover, the newer triptans have an increased bioavailability over sumatriptan, though it is not now certain whether this will translate into clinically important advantages. Naratriptan is metabolized alone by MAO, thus perhaps reducing risk (serotonin syndrome, see Chapter 7) if used with an MAO-inhibitor, though this is not recommended.

See Table 6.10 for a comparison of sumatriptan, zolmitriptan, naratriptan, and rizatriptan.

2. Proposed mechanisms

As a group, the "triptans" are likely to affect migraine via one of the following mechanisms:

- Neuronal inhibition, which blocks depolarization of sensory afferents at the trigeminal nerve, thus blocking vasoactive peptide release and neurovascular inflammation of the meningeal and dural vasculature;
- Central neuronal inhibition within the trigeminal nuclei in

TABLE 6.10. **TRIPTAN COMPARISON**

Usual dose	Sumatriptan Oral	Sumatriptan Nasal	Sumatriptan Injectable	Zolmitriptan	Naratriptan	Rizatriptan
	25/50 mg, MR in 2 hours	5/20 mg, MR in 2 hours	6 mg, SQ, MR in 1 hour	2.5/5 mg, MR in 2 hours	2.5 mg, MR in 4 hours	10–20 mg, MR in 2 hours
Max dose/d	200–300 mg	40 mg	12 mg	10 mg	5 mg	40 mg
Bioavailability (%)	15%	17%	97%	48%	63–74%	40%
$T_{1/2}$	2 hours	2 hours	2 hours	3 hours	6 hours	2 hours
T_{max}	2 hrs	1–1.5 hrs	5–20 min	1 hour	2–3 hours	1 hour
Onset of action	0.5–1.5 hrs	15 min–1.5 hrs	10 minutes	1 hr	1–3 hrs	1/2–2 hours
Metabolism	MAO	MAO	MAO	P450/MAO	P450	MAO
Dose adjust in renal impairment	NO	NO	NO	NO	YES	NO
Lipophilicity	–	–	–	+	+ +	+

the brainstem (there is uncertainty as to whether sumatriptan crosses the blood brain barrier, but naratriptan, rizatriptan (minimally), and zolmitriptan do); and

- Vasoconstriction of meningeal, dural, and cerebral arteries (without affecting regional cerebral blood flow), since the small vessels controlling cerebral blood flow are not constricted.

3. Recommended use
a. Acute, moderate to severe migraine
b. Cluster headache
c. Menstrual migraine

4. Principles of use
The "triptans" should be used early in the course of the headache but not (at least with sumatriptan) during the aura. They should be avoided in individuals with contraindications to their use, and administration should only occur after appropriate historical detail regarding cardiovascular history, risk factors, and family history has been obtained (see Contraindications/cautionary warnings section).

5. Drugs in this group (see Table 6.21 for dose details)
Currently, sumatriptan (Imitrex), zolmitriptan (Zomig), rizatriptan (Maxalt), and naratriptan (Amerge) are available. Other triptans are expected to be available within the next year or two.

a. Sumatriptan (Imitrex)
Sumatriptan, the current gold standard among the triptans, has been well studied, and more clinical information is available for Sumatriptan than other products. For oral administration, the 50 mg tablet is recommended over the 25 mg size, and recent introduction of the nasal spray formulation has prompted increasing emphasis on this form of delivery. Efficacy of the intranasal form is reported to be between 75% and 78% compared to 32% for placebo (and higher than DHE nasal spray). The subcutaneous form is superior to intranasal DHE in terms of speed and degree of relief. Subcutaneous sumatriptan was superior to subcutaneous DHE in aborting attacks at 2 hours, and sumatriptan showed a faster onset but a shorter duration of action than DHE (Winner, 1996). A high level of sumatriptan efficacy is maintained on repeated and long-term use, and the adverse effect profile is unchanged. Rebound headaches may occur. The drug should not be used concomi-

tantly with MAOIs or other vasoconstrictor drugs, particularly ergot derivatives, including the preventive agents (methysergide and methylergonovine), as well as DHE and ergotamine tartrate.

A possible advantage of sumatriptan is its "portfolio" of available delivery systems, ranging from the subcutaneous to the oral to the nasal spray preparations. Thus, the clinician has a range of available delivery options with varying degrees of convenience, efficiency, and speed of action.

b. Zolmitriptan (Zomig)

Zolmitriptan, recently introduced in the United States, has a longer half-life than sumatriptan and a more rapid T_{max}. These characteristics are likely to imply faster onset of action and greater early efficacy, although extensive post-marketing experience is not yet available. Zolmitriptan has a high affinity for 5-HT_{1d} and 5-HT_{1b} receptors as well as moderate affinity for 5-HT_{1f}. Early post-marketing experience suggests wide acceptance and patient satisfaction. Anecdotally, some patients who have not responded to sumatriptan do respond to zolmitriptan; the reverse is true as well.

c. Naratriptan (Amerge)

Naratriptan may (uncertain) have a milder side effect profile than sumatriptan and perhaps the others, and, if true, can be characterized as the "kinder and gentler" triptan. Its longer half-life suggests a reduced recurrence rate, but its delayed onset of action (2–3 hours) offers a modest disadvantage. Naratriptan, like zolmitriptan, comes only in tablet form at this time. Short-term daily use for menstrual migraine and analgesic rebound headache is being studied.

d. Rizatriptan (Maxalt)

Rizatriptan is the most recent triptan to be approved for migraine in the United States. Its advantage appears to be very early onset of action and headache reduction compared to sumatriptan at two hours. Its half-life is 2–3 hours, and its T_{max} is reached in 1 hour, similar to that of zolmitriptan. It is primarily eliminated by MAO. It is marketed both in tablet and dissolvable "wafer" forms, which offer enhanced convenience of administration. Rizatriptan, like the other triptans, has high affinity for the 5-HT_{1d} receptor.

6. Major untoward reactions and contraindications

a. The major untoward reactions of this group of medications include the following:

- Chest pressure, heaviness
- Flushing/dizziness
- Paresthesia (tingling, flushing)
- Drowsiness
- Nausea
- Neck pain or stiffness

More serious adverse effects include vasospasm, arrhythmias, and myocardial pain and infarction.

In the majority of patients, the intensity of the adverse effects is mild, with generally short duration. Chest symptoms are reported by up to 40% of patients taking sumatriptan and are characterized as short-lived heaviness and sometimes as pressure in the arms and chest. Shortness of breath, anxiety, and palpitations are noted. In patients with preexisting cardiovascular disease, sumatriptan has been associated with ischemia, infarction, and ventricular fibrillation.

It remains uncertain whether all of the triptans will, after postmarketing experience accumulates, demonstrate the same general risks and adverse effect profiles as sumatriptan. Comparative studies at this point remain incomplete. It is likely that with widespread use and without the protocol restrictions of premarketing investigations, all triptans will share similar risk and adverse effect features.

b. The class contraindications for the triptans include:

- Coronary artery disease
- Prinzmetal's angina
- Complicated/hemiplegic migraine
- Breastfeeding
- Diabetes
- Hepatic disease
- Hypercholesterolemia
- Severe, uncontrolled hypertension
- Pregnancy
- MAOI use (sumatriptan, rizatriptan, zolmitriptan) concurrently or within 2 weeks of discontinuing MAOIs
- Use with other vasoconstrictors/ergots concurrently or within 24 hours

Patients who are at risk for coronary artery disease, such as those with hypercholesterolemia, obesity, diabetes, or smoking, should be screened for subclinical cardiovascular disease prior to the administration of all triptans.

c. The triptans should not be used in conjunction with ergot derivatives, and a 24-hour waiting period must ensue. Serotonin specific reuptake inhibitor (SSRI) use is relatively contraindicated because of a potential for the serotonin syndrome (see Chapter 7). MAOIs should be avoided in patients using sumatriptan, zolmitriptan, and rizatriptan, particularly. To date no evidence of teratogenicity in humans has been found, but there is minimal data in pregnant women and use in pregnancy is not recommended. Hepatic disease may increase bioavailability and peak concentrations. Renal impairment, coupled with hepatic insufficiency, may increase bioavailability and should be used cautiously in patients with hepatic and renal disease.

The safety of the triptans in children remains uncertain. Studies are underway. Some adverse effects have been noted, but cautious use is undertaken in certain clinical settings.

F. Corticosteroids
1. General comments

Corticosteroids have long been considered effective in the treatment of many headache conditions but are most appropriate for cluster headache and prolonged, intractable attacks of migraine. In addition to the well-known risks of corticosteroid therapy, increasing concern is noted regarding the possible development of avascular necrosis, particularly, but not exclusively, of the hip. Though extremely rare when considering the frequency with which steroids are administered, the condition has been reported with both occasional, low-dose and prolonged, high-dose usage. Proper informed consent is advisable.

2. Proposed mechanisms

The mechanism by which steroids influence headache remains uncertain. The following are possible:

a. Anti-inflammatory effect on neurogenic inflammation
b. Reduction of vasogenic edema
c. Effects on central aminergic/serotonergic mechanisms
d. Calcium channel blocking effect on cerebral blood vessels
e. Inhibitory effect on dorsal raphe nuclei (Peroutka, 1993)

3. Recommended use

a. Cluster headache

- When refractory to other agents (should not use for more than two weeks at a time and ideally for much shorter periods)
- For a series of breakthrough attacks
- When immediate control is necessary

b. Intractable migraine (should be limited to most severe refractory cases, because of risks)
c. Altitudinal headache
d. Headaches associated with increased intracranial pressure/edema

When used for cluster headache or intractable migraine, it is recommended that a short "tapering" course of oral steroids be used (see Table 6.11).

4. Principles of use (see Table 6.21)

Steroids should be used according to general prescribing guidelines and restrictions. For intractable, severe headaches (migraine or cluster headache), intravenous regimens are available (see Chapter 9). Steroid treatment is best reserved

TABLE 6.11. **RECOMMENDED PREDNISONE PROGRAM FOR 7- AND 10-DAY TREATMENT**[a]

	7-Day Prednisone Program (5 mg tablets—dispense 60 tablets)		
Day	**Breakfast (mg)**	**Lunch (mg)**	**Dinner (mg)**
1	20 (4 pills)	20	20
2	20	20	20
3	20	15 (3 pills)	15
4	15	15	10 (2 pills)
5	10	10	10
6	10	5 (1 pill)	5
7	5	5	
	10-Day Prednisone Program (5 mg tablets—dispense 80 tablets)		
Day	**Breakfast (mg)**	**Lunch (mg)**	**Dinner (mg)**
1	20 (4 pills)	20	20
2	20	20	20
3	20	20	20
4	20	20	20
5	20	15 (3 pills)	15
6	15	15	10 (2 pills)
7	10	10	10
8	10	5 (1 pill)	5
9	5		5
10	5		

[a]Prednisone should not be used if infection, an ulcer, or pregnancy is present. (Consult standard references for contraindications.) Aspirin and other nonsteroidal anti-inflammatory drugs should be avoided while taking prednisone.
WARNING: Steroid use has been associated in rare instances with avascular necrosis.

for circumstances in which other appropriate agents have failed or are contraindicated and in patients with severe, acute, protracted conditions.

5. **Selected drugs in this group (see Tables 6.12 and 6.13)**

6. **Selected major untoward reactions and contraindications**
   Contraindications

   1) Osteoporosis (with prolonged use)
   2) Diabetes (aggravation)
   3) Hypertension (aggravation)
   4) Diverticulosis/diverticulitis (may cause perforation even with short-term use)

TABLE 6.12.   **SELECTED STEROIDS AND DOSE***

Prednisone	PO 40–100 mg per day, then taper
Dexamethasone (Decadron)	PO, IM, or IV 8–20 mg per day
Hydrocortisone	IV 100–500 mg per day. See Treatment Chapter 6.
Methylprednisolone (Solu-Medrol)	IV 100–500 mg per day

*Avoid prolonged, repetitive use.

TABLE 6.13.   **COMPARISON OF SELECTED CORTICOSTEROID DRUG PROFILES**[a]

Drug	Potency	Na⁺ Retention[a]	Duration of Action[b]	Equivalent Dose (mg)[e]
6-α-methyl-prednisolone	5	0.5	I	4
β-methasone	25	0	L	0.75
Corticosterone	0.35	15	S	—
Cortisol (hydrocortisone)	1	1	S	20
Cortisone (11-Dehydrocortisol)	0.8	0.8	S	25
Dexamethasone	25	0	L	0.75
Paramethasone	10	0	L	2
Prednisolone	4	0.8	I	5
Prednisone	4	0.8	I	5
Triamcinolone	5	0	I	4

[a]Modified and abstracted from Timothy Covington, Pharm. D. et al. Drug facts and comparisons, 1989 ed. The pharmacological basis of therapeutics. 8th ed. J. B. Lippicott & Co. St. Louis, MO, p. 1447.
[b]Relative anti-inflammatory potency.
[c]Relative mineralocorticoid (sodium-retaining) potency.
[d]Duration of action: S = Short-acting (8–12 hrs)
                    I = Intermediate-acting (18–36 hrs)
                    L = Long-acting (36–54 hrs)
[e]Approximate equivalent dose (mg), as applied to oral or intravenous administration

Untoward reactions

1) Anorexia/increased appetite/GI distress
2) Behavior/personality changes
3) Psychosis/hallucinations/agitation
4) Hypothalamic/pituitary/adrenal axis suppression (with long-term use)
5) Cataract formation (with long-term use)
6) Myopathy
7) Avascular necrosis of femoral and humeral head (rare but reported)
8) Steroid dependence and Cushing's syndrome (long-term use)

See standard references for additional untoward reactions, guidelines, contraindications, and warnings.

G. Neuroleptics
1. General comments

Neuroleptics are generally used for symptomatic relief of pain and for the treatment of nausea and vomiting. Neuroleptics are available in oral, rectal, and parenteral forms. Metoclopramide and domperidone have the additional advantage of enhancing gut motility and promoting absorption, thus increasing the effectiveness of orally administered agents for headache. (Domperidone, currently an investigational antiemetic in the United States, is used in cancer chemotherapy. It has shown efficacy in the treatment of gastroesophageal reflux disease and has antiemetic and prokinetic effects. It is antagonistic at the D_1 and D_2 dopaminergic receptors, but unlike phenothiazines and metoclopramide it is devoid of central effects, since it penetrates the central nervous system [CNS] poorly.)

2. Proposed mechanisms

Traditionally, the value of neuroleptics in headache patients was via the control of nausea, but the possible importance of dopaminergic mechanisms in migraine and the clinical utility of certain neuroleptics in controlling migraine have increased the scope of interest. Most neuroleptics used in migraine are antagonistic at D_2 receptors. Both metoclopramide and domperidone, administered prior to the analgesic (approximately 30 minutes), have been shown to improve oral absorption of acetaminophen and aspirin, though there is little evidence to suggest that improved antimigraine efficacy occurs (Ferrari, 1997). Metoclopramide and domperidone also enhance gastric motility and absorption. An influence on histaminic receptors may be of value as well.

3. Recommended use
a. Control of nausea/vomiting
b. Symptomatic therapy of migraine and cluster headache

4. Principles of use (see Table 6.21)

Drugs in this group should be given by rectal or parenteral route for nausea and vomiting. They also may be useful for symptomatic treatment of pain by oral, rectal, or parenteral route. Metoclopramide, like many of the other neuroleptics, may cause acute dystonia (perhaps greater in adolescents and children), whereas domperidone does not easily cross the blood brain barrier and may be a lesser risk for these adverse effects (Ferrari, 1997). (See Chapter 9 for intravenous protocols using chlorpromazine and prochlorperazine in the treatment of acute migraine.)

5. Selected drugs in this group

a. Phenothiazines

1) Chlorpromazine (Thorazine)
2) Prochlorperazine (Compazine)
3) Perphenazine (Trilafon)
4) Pimozide (Orap)—recently recommended for facial neuralgia
5) Promethazine (Phenergan)
6) Trimethobenzamide (Tigan)

b. Butyrophenones

1) Haloperidol (Haldol)
2) Droperidol (Inapsine)

See page 91 for a discussion of olanzapine (Zyprexa), risperidone (Risperdal), and quetiapine (Seroquel), as well as droperidol (Inapsine).

6. Selected major untoward reactions and contraindications

a. Common untoward reactions of most neuroleptic agents

1) Extrapyramidal reactions (acute dystonia, tardive dyskinesia, akathisia, Parkinsonism, etc.)
2) Hypotension (particularly with parenteral usage)
3) Sedation/confusion
4) Anticholinergic effects

b. Contraindications/cautionary warnings

1) Severe hypotension
2) Particular vulnerability to extrapyramidal reactions

3) Previous adverse reactions
4) Conditions worsened by anticholinergic effects

- narrow-angle glaucoma
- prostatism, benign prostatic hypertrophy
- some cardiac arrhythmias
- concomitant use of CNS depressants
- others

See standard references for additional untoward reactions, guidelines, contraindications, and warnings.

7. Special considerations

Extrapyramidal reactions (dystonia or akathisia) may respond to diphenhydramine (Benadryl, 25–50 mg), via oral, intramuscular, or intravenous route.

While useful for acute headache treatment, and even prevention in some instances, neuroleptic agents should be used cautiously. Their effect on pain as well as on nausea may be significant in some, but not all, individuals, and evidence-based efficacy data are limited.

Recently three neuroleptic agents, risperidone (Risperdal), olanzapine (Zyprexa), and quetiapine (Seroquel), became available. These drugs are currently used as antipsychotic agents. Risperidone is a selective monoaminergic antagonist with high affinity (antagonism) for blockade at both serotonergic 5-HT_2 and dopaminergic D_2 and lesser at H_1 and H_2 histaminic receptors. (Blockers of 5-HT_2 receptors may have value in migraine prophylaxis.) At therapeutic dosages, risperidone's action as a serotonin and dopamine antagonist may be responsible for its effectiveness on positive and negative symptoms of schizophrenia. Its relative lack of extrapyramidal adverse reactions (relatively less than other D_2 antagonists) may result from its reduced influence on dopamine receptors in the nigrostriatal pathway, thereby limiting the extrapyramidal effects. Olanzapine is an atypical antipsychotic agent and has an affect at $alpha_1$ adrenergic, dopaminergic ($D_{1,2,4}$), histaminic (H_1), muscarinic, and serotonin type 2 (5-HT_2) receptors. It also has a reduced incidence of extrapyramidal reactions and has a low potential for drug interactions in general. Quetiapine (Seroquel) similarly is an antipsychotic agent with reduced extrapyramidal effects. It is antagonistic at 5-HT_2 and D_2 receptors and has substantial histamine H_1 blocking effects. It has no antimuscarinic effects (no anticholinergic effects) and also blocks adrenergic $alpha_1$ and $alpha_2$ receptors. The role of these drugs in the treatment of headache remains unstudied, but anecdotal experience suggests possible value in patients with borderline personality disorders and intractable headaches (see Chapter 20).

Droperidol (Inapsine) is a butyrophenone derivative that has been used as an inducing agent and as an adjunct medication during general anesthesia. It has antiemetic properties that are presumed to be the result of dopamine blockade in the chemoreceptor trigger zone of the brain. The drug antagonizes dopamine-mediated neurotransmission at the synapse and may block postsynaptic dopamine receptor sites as well. It may have analgesic properties and can cause extrapyramidal reactions. Wang (1997) and colleagues conducted a pilot study of droperidol, administered intravenously to treat status migrainosis, and concluded that it was effective and safe for the treatment of refractory migraine. Sedation and akathisia were common adverse effects.

Several of the neuroleptics, including prochlorperazine, promethazine, and others (see above), have antihistaminic effects, as do the primary antihistaminic drugs, such as diphenhydramine and hydroxyzine. Theoretically, histamine, which stimulates cerebral endothelial H_1-receptors, may have a role in the pathophysiology of migraine because it may be capable of activating nitrous oxide (NO) synthase that catalyzes the formation of nitrous oxide. NO may cause muscular relaxation and excite perivascular trigeminal axones that can initiate neurogenic inflammation (Lassen, 1996).

H. Other Symptomatic (and/or Preventive) Agents
1. Magnesium

Increasing interest in the possible role of magnesium in the mechanism and treatment of headache has emerged in the past several years. Decreased serum and intracellular levels of magnesium have been reported in migraine, and reduced intracerebral magnesium has been noted in migraineurs (Lodi, 1997; Mazzotta, 1996; Mishima, 1997; Ramadan, 1989). A placebo-controlled study of women with premenstrual syndrome (PMS) and migraine has shown a reduction in the intensity and duration of symptoms of PMS and headache when magnesium was given in advance of menstruation (Facchinetti, 1991). Mauskop (1996) has reported the efficacy of intravenous infusion of 1 gm of magnesium sulfate (Mg So_4) with migraine and correlates the response to a low basal serum ionized magnesium level. He suggests that intravenous infusion of 1 gm of Mg So_4 results in rapid relief of headache in patients with low serum magnesium levels.

Peikeart (1996) gave oral magnesium (trimagnesium dicitrate) at a dose of 600 mg for 12 weeks vs. placebo in an attempt to prevent headache and suggests that it is marginally effective in migraine prophylaxis. Pfaffenrath (1996), in a multicenter study, found equivocal results.

2. Riboflavin

Schoenen (1998) has compared riboflavin (400 mg/day) and placebo in 55 patients with migraine and demonstrated efficacy, tolerability, and low cost. He suggests that the drug may have value for migraine prophylaxis, based upon the theory that a deficit of mitochondrial energy metabolism may play a role in migraine pathogenesis. Side effects included diarrhea and polyuria.

III. Preventive Drugs Used to Treat Headache and Face Pain

Preventive treatment of headache is aimed at reducing the frequency, severity, and duration of attacks. Many of the drugs used have known uses in the treatment of illnesses considered comorbid with primary headaches. It may turn out to be that the same or related neurotransmitter and receptor mechanisms related to emotion, personality, and perception are the same in migraine and those illnesses that are comorbid with it. Preventive medications are not generally necessary if effective and safe symptomatic medication can be provided at a frequency that is acceptable. Preventive medications should be considered when this is not possible. Initiation of treatment should begin at low doses and be titrated upward slowly. It is desirable for preventive medications to be challenged every 6 months or sooner and withdrawn if there is reason to believe that the headache has entered remission. When withdrawn, treatment should be discontinued gradually. Some drugs require a longer period of use before efficacy can be measured. At this time it does not appear that any single preventive drug is superior to the others when measures of efficacy and the potential for adverse effects are considered simultaneously.

The major groups used for the prevention of primary headaches include:

- Beta-adrenergic blockers;
- Calcium channel antagonists;
- Antidepressants;
- Ergot derivatives (methysergide and related agents);
- Anticonvulsants;
- Nonsteroidal anti-inflammatory agents;
- Lithium (cluster headache); and
- Others (see end of chapter).

All or most preventive agents influence serotonin or serotonin receptor function (particularly 5-HT$_2$), although exceptions exist. Several bind to one or more 5–HT or other receptor sites and may "downregulate" the receptors. More recently it has become apparent that influence on various other receptor/neurotransmitter systems or other mechanisms may also be important in migraine prophylaxis, including but not limited to the following systems: gamma-aminobutyric acid (GABA), histaminic, noradrenergic, dopaminergic, and prostaglandin.

Guidelines for the use of preventive agents include:

- Administering a full course for 1–6 months, if effective;
- Ideally, allowing at least 1 month usage at therapeutic, tolerable dosage before evaluating effectiveness;
- Using concurrent symptomatic medication carefully and being aware of additive potential adverse effects, which should be avoided or monitored carefully (e.g., methysergide when used together with ergotamine tartrate for symptomatic treatment: both are vasoconstrictive; beta blockade with neuroleptics or tricyclic antidepressants (TCAs): can cause hypotension; SSRIs and sumatriptan: both can enhance serotonin influence; antidepressants and neuroleptics: both cause anticholinergic effects; etc.; and
- Avoidance during pregnancy, if possible, and encouraging effective birth control in fertile women.

A. Beta-Adrenergic Blockers
1. General comments
This is the most widely used group of prophylactic agents for migraine and related headache. In 60–80% of cases they are effective in reducing frequency of headache at least 50%. They are not generally effective in the treatment of cluster headache. The beta blockers *without* intrinsic sympathomimetic (agonist) activity appear more likely to benefit migraine. Beta blockers should be avoided in patients with significant focal neurological symptoms or prolonged aura, since stroke during migraine attacks has rarely occurred when these drugs have been administered (causal relationship not established). They should be avoided when possible and used cautiously when other vasoconstrictive drugs are used regularly. The following beta blockers are considered useful for migraine:

- Propranolol
- Timolol
- Nadolol

- Metoprolol
- Atenolol

Unlike the other beta-adrenergic blockers, nadolol is not primarily metabolized in the liver but excreted principally by the kidneys. This makes nadolol particularly appropriate when used in combination with agents primarily metabolized in the liver, which have hepatotoxic effects, or in patients who have liver disease. Some beta blockers, those that have lipophilic qualities such as propranolol and metoprolol, are influenced by drugs that inhibit the P-450 cytochrome system (see page 141). Prozac is such a drug. When fluoxetine, for example, is administered to a patient on a stable dose of propranolol, the serum level of propranolol increases as a result of decreased metabolism, thereby resulting in potential adverse effects, such as hypotension and heart block. By contrast, nadolol and atenolol (hydrophilic) are not affected by this drug interaction.

2. **Proposed mechanisms**

It is not clear whether the beta adrenergic blockers act through beta blockade or through an agonist affect on 5-HT receptors or other mechanisms.
   a. Inhibition of norepinephrine release by blocking prejunctional beta-receptors.
   b. Delayed reduction in tyrosine hydroxylase activity, which is the rate-limiting step in norepinephrine synthesis.
   c. Delayed reduction of locus ceruleus neuron firing rate.
   d. Agonist effects at 5-HT$_1$ receptors; 5-HT$_2$ antagonistic effects.

3. **Recommended use**
   a. Migraine
   b. Chronic daily headache
   c. Other related headache disorders (but not cluster headache)

4. **Principles of use (see Table 6.21)**

Beta-adrenergic blocking agents should be initially administered in small, divided dosages, titrating upward to tolerance.

Experience with the sustained action drugs, such as Inderal LA and Corgard, suggests that b.i.d. dosing is superior to once-a-day dosing. Bioavailability of Inderal LA is less than the short-acting forms, thus requiring increased total daily dosage.

5. **Selected drugs in this group**

See Table 6.14.

TABLE 6.14.   BETA BLOCKERS IN THE TREATMENT OF HEADACHE

Drug	Trade Name	Cardio-Selectivity	ISA	Lipid Solubility	Oral% Bioavial	T$_{1/2}$ hours	Dose
Atenolol	Tenormin	+	−	−	50.00	5–8	50–100mg/day
Metoprolol	Lopressor	+	−	+ +	40.00	3–4	50–200mg/day
Nadolol	Corgard	−	−	−	35.00	10–20	80–240mg/day
Propranolol	Inderal	−	−	+ + +	25.00	3–5	80–240mg/day
Timolol	Blocadren	−	−	+ +	50.00	3–5	10–30mg/day

ISA = Instrinsic Sympathomimetic Activity.

In general, the more lipid soluble agents have high GI absorption, high first-pass metabolism, high CNS distribution and a short duration of action. The less lipid soluble agents, conversely have little first pass metabolism, low CNS distribution, long duration of action and are primarily renally excreted. Lipid insoluble agents should be used in patients with severe depression, nightmares, or fatigue due to their decreased CNS side-effect profile. On the other hand, lipid-soluble agents are preferred in patients with renal disease due to the hepatic metabolism of the agents.

6. Selected major untoward reactions and contraindications

a. Adverse responses

1) Fatigue
2) Depression and memory disturbances
3) Impotence
4) Reduced tolerance for physical activity
5) Hypotension/bradycardia
6) Weight gain
7) Peripheral vasoconstriction
8) Masking of sympathetic-induced hypoglycemic symptomatology
9) Adverse influence on cholesterol and lipid metabolism
10) Bronchospasm

b. Contraindications/cautionary warnings

1) Congestive heart failure (low dose beta-blockers are now used in treatment of some cases of congestive heart failure)
2) Asthma
3) Significant diabetes/hypoglycemia
4) Bradycardia
5) Hypotension
6) Moderate to severe hyperlipidemia
7) Moderate to severe peripheral vascular disease
8) Vertebrobasilar migraine/complicated migraine
9) Significant cerebrovascular disease

See standard references for additional untoward reactions, guidelines, contraindications, and warnings.

7. Special considerations

Beta-blocker therapy must be individualized. If one agent fails, use of another is advisable. *Underdosing is a major cause of therapeutic failure. When discontinuing after extended usage, a gradual reduction program is necessary.*

B. Calcium Channel Antagonists

1. General comments

Calcium channel antagonists (CCA) belong to four different chemically heterogenous groups: dihydropyridines (nifedipine, nimodipine, and nicardipine); phenylalkylamines (verapamil); benzothiazepines (diltiazem); and diphenylpiperazines (flunarazine).

Verapamil is the most widely used CCA for the treatment of headache. Verapamil may require several weeks of therapeutic dose administration before beneficial effects are noticeable. Nifedipine may produce a worsening of headache in up to 30% of cases.

Flunarizine, a calcium-channel antagonist that may inhibit neurogenic inflammation by preventing release of substance P, is not available in the United States. It also influences the dopaminergic system and can induce extrapyramidal adverse effects, while also increasing basal prolactin levels. While most widely used as a preventive agent, flunarizine has been used in the treatment of acute migraine attacks through intravenous administration (Soyka, 1989).

Currently, except for flunarazine, CCAs are not as well established for migraine as the beta-adrenergic blockers, but verapamil is clearly more effective than the beta-adrenergic blockers in the treatment of cluster headache.

CCAs are more appropriate, but not generally as effective, as beta blockers in the treatment of migraine in the following circumstances:

- When bradycardia limits the use of beta-adrenergic blockers (CCAs such as verapamil generally do not slow pulse rate significantly);
- In the presence of asthmatic-like conditions;
- In the presence of peripheral or cerebrovascular disease; and
- In the presence of moderate to severe diabetes, hypoglycemia, hyperlipidemia, or complicated migraine.

2. Proposed mechanisms

The mechanism of action on headache remains uncertain. The following actions have been proposed:

a. Altering calcium flux, thereby preventing vasoconstriction and release of substance P
b. Effects at the 5-HT receptor site
c. ? Interference with neurovascular inflammation
d. ? Interference with initiation and propagtion of spreading depression
e. ? Inhibition of calcium-dependent enzymes involved in prostaglandin formation
f. ? Prevention of hypoxia on cerebral neurons

3. Recommended use

a. Migraine

b. Cluster headache (verapamil, nimodipine)

c. Daily chronic headache

4. Principles of use (see Table 6.21)

As with beta-adrenergic blockers, a small, divided dose should be used initially and then titrated upward to tolerance. High-dose verapamil (160 mg t.i.d. or q.i.d.) appears necessary for beneficial effects in many patients, particularly cluster headache patients. As with long-acting beta-adrenergic blockers, the sustained-release forms of calcium antagonists appear to have reduced bioavailability, and increased dosing may be necessary. Recent concern (though controversial) regarding cardiovascular risks in patients taking short-acting CCAs for hypertension has raised the question as to the appropriateness of widespread use in headache treatment. A cancer risk has also been raised in the literature, though this too has not been fully substantiated. The clinician is advised to maintain vigilance and be aware of additional information on risks related to the use of calcium channel antagonists.

5. Drugs in this group (selected)

a. Verapamil (Calan, Isoptin)

b. Nifedipine (Procardia)

c. Nimodipine (Nimotop)

d. Diltiazem (Cardizem)

e. Flunarazine (Sibelium) (not available in the United States)

6. Selected major untoward reactions and contraindications

a. **Untoward reactions**

1) Cardiovascular (hypotension, peripheral edema, palpitations, syncope/AV block/bradycardia, congestive heart failure)

2) Dermatologic (rash, hair loss, erythema, Stevens-Johnson syndrome, etc.)

3) Hematologic (anemia, leukopenia, thrombocytopenia, etc.)

4) Miscellaneous (flushing, gum hyperplasia, sexual dysfunction, gynecomastia, hyperglycemia, etc.)

5) Elevated liver enzymes

b. **Contraindications/cautionary warnings**

1) Congestive heart failure

2) Heart block (second or third degree AV block)

    3) Moderate to severe bradycardia

    4) Hypotension

    5) "Sick sinus" syndrome

    6) Other cardiac arrhythmias

    7) Severe constipation

    8) Moderate to severe hepatic disease

See standard references for additional untoward reactions, guidelines, contraindications, and warnings.

C. Tricyclic Antidepressants (TCA)

See next sections for newer antidepressants and MAOIs

1. General comments

TCAs are particularly valuable in patients with daily chronic headache, atypical facial pain, neuropathic pain syndromes, fibromyalgia, and neck pain disorders, with or without depression. They are also effective in many patients with intermittent migraine and related headache forms. Patients with sleep onset difficulties may benefit from a sedating TCA given at night. Ziegler (1993) demonstrated that both amitriptyline and propranolol have beneficial prophylactic effects on migraine, and that the benefits neither directly correlate with blood levels nor with an alteration in autonomic function. Amitriptyline reduced the severity, frequency, and duration of headaches, whereas propranolol reduced only the severity of the attacks.

2. Proposed mechanisms

- Inhibition of central reuptake of 5–HT and norepinephrine;
- "Downregulation" of 5–TH$_2$ receptors and decreased beta-receptor density; and
- Enhancement of opioid mechanisms.

The effect of antidepressants on mood may be related but not fundamental to the effect on headache (mood may in and of itself improve with headache control). TCAs may be particularly beneficial in patients with comorbid illness, particularly depression, anxiety, and sleep disturbances. When effective for pain, the benefit may occur within days of proper dose administration, whereas depression treatment generally requires several weeks of therapy. Individual sensitivity to the adverse effects of these agents varies greatly. At least 1–2 weeks and maybe more are required for appreciation of efficacy, and individual dose titration is necessary. The synaptic effects may be responsible for pain control, and these include norepinephrine and 5-HT receptor blockade, particularly that of 5-HT$_2$ receptor, which is excitatory and may induce perivascular inflammation.

3. **Recommended use**
   a. Migraine and related headaches
   b. Episodic and chronic "tension-type" headache, daily chronic headache, and transformed migraine (may be benefited by concurrent beta blocker administration) (Mathew, 1981)
   c. Post-traumatic headaches, myofascial pain, and fibromyalgia
   d. Facial pain syndromes
   e. Pain syndromes accompanied by sleep disturbance, depression, and/or anxiety
   f. Neuralgic/neuropathic pain syndromes

4. **Principles of use (see Table 6.21)**
   Generally, TCAs should be initially administered as a single dose at bedtime. Exceptions include those drugs that have an activating or stimulating effect, e.g., desipramine, nortriptyline, and protriptyline. If daytime sedation is present even when a TCA is given at bedtime, switching from a tertiary TCA (amitriptyline or doxepin) to a secondary TCA (nortriptyline or protriptyline) may be beneficial. If insomnia or nightmares develop, lowering the dose and/or administering earlier in the day may be helpful. Divided, small dose daytime administration may be useful for control of anxiety and pain. *Caution should be used when using in the elderly, in those with a history of cardiac arrhythmias, and in children under the age of 12.*

   A therapeutic window may exist below and above which these drugs are ineffective. Thus, individual dosing and monitoring are essential. Moreover, because of the long half-life, drug accumulation is common and down-dosing is often necessary.

5. **Selected drugs in this group**
   The following drugs are the major TCAs used for headache:

   - Amitriptyline (Elavil, Endep)
   - Nortriptyline (Pamelor, Aventyl)
   - Doxepin (Sinequan, Adapin)
   - Desipramine (Norpramin)
   - Protriptyline (Vivactil)
   - Others

   Other tricyclics and atypical tricyclics are available, such as clomipramine (Anafranil) (see next sections for newer antidepressants and MAO inhibitors). The benefit of clomipramine for headache, as with many other TCAs, has yet to be established or has been found to be of relatively little value (as in the case of trazodone (Desyrel)) See Table 6.15 for a comparison of selected, available antidepressants.

6. **Selected major untoward reactions and contraindications**

   a. **Untoward reactions include**

      1) Weight gain
      2) Dizziness
      3) Tremor/hypomania
      4) Confusion/delirium
      5) May lower seizure threshold
      6) Anticholinergic symptoms, such as
         a) Drowsiness
         b) Dry mouth
         c) Constipation
         d) Urinary retention
         e) Blurred vision
         f) Tachycardia
         g) Others
      7) Akathesia
      8) Priapism (trazodone)

   b. **Contraindications/cautionary warnings**

      1) Significant cardiac arrhythmia
      2) Glaucoma (anticholinergic-sensitive, angle closure)
      3) Urinary retention (avoid those with strong anticholinergic effects)
      4) Moderate to severe hypotension
      5) Other

     See standard references for additional untoward reactions, guidelines, contraindications, and warnings.

7. **Special considerations**

   Blood level monitoring is advisable in patients using TCA. The drugs accumulate and have an impact upon cardiac function and lower the seizure threshold. Electrocardiogram monitoring to evaluate the QRS interval (should be shorter than 100 msec) is recommended. Monitoring liver function is advisable. In patients with a vulnerability toward seizures or when high dosages are required, electroencephalogram monitoring is advisable. Use in younger children should be under-

TABLE 6.15. **COMPARISON OF THE ANTIDEPRESSANTS**

Drug	Receptor-related Side Effects			Reuptake Blocking Activity		$T_{1/2}$ (hours) parent	Time to steady state (days)	Special Considerations
	Muscarinic (Anticholinergic)	Histamine$_1$ (Sedation)	Alpha Adrenergic (Orthostatic hypotension)	NE	5-HT			
Tertiary Amines								
Amitriptyline (Elavil)	VH	VH	M	M	VH	31–46	4–10	Lower clearance of metabolite nortriptyline in the elderly
Clomipramine (Anafranil)	H	H	M	M	VH	19–37	7–14	
Doxepin (Sinequan)	M	H	M	S	M	8–24	2–8	histamine H$_1$- and H$_2$-receptor agonist
Imipramine (Tofranil)	M	M	H	M	VH	11–25	2–5	
Secondary Amines								
Desipramine (Norpramin)	S	S	S	VH	M	12–24	2–11	
Nortriptyline (Pamelor)	M	M	S	VH	M	18–44	4–19	Reduced clearance with low creatinine; effective serum conc 50–150 ng/mL
Triazolopyridine								
Trazodone (Desyrel)	S	M	M	O	H	4–9	3–7	Metabolite is 5-HT agonist; given at bedtime; causes confusion in some patients

continued

TTABLE 6.15. COMPARISON OF THE ANTIDEPRESSANTS

Drug	Receptor-related Side Effects			Reuptake Blocking Activity		$T_{1/2}$ (hours) parent	Time to steady state (days)	Special Considerations
	Muscarinic (Anti-cholinergic)	Histamine$_1$ (Sedation)	Alpha Adrenergic (Orthostatic hypotension)	NE	5-HT			
Aminoketone Bupropion (Wellbutrin)	O	S/O	S/O	S/O	S/O	8–24	1.5–5	Dopamine uptake blocker, causes seizures at higher doses
Phenytylamine Venlafaxine (Effexor)	O	O	O	H	H	5–11	3–4	Modulates for NE, 5-HT, DA. Monitor pulse rate, blood pressure, heart rate
Selective Serotonin Reuptake Inhibitors Fluoxetine (Prozac)	S	S/O	S	S	MX	85	28–35	Zero order kinetics; alters hepatic metabolism of other drugs
Fluvoxamine (Luvox)	O	O	O	S/O	MX	15.00	7.00	Alters hepatic metabolism of other drugs
Paroxetine (Paxil)	O	O	O	S/O	MX	24.00	5–10	Alters hepatic metabolism of other drugs
Sertraline (Zoloft)	O	O	O	S/O	MX	25.00	7–70	Alters hepatic metabolism of other drugs

*Active metabolite norfluoxetine 7–9 days.
# N-desmethyl sertraline 2–4 days.
O = none; S-slight; VH = very high; MX-maximum
Adapted from: Barkin RL, et al. Management of chronic pain: Part 1 Dis Mon 1996; 0 42:389–454

taken with caution, since fatal consequences, mainly due to cardiac arrhythmias, have been reported.

D. Newer Antidepressants

1. General comments

Fluoxetine, the first of a wave of newer antidepressants, is an atypical, nontricyclic antidepressant with potent specific 5–HT reuptake inhibitory properties. As a group the SSRIs are chemically unrelated to TCAs, heterocyclics, or other antidepressants. In addition to neuronal serotonin reuptake inhibition, they have weak noradrenalin and dopamine effects. They have limited affinity at alpha$_1$, alpha$_2$, and beta-adrenergic, benzodiazepine, dopamine$_2$, GABA, histamine, and muscarinic receptors. They are free of many of the side effects associated with other antidepressants, such as cardiovascular, sedative, and anticholinergic effects. These agents can be used carefully in combination with TCAs, but combination therapy often results in enhanced blood levels of TCAs. Toxic responses, including headaches, arrhythmias, and seizures, are more likely at high doses, and when possible, blood levels should be carefully monitored, particularly in "at risk" patients, such as those with cardiac arrhythmias and seizure disorders.

2. Proposed mechanisms

a. Potent selective serotonin reuptake inhibitors
b. Similar mechanism to other antidepressants

3. Recommended use

At the time of this edition, little in the way of efficacy in the control of headache has been demonstrated. A controlled study using fluoxetine (Saper, 1994) showed no effect on migraine and only modest effect on daily chronic headache. The dosages were generally low (40 mg or less), and treatment was implemented for only 3 months. A longer trial at higher dosages might have had different results. An open label trial using paroxetine showed modest improvement in daily headache control. Thus, although widely used, there is little to suggest their value beyond the treatment of migraine comorbidities, although further study might offer different conclusions. The newer antidepressants are used in a variety of possibly related neuropsychiatric conditions, including obsessive-compulsive disease, bipolar disease, eating disorders, panic attacks and anxiety disorders, and, of course, depression.

4. Principles of use (see Table 6.21)

Individual dose titration is necessary. Fluoxetine, and perhaps others, may interfere with sleep, even when given early in the day. Gradual increase in dose is recommended. *Synergistic and enhancing effects with other medications may occur, and downward dosing of other medications, particularly TCAs, neuroleptics, and anticonvulsants, must be considered.* Caution must be used when adding fluoxetine or other P-450 enzyme inhibitors to an existing treatment with a lipophilic beta blocker, such as propranolol or metoprolol. Fluoxetine, through inhibition of the P-450 enzyme system (see page 141), will raise the serum level of the beta blocker, thus causing a potential for hypotension and cardiac effects. These drugs cannot be used with MAO inhibitors. Death has occurred as a result of the serotonin syndrome (see Chapter 7).

5. Selected drugs in this group

- Fluoxetine (Prozac)
- Sertraline (Zoloft)
- Paroxetine (Paxil)
- Fluvoxamine (Luvox)

6. Selected major untoward reactions and contraindications

a. Untoward reactions (as a group)

1) Agitation/tremor
2) Nausea
3) Headache
4) Hypomania/delirium/other psychiatric syndromes
5) Insomnia
6) Lower seizure threshold
7) Akathesia/tremor/other extrapyramidal reactions
8) Nausea/diarrhea
9) Anorgasmia/sexual dysfunction
10) Questionable suicidal preoccupation/impulsive behavior
11) Inappropriate secretion of antidiuretic hormone
12) Serotonin syndrome

Certain drugs have specific characteristics. Fluoxetine and sertraline are more likely to be associated with weight loss. Paroxetine has greater anticholinergic and sedating adverse effects. Fluoxetine and fluvoxamine are contraindicated in patients taking terfenadine, cisapride, or astemizole. Except for fluoxetine, which has an extended half-life, gradual reduction in dosing, rather than sudden discontinuance, is advisable to avoid withdrawal symptomatology.

Unlike certain other antidepressants, SSRIs do not generally (but can) cause orthostatic hypotension or cardiac conduction defects (interaction with other drugs must be monitored). However, fatal reactions have occurred when treatment with MAOIs and fluoxetine has overlapped. *It is strongly recommended that MAOIs be discontinued for at least 3 weeks before fluoxetine is added; fluoxetine should be discontinued for at least 5 weeks (other SSRIs, 2–3 weeks) before an MAO inhibitor is added to a treatment regimen.*

Moreover, adverse behavioral and neurological effects have occurred when fluoxetine has been used simultaneously with lithium, haloperidol, tryptophan, or carbamazepine. Because fluoxetine is strongly bound to protein, its use with warfarin and digoxin is of concern, since these drugs may be displaced.

Fluoxetine in combination with other SSRIs, TCAs, or anticonvulsants may have a synergistic or enhancing effect, along with increased blood levels. Avoidance or careful monitoring is recommended. The combined use of fluoxetine and nortriptyline has resulted in seizures, even in patients without a previous history. When adding fluoxetine to an existing treatment of antidepressants or anticonvulsants, it is prudent to reduce the preexisting treatment and then increase both drugs slowly over time, if combined treatment is required.

b. Selected contraindications/cautionary warnings

1) Seizure disorders
2) A strong history of akathesia or extrapyramidal reactions to SSRIs, TCAs, or neuroleptics
3) Hepatic disease
4) Mania
5) MAO inhibitor therapy
6) Others

See standard references for additional untoward reactions, guidelines, contraindications, and warnings.

c. Treatment of sexual dysfunction with antidepressants

Sexual dysfunction represents a major disadvantage of SSRIs. A variety of disturbances are possible (Gitlin, 1995). For short-acting SSRIs, such as sertraline and paroxetine, short-term discontinuance prior to sexual activity can be of value. Because of fluoxetine's longer influence (up to 5 weeks), short-term discontinuation is of little value. Other possible aids include pretreatment with psychostimulants, such as dextroamphetamine and methylphenidate. These appear to counteract the sexually inhibiting effects of SSRIs while also enhancing sexual responsiveness (Bartlik, 1995). These drugs should be administered several hours before sexual activity. OTC drugs may be of benefit, and these include caffeine and a combination of pseudoephedrine and chlorpheniramine maleate. Other antidotal interventions include cyproheptadine, yohimbine, dopamine agonists, bupropion, and buspirone, as well as others. Cyproheptadine, an antihistamine that interferes with serotonergic effects, reverses the antidepressant effect of SSRIs and also may reduce sexual dysfunction. Yohimbine is a presynaptic alpha-$_2$ blocker reported to reverse antidepressant-induced sexual side effects in several reports. Amantadine, a mild dopamine agonist used as an antiviral agent and in the treatment of neuropathic pain and Parkinson's disease, has been reported to reverse anorgasmia in patients taking fluoxetine. The dose is 100 mg a day or 100 mg b.i.d. Bupropion (Wellbutrin) at a dose of 75 mg a day was also found in one study to decrease fluoxetine-induced sexual dysfunction. Buspirone suppresses serotonin activity while enhancing noradrenergic and dopaminergic cell firing, has some inhibitory actions on GABAergic pathways, and has a high affinity for serotonin (5-HT$_{1a}$ receptors). It may be useful preventively or "as needed" (Topics in Pain Management, 1997).

E. Other Antidepressants

Other antidepressants are currently available, and their use in headache is currently under investigation. These include nefazodone (Serzone), venlafaxine (Effexor), and mirtazepine (Remeron). Venlafaxine and mirtazepine are unrelated to other antidepressants. Nefazodone is structurally similar to trazodone but with less sedation and orthostatic hypotension associated with use. At the time of this writing, these drugs have not been established as effective in the treatment of headache, though some authorities believe their value will be demonstrated from pending studies, particularly those involving nefazadone.

F. Antidepressants: MAOIs

1. General comments

MAOIs are appropriate for patients with refractory, recurring headache, particularly migraine and certain migraine variant forms. They are also helpful in patients with severe depression and headache and might be helpful in headache patients with phobic (panic) elements. Their use with the triptans and other agents that enhance serotonin transmission must be undertaken with caution as a result of the possible development of the serotonin syndrome (see Chapter 7). Sumatriptan, zolmitriptan, and rizatriptan must not be used with MAOIs because these triptans are metabolized primarily by MAO.

Two MAOI subtypes exist:

- Phenelzine and tranylcypromine preferentially deaminate norepinephrine and 5–HT via inhibition of MAO–A.
- L–deprenyl preferentially deaminates dopamine via inhibition of MAO–B. (Inhibition of MAO–B has not yet been shown to assist in the control of headache.)

Phenelzine (Nardil) is a nonspecific inhibitor of MAO-A. Phenelzine can be combined with amitriptyline, nortriptyline, and doxepin in cases of refractory headache, but careful and precise administration is required. (See Table 6.16.) *Phenelzine and related agents cannot be combined with imipramine, desipramine, fluoxetine, and several other agents. The use of SSRIs and MAO inhibitors is contraindicated, and combining MAO inhibitors and the other newer antidepressants should be avoided until safety can be demonstrated. At least 3 weeks should pass after MAO inhibitor discontinuance before initiating therapy with these agents. Five weeks must pass after fluoxetine discontinuance before initiating MAO inhibitor therapy, and 3 weeks must pass when switching from one MAOI*

TABLE 6.16 **GUIDELINES FOR COMBINED MAOI AND TCA USAGE**[a]

1. Begin both phenelzine and TCA (amitriptyline, nortriptyline, or doxepin only) simultaneously, or
2. Add phenelzine to existing program of the above.
3. Do not add TCA to existing treatment of phenelzine.
4. Avoid MAOI usage with imipramine, desipramine, or SSRIs, and certain others. MAOI must be discontinued for at least 3 weeks before any of these agents is administered; fluoxetine must be discontinued for at least 5 weeks prior to the administration of MAOI.
5. When switching from one MAOI to another, at least 3 weeks must separate the administration of the second agent from the discontinuation of the first.
6. Informed consent is advisable.

[a]The combined use of MAOI and certain TCA has historically been discouraged. However, this practice is reasonably well established in the treatment of severe, intractable depression. Effective and safe combined usage has been anecdotally reported for a small percentage of patients with severe, intractable headache, some with elements of depression. The reader is strongly advised to employ extreme caution if this program is being considered. Detailed patient education is required. Proper administration is essential and patient selection critical. Avoid use in noncompliant patients or in those who take instruction poorly.

to another. Patients taking MAOIs cannot use isometheptene (Midrin and Isocom), meperidine, sumatriptan, zolmitriptan, rizatriptan, and several other agents.

2. **Proposed mechanisms**
   a. Enhancement of synaptic norepinephrine and 5–HT
   b. Others
3. **Recommended use**
   a. Severe, resistant migraine
   b. Severe, resistant, nonneuralgic facial pain syndromes
   c. Severe, resistant, chronic daily headache and related forms
   d. Severe headache in the presence of depression, panic disorder, or obsessive-compulsive disorder
4. **Principles of use (see Table 6.21)**
   a. Patients should be placed on a specific MAOI diet in advance of treatment (see Table 6.17) and continue for 3 weeks after discontinuance.
   b. Patients must carefully adhere to restrictions regarding the use of other drugs, including OTC drugs, cold preparations, etc. (Tables 6.18 and 6.19.)

TABLE 6.17.   **FOODS TO AVOID WHILE ON MAO INHIBITORS**

1 Foods that have a high tyramine content (most common in foods that are aged, fermented, or smoked to increase their flavor), such as cheeses, sour cream, yogurt, pickled herring, chicken livers, bananas, avocados, soy sauce, broad bean pods (fava bean pods), yeast extracts, meats prepared with tenderizers, or dry sausage.
2. Alcoholic beverages, including beer and wines (especially Chianti and other hearty red wines).
3. High caffeine-containing foods or beverages, such as coffee, chocolate, tea, or cola.

TABLE 6.18.   **SELECTED CATEGORIES OF MEDICATIONS TO BE AVOIDED WITH MAOI**

- Appetite suppressants
- Certain asthma medications
- Decongestant cold medications (including those with dextromethorphan)
- L-tryptophan-containing preparations
- Isometheptene-containing drugs
- Most other antidepressants, particularly SSRIs, imipramine, desipramine, others
- Mixed allergy drugs (except simple antihistamines)
- Nasal sprays (except steroids only)
- Stimulants and weight-reducing preparations
- Anticonvulsants (specifically carbamazepine)
- Opioid preparations containing meperidine
- Other MAOIs

TABLE 6.19.   **SELECTED OVER-THE-COUNTER PRODUCTS CONTAINING EITHER PSEUDOEPHEDRINE, PHENYLEPHRINE, OR PHENYLPROPANOLAMINE**

Pseudoephedrine	
Actifed	Robitussin-PE
Contac	Sine-Aid
CoTylenol	Sinutab
Vicks Formula 44M	Tylenol Maximum Strength
Vicks Formula 44D	Sinus Medication
Vicks Nyquil	
Phenylephrine	
Dimetane Decongestant	Nostril
Dristan Advanced Formula Tablets and Coated	Vicks Sinex
Caplets	Robitussin Night Relief
Neo-Synephrine	
Phenylpropanolamine	
Alka-Seltzer Plus	Coricidin
Acutrim	Dexatrim
Allerest	Sine-Off
Cheracol Plus	Triaminic

5. Selected drugs in this group

   a. Phenelzine (Nardil)

   b. Tranylcypromine (Parnate)

6. Selected major untoward reactions and contraindications

a. Major untoward reactions

   1) Orthostatic hypotension (gradual onset)

   2) Severe hypertension when combined with a contra-indicated drug or food substance

   3) Serotonin syndrome (see Chapter 7)

   4) Sexual dysfunction

   5) Constipation

   6) Insomnia

   7) Weight gain

   8) Peripheral edema

   9) Hypomania and agitation

   10) Anticholinergic effects

b. Contraindications/cautionary warnings

   1) Pheochromocytoma

   2) Certain drugs, among which are:

   a) Sumatriptan, zolmitriptan, and rizatriptan

   b) Fluoxetine, other SSRIs, and newer antidepressants (until studies confirm safety)

   c) Imipramine, clomipramine, desipramine, etc.

   d) Isometheptene (Midrin)

e) Carbamazepine
f) Agents with sympathomimetic effects (deconges tants, stimulants, etc.) (See Tables 6.18 and 6.19)
g) Pizotifen
h) Stimulants
3) Certain foods (see Table 6.17)
4) Severe liver or cardiac disease
5) Closed angle glaucoma
6) Severe prostatic disease

See standard references for additional untoward reactions, guidelines, contraindications, and warnings.

7. Special considerations

MAOI therapy can be very effective but requires close medical supervision by experienced physicians. Patients must be compliant and well informed. These agents should be administered by physicians with full knowledge of prescribing data who are treating resistant cases of severe headache. Casual use is discouraged.

F. Ergot Derivatives and Other Drugs Acting on 5-HT Receptor Mechanisms

1. General comments

Methysergide, methylergonovine, pizotifen, and cyproheptadine are agents used in the prevention of migraine and which act on serotonergic mechanisms. Methysergide and methylergonovine, because of their adverse effect profile, are generally reserved for resistant cases or those in which other agents are not effective or cannot be used. This section will review the ergot derivatives. Pizotifen is not available in the United States (see page 124), and cyproheptadine is reviewed on page 121.

Methysergide is the oldest of the prophylactic agents for migraine, cluster, and related headaches. It is effective in migraine prophylaxis in 60% or more of cases.

The historic concern for the development of fibrotic reactions (retroperitoneal fibrosis, pleuropulmonary fibrosis, and cardiac valvular changes) after prolonged use of ergot derivatives still exists. However, current belief regarding methysergide is that these responses reflect an *idiosyncratic reaction,* rather than a dose-time-related factor. As such, dose or length of use may not be the primary factors in determining risk.

Ergonovine maleate is no longer commercially available. However, a closely related drug, methylergonovine, which is a metabolite of methysergide, is available as Methergine. The two drug profiles (ergonovine and methylergonovine) are similar and will be considered together. Both are ergot alkaloids. They generally lack the degree of arterial constricting effects of methysergide but have greater oxytocic effects than methysergide or ergotamine tartrate.

2. **Proposed mechanisms**
   - $5-HT_2$ receptor antagonist
   - $5-HT_1$ agonist
   - $5-HT_{1c}$ agonist
   - Other central effects

   The receptor influences of these drugs appear to mediate neuronal depolarization. 5-HT receptors are important in perivascular inflammation.

3. **Recommended use**
   a. Resistant migraine, including menstrual migraine (episodic prophylaxis)
   b. Cluster headache
   c. Resistant daily chronic headache
   d. Resistant atypical facial pain syndromes
   e. Patients placed on these agents should be those in whom more standard medications have failed or could not be used

4. **Principles of usage (see Table 6.21)**
   a. **Methysergide**

      1) 2 mg 3–5 times per day
      2) Maximum daily dose is 14 mg per day (preferably 8–10 mg per day)
      3) Do not use for more than 6 months without a 1-month interruption ("drug holiday") and appropriate evaluation for fibrotic reactions (see below)

   b. **Methylergonovine**

      1) 0.2–0.4 mg t.i.d. to q.i.d.
      2) Not advisable to use for more than 6 months without a 1-month "drug holiday" and appropriate evaluation for fibrotic reactions (see below)

5. **Drugs in this group (drugs active on 5-HT receptor mechanisms)**
   a. Methysergide (Sansert) (ergot)
   b. Methylergonovine (Methergine) (ergot)
   c. Pizotyline (Pizotifen) (see page 124) (nonergot)

    d. Cyproheptadine (Periactin) (see Section I, page 121)
       (nonergot)

6. Selected major untoward reactions and contraindications

Fibrotic reactions, well known with methysergide, also occur with methylergonovine. Two cases have been personally encountered in patients taking methylergonovine despite the appropriate drug holiday every 6 months. With methysergide, fibrotic reactions are estimated to occur in 1 in 2000 cases. Reactions, most recognized in the retroperitoneal region, may also occur in pulmonary and cardiovalvular tissue. Both cardiac valvular disease and retroperitoneal fibrosis have been reported with excessive use of ergotamine tartrate as well. In addition to the ergot derivatives, agents such as analgesics may cause fibrotic reactions. In a retrospective study of seven patients with retroperitoneal fibrosis, none had ever taken methysergide, but four of the seven used excessive amounts of analgesics (Lewis, 1975). Several case reports have now confirmed the likelihood that methysergide, as well as possibly ergotamine tartrate, can affect heart valves as well as the retroperitoneal and pulmonary tissue. Pathology from the valvular fibrosis in methysergide-treated patients appears similar to that seen in carcinoid syndrome, a disorder also related to serotonin.

It is uncertain whether the 1-month holiday provides any protection against the development of progressive fibrosis. In at least one case, short-term use appears to have been associated with fibrotic reactions, although the use of analgesics and other agents that can cause fibrosis could not be excluded.

Diagnostically, prior to the development of MR and CT scanning, intravenous pyelography was the diagnostic treatment of choice. More recently reliance on enhanced CT and MR imaging has lessened the utilization of the intravenous pyelogram. Unfortunately, CT scanning and perhaps even MR imaging may not be entirely reliable in assessing retroperitoneal fibrosis (personally observed case, J.R.S. and D.G.).

Recently Bucci (1997) described a 24-year-old woman with manifestations of retroperitoneal fibrosis while taking methysergide whose laboratory studies yielded substantially increased serum procollagen III levels and anticardiolipin antibodies accompanied with anti-beta$_2$ glycoprotein I (GPI) levels. These findings were not previously described with this disorder. These abnormalities resolved after cessation of methysergide therapy. The author concluded that measurement of serum procollagen III levels may be a useful marker of the fibrotic process in patients with retroperitoneal fibrosis.

At this time, the following are recommended: warn patients about the possibility of a fibrotic reaction, document the warning, provide a 6-month course of treatment with a 1-month drug holiday, and remain vigilant for signs of renal disease and urinary obstruction, cardiac valvular murmurs, or other signs of fibrotic disease. Every 6 months for at least the first several years, MR or CT imaging with enhancement, cardiac auscultation, and chest x-ray are indicated. IVP should be undertaken if signs of back pain or abdominal complaints occur (see Table 6.20). The validity of serum studies remains to be determined.

a. **Major untoward reactions**

1) Nausea
2) Muscle aches (chest, abdomen, or legs)
3) Hallucinations
4) Weight gain
5) Frank claudication
6) Fibrotic lesions

b. **Contraindications/cautionary warnings**

1) Peripheral, cerebral, or cardiovascular disease
2) Thrombophlebitis (deep vein)
3) Severe hypertension
4) Pregnancy
5) Significant renal, hepatic disease
6) Previous fibrotic reactions

TABLE 6.20. **RECOMMENDED EVALUATION TO MONITOR FIBROTIC REACTIONS (RF)[a]**

1. Cardiac and carotid auscultation for new murmurs or bruits or change from known abnormalities. (Echocardiogram, carotid ultrasound testing recommended if suspected abnormality.)
2. Palpation of peripheral vascular and carotid pulsations. (Ultrasound testing recommended if abnormality suspected.)
3. Enhanced abdominal CT and/or enhanced MR imaging for retroperitoneal fibrosis.
4. Chest x-ray for pleuropulmonary fibrosis.
5. IVP—for patients with suspected symptoms of RF, even if CT or MR imaging is normal.

[a]Recommended for patients on continuous ergot therapy for 6 months or more.

See standard references for additional untoward reactions, guidelines, contraindications, and warnings.

7. Special considerations

These agents should be administered by physicians who are treating resistant cases of severe headache. A thorough understanding of these drugs is required, and casual use is discouraged.

Table 6.20 provides a recommended evaluation for fibrotic reactions.

G. Anticonvulsants: Divalproex (Depakote)

1. General comments

Divalproex has emerged as an important and primary treatment for the prevention of both migraine and daily headache. Double-blind, controlled clinical trials demonstrate divalproex's effectiveness in reducing migraine frequency as well as severity and duration of attacks (Hering, 1995; Jensen, 1994; Mathew, 1995). It may also have an important role in the prevention of cluster headache (Hering, 1989). The FDA has approved divalproex for migraine prophylaxis.

Because of its side effect profile, divalproex is recommended as a first-line preventive agent, when other treatments, such as beta blockers and antidepressants, cannot be used. Also, divalproex may be the treatment of first choice in patients with migraine comorbidities, such as seizures, bipolar disease, and those with personality disorders, such as the borderline personality (see Chapter 20).

2. Proposed mechanisms

a. Increased GABA levels in synaptosomes

b. Enhanced postsynaptic response to GABA

c. Increased potassium conductance producing neuronal hyperpolarization

d. Inhibits "firing" of 5–HT neurons of the dorsal raphe

e. Influence on voltage-dependent calcium and sodium channels

f. Decreased plasma extravasation following substance P administration

3. Recommended use

a. Migraine

b. Daily chronic headache

c. Cluster headache

d. Atypical facial plain syndromes

e. In headache patients with "rapid cycling," bipolar-like illness

f. In patients with borderline personality and migraine

4. Principles of use (see Table 6.21)

Divalproex therapy should be initiated at a dose of 125–250 mg 2–4 times per day. Syrup and "sprinkle" formulations are available. Divalproex (Depakote) is available in 125-, 250-, and 500-mg tablet sizes, and a 125 mg sprinkle capsule size. Optimum effectiveness for headaches may occur anywhere above 1000 mg per day and serum levels between 50 and 100 μg/ml.

Dosages should be increased gradually to a maximum dose of 1–2 grams per day. Efficacy has been demonstrated at dosages of 500 mg per day, but generally a higher dose is required.

5. Drugs in this group

Depakote

6. Selected major untoward reactions and contraindications

a. Major untoward reactions

1) Nausea and GI upset
2) Sedation
3) Thrombocytopenia
4) Hair loss
5) Tremor
6) Change in cognition
7) Hepatotoxicity (should be avoided in very young children unless considered absolutely necessary)
8) Weight gain

In young children, generally under the age of 2, hepatic dysfunction with fatal outcome has been reported. The drug is also potentially teratogenic. Thrombocytopenia can occur, and monitoring is necessary.

b. Contraindications/cautionary warnings

1) Pregnancy
2) Significant hepatic disease
3) Childhood (relative contraindication. Generally, the drug is inadvisable in very young children (2 years and younger). Careful monitoring is required if the drug is administered.)

4) Concurrent barbiturate/benzodiazepine use (relative contraindication), due to excessive sedation when used concurrently

5) Use carefully with other drugs metabolized by the liver

See standard references for additional untoward reactions, guidelines, contraindications, and warnings.

7. Special considerations

It is advisable to evaluate hematological and liver function studies before beginning treatment because most serious adverse effects occur in the first 4 months, shortly after treatment initiation. Periodic hematological studies to assess for thrombocytopenia is recommended by some authorities. Blood level monitoring is optional. A higher-than-expected potential for adverse effects is present when combined with antidepressants or other anticonvulsants, particularly barbiturates and other liver metabolized drugs, such as verapamil.

Because of its effects on fetal development, divalproex should be used cautiously in fertile women. Warnings and appropriate methods of contraception are necessary.

Severe sedation and coma have occurred when valproate is combined with barbiturates. (Benzodiazepines may also pose an increased sedative risk.) In the headache population, strong warning and careful monitoring are necessary because analgesic agents containing barbiturate are frequently prescribed. Because the reaction may be idiosyncratic, risks cannot be predicted or easily anticipated. Some patients are apparently able to use these agents concurrently, but this cannot be predicted in advance of usage.

H. The Other Anticonvulsants: (Phenytoin, Carbamazepine, and Gabapentin)

1. General comments

In addition to divalproex, which is the only anticonvulsant demonstrated with certainty to benefit migraine and other headaches, other anticonvulsants have been used in the treatment of selected cases of migraine, cluster headache, and facial pain conditions, including true neuralgias and atypical facial pain syndromes. It is not known whether they are more effective in children and adults with paroxysmal EEGs, but at least one report suggests greater efficacy in the presence of disturbed electroencephalographic patterns.

Phenytoin and carbamazepine can reduce the efficacy of oral contraceptives and, therefore, specific warnings are necessary.

Gabapentin was developed as a GABA agonist. It has high lipid solubility, is not metabolized by the liver, and has no protein binding and is thus devoid of the usual drug interactions. These actions appear to be that of a GABA analog. Gabapentin has been increasingly utilized successfully in the treatment of a variety of painful states, including neuropathic pain, but its value in the treatment of headache remains uncertain. Although generally devoid of major adverse effects, reports suggest that it may enhance hyperactivity in pediatric patients with pretreatment hyperactive disorders. In addition, a variety of subtle and more obvious movement disorders have occurred in patients taking gabapentin. These include retrocollis, oculogyric crises, opisthotonos, myoclonus, and jaw clenching. In another report choreiform movements were noted (Beutefisch, 1996; Reeves, 1996; Tallian, 1996; Wolf, 1995).

2. Proposed mechanisms

a. Membrane stabilization (phenytoin, carbamazepine)
b. Gabapentin may work through its characteristic as a GABA analog

3. Recommended use

Except for the early reports on phenytoin in pediatric migraine, these agents have not been shown to be specifically useful for headaches. Anecdotal reports have prompted their use in certain instances, and studies are currently underway assessing the value of gabapentin in the treatment of headache. These agents may have a role in atypical pain disorders, neuralgic pain, the cluster-tic syndrome (see Chapters 12 and 16), headache associated with neuralgia, and cases of refractory migraine, cluster, or daily chronic headache.

4. Principles of use (see Table 6.21)

Phenytoin is administered in dosages of 200–400 mg per day. Phenytoin in the form of Dilantin, which is a sustained-release preparation, can be given as a single dose per day (usually at night), *but generic forms must be given in divided dosages.*

Carbamazepine (Tegretol) should be given in dosages beginning at 100–200 mg 2–3 times per day, with gradual increase to tolerance or efficacy. A sustained release formulation is now available and is administered twice daily.

Gabapentin is rapidly distributed to the CNS. Its half-life is 5–7 hours and is not altered with increasing or multiple doses. It does not generally react with other drugs, but Maalox, though not food, reduces the bioavailability, and gabapentin should be taken at least two hours after Maalox administration. Dosages range from 900 to 3600 mg per day in three divided dosages in children over the age of 12. Titration should occur at a moderate rate, and reduction should occur gradually so as not to induce withdrawal symptomatology. It is available in a 100, 300, and 400 mg capsule.

5. **Selected major untoward reactions and contraindications**

   a. **Untoward reactions**

      1) Phenytoin: dizziness, drowsiness, rash, insomnia, ataxia, severe drug reactions, leukopenia, etc.
      2) Carbamazepine: leukopenia, dizziness, ataxia, drowsiness, diplopia, and severe drug reactions
      3) Concurrent administration with fluoxetine may result in toxicity (carbamazepine, phenytoin)
      4) Fetal deformity is a risk (phenytoin and carbamazepine)
      5) Gabapentin: movement disorders, myoclonus, enhanced behavioral disturbances in hyperactive children, and tremor

   b. **Contraindications/cautionary warnings**

      1) Verapamil (and other CCAs) potentiate the effects of carbamazepine and perhaps other anticonvulsants
      2) Pregnancy
      3) Known allergies to the medication
      4) Oral contraceptive use, unless special warnings are given (carbamazepine and phenytoin)
      5) Carbamazepine cannot be used concurrently with MAOIs

      See standard references for additional untoward reactions, guidelines, contraindications, and warnings.

6. **Special considerations**

   Blood level monitoring is advisable for carbamazepine and phenytoin. Also, periodic evaluation for hematological and liver function is recommended, per standard protocol. Inappropriate secretion of ADH has been reported and was likely responsible for hyponatremia producing headaches and nausea in a patient with headache and seizures who had been taking carbamazepine for years (personal observation).

   Because of the interference with oral contraceptives, women in childbearing years who are administered carbamazepine or phenytoin should be informed of the reduced contraceptive efficiency and warned of the possible teratogenic effects.

Recently, the anticonvulsant lamotrigine (Lamictal) was introduced. This drug inhibits the release of excitatory neurotransmitters (primarily glutamate) by blocking the voltage-dependent sodium channels, thereby stabilizing the presynaptic membrane. Its use in headache has not been established and cannot be recommended at this time, except in investigative trials. Another agent, topiramate (Topamax), is available and also inhibits sodium and calcium channels and potentiates GABA-mediated chloride currents. It too has not been demonstrated as effective in the treatment of headache. Vigabatrin (Sabril) is a synthetic derivative of GABA and inhibits GABA transaminase, which is the enzyme responsible for catabolism of GABA. It has not yet been shown to be effective in the treatment of headache.

I. Antihistamines (Cyproheptadine, Hydroxyzine)

1. General comments

Antihistamines may be helpful in the symptomatic and preventive treatment of head pain. Historically, cyproheptadine has been used in the preventive treatment of migraine and cluster headache and in treating the serotonin syndrome (see Chapter 7). Cyproheptadine has potent H_1 and 5-HT_2 antagonistic effects, as well as calcium channel blocking properties. In addition to their antihistaminic effects, these drugs also possess anticholinergic, antipruritic, and sedative effects. Hydroxyzine has been used as a symptomatic agent. These drugs are generally considered safe, but sedation, weight gain, and anticholinergic effects have limited their usefulness in some patients.

2. Proposed mechanisms

a. Antagonist at 5–HT_2 (cyproheptadine)
b. Antagonistic histamine H_1 and muscarinic receptor influence
c. A primary analgesic effect?

3. Recommended use

a. Migraine (cyproheptadine may be particularly useful in children, symptomatically and preventively)
b. Cluster headache?
c. Serotonin syndrome (cyproheptadine) (see Chapter 7)
d. As backup symptomatic medication when analgesics are overused (hydroxyzine)
e. To reverse dystonic reactions from neuroleptics (diphenhydramine).

4. Principles of use

For prevention, small daily dosages should be started, increasing to tolerance or efficacy.

5. Selected drugs in this group

a. Cyproheptadine (Periactin)

b. Hydroxyzine (Vistaril and Atarax)

6. Selected major untoward reactions and contraindications

a. Major untoward reactions

1) Sedation
2) Weight gain
3) Anticholinergic effects
4) Cyproheptadine has been known to reverse the effects of antidepressants, resulting in a reversal of the antidepressant influence

b. Contraindications/cautionary warnings

1) Closed-angle glaucoma
2) Prostatic hypertrophy/bladder neck obstruction
3) Stenosing peptic ulcer
4) MAOI use (with cyproheptadine only)
5) Should be used cautiously in patients with depression on standard antidepressants

See standard references for additional untoward reactions, guidelines, contraindications, and warnings.

7. Special considerations

These drugs may have special application in children with migraine, particularly cyproheptadine. In dosages of 2–4 mg b.i.d. to t.i.d. or 2–4 mg h.s., cyproheptadine may provide effective migraine prophylaxis. Cyproheptadine may also be used in adults with migraine and cluster headache, except that weight gain and sedation often interfere with patient compliance. Nighttime sedation, however, may be of value in some instances. The benefits of hydroxyzine remain anecdotal for migraine prevention as well as symptomatic usage. Certain patients appear to respond both prophylactically and symptomatically. Cyproheptadine may reverse the antidepressant effects of various antidepressants and should be used cautiously in patients with severe depression.

J. Lithium Carbonate

1. General comments

Lithium carbonate is one of the primary therapies for cluster headache and may have application for other refractory headache conditions as well, including cyclic migraine. It may have added value in patients with migraine and depression, bipolar-like illness, or a family history of bipolar illness. Lithium is the treatment of choice for hypnic headaches (see Chapter 12).

2. Proposed mechanisms
a. Depletes inositol with resulting dampening of second messenger system
b. Effects on hypothalamus
c. Increase neuronal release of norepinephrine (minor)

3. Recommended use
a. Cluster headache
b. Cyclic migraine
c. Atypical facial pain
d. Headache syndromes with significant depression or family history of depression (bipolar or bipolar-like symptoms)
e. Hypnic headache (severe, nocturnal headache, usually in older individuals) (see Chapter 12)

4. Principles of use (see Table 6.21)
a. For cluster headache, at dosages of 150–300 mg b.i.d. to t.i.d.
b. Patients should avoid excessive salt intake (reduces effect) or reduced salt intake (enhances effect).
c. Careful monitoring during periods of increased perspiration (salt loss) is advisable.
d. Blood levels do not correlate with therapeutic benefit for headache but should be monitored to avoid toxicity.
e. Reduce dose when used simultaneously with verapamil and other CCAs, carbamazepine, NSAIDs, and fluoxetine.
f. Monitor thyroid and renal function periodically.
g. For hypnic headache, 100–450 mg at h.s. to control nocturnal attacks

5. Drugs in this group
Various forms of lithium carbonate are available, in slow-release, regular, and syrup formulations.

6. Selected major untoward reactions and contraindications
a. **Major untoward reactions**

    1) Tremor/imbalance
    2) Polyuria
    3) Thirst
    4) Edema

5) Mental changes
6) Increase in white blood count (leukocytosis)

Long-term usage may induce hypothyroidism, oliguric renal failure, and diabetes insipidus.

Careful monitoring when used with CCAs is required. Toxic effects of lithium may appear despite normal serum levels and at standard lithium doses when concurrently used with CCAs, carbamazepine, NSAIDs, and fluoxetine. Concurrent use with diuretics is not advisable, since sodium depletion or renal changes are possible.

b. Contraindications/cautionary warnings

1) Significant renal or cardiovascular disease
2) Dehydration
3) Sodium depletion
4) Hypothyroidism

See standard references for additional untoward reactions, guidelines, contraindications, and warnings.

K. Pizotifen (Sandomigrin)
1. General comments
Pizotifen is not available in the United States but is widely used in Canada and Europe. It is reported to be of value in patients with migraine. Pizotifen, like cyproheptadine, has both 5-HT$_2$ and histamine antagonistic properties and shares many of the same side effects such as drowsiness, increased appetite, and weight gain.

2. Proposed mechanisms
a. 5–HT$_2$ antagonist
b. H$_1$ antagonist

3. Recommended use
a. Migraine
b. Cluster headache

4. Principles of use
The drug is started at 0.5 mg at h.s., gradually increasing to 0.5 mg t.i.d. The entire dose can be given at night, up to 6 mg per day.

5. Drugs in this group
Sandomigran

6. Selected major untoward reactions and contraindications
Untoward reactions include drowsiness, abnormal liver function test, and weight gain. Contraindications include pa-

tients simultaneously using MAOIs or within 3 weeks of MAOI discontinuance.

See standard references for additional untoward reactions, guidelines, contraindications, and warnings.

L. Other Drugs
1. NSAIDs

While the nonsteroidal anti-inflammatory drugs are well known for their symptomatic relief of headache, they are used only occasionally in prophylaxis. Short-term usage at the time of menses (naproxen) was better than placebo (Welch, 1986). Because of their effects on the GI and renal systems, long-term preventive use should be restricted. Indomethacin is the treatment of choice for chronic paroxysmal hemicrania, hemicrania continua, and benign exertional headaches (see Chapters 12 and 15).

2. Feverfew

Feverfew (tanacetum parthenium) inhibits the release of 5-HT from platelets and may have some anti-inflammatory properties. One double-blind study measuring its effect against placebo confirmed that daily use was effective in reducing frequency and severity of headaches (Murphy, 1988).

3. Clonidine (Catapres)

The value of clonidine, an alpha-2-adrenergic receptor agonist, for migraine and cluster headache is uncertain. Initial studies were promising, but subsequent studies have failed to reveal efficacy. In selected cases of migraine, however, the drug appears to be useful. Recently in an uncontrolled trial, the drug was found to be helpful in the treatment of episodic cluster headache (Leone, 1997). It may have particular value in treating withdrawal symptoms from narcotics in headache patients and may enhance the analgesic effects of opioids. Nicotine withdrawal symptomatology may be similarly reduced with clonidine treatment. Its specific value for headache remains debatable.

Clonidine is available in two forms. In addition to tablets of 0.1, 0.2, and 0.3 mg, Catapres patches deliver 0.1, 0.2, or 0.3 mg per day of the drug.

Major untoward reactions include dry mouth, drowsiness, dizziness, constipation, and sedation. *When used simultaneously with beta-adrenergic blockers, careful reduction of either agent is required, since hypertensive reactions are possible.*

See standard references for additional untoward reactions, guidelines, contraindications, and warnings.

4. Baclofen (Lioresal)

Baclofen (Lioresal) is a muscle relaxant and antispasmodic. The precise mechanism of action is unknown. It inhibits both monosynaptic and polysynaptic reflexes at the spinal level, is an analogue of the putative inhibitory neurotransmitter gamma-aminobutyric acid (GABA), and has central CNS depressant properties including sedation, somnolence, ataxia, and respiratory and cardiovascular depression.

In pain treatment, baclofen is of greatest value in the treatment of neuralgic syndromes, such as trigeminal neuralgia. It may be added to other antineuralgic therapies, administered at 10 mg b.i.d. to t.i.d., with upward titration to 60–80 mg per day. Tolerance usually develops to its untoward reactions, but very slow, upward dosing is recommended. Anecdotal use for migraine prophylaxis has been reported, and occasional patients may respond to baclofen for both symptomatic or preventive usage. When discontinuing, the drug should be tapered to avoid withdrawal symptomatology, such as seizures.

See standard references for additional untoward reactions, guidelines, contraindications, and warnings.

5. Muscle relaxants

A variety of other "muscle relaxants" are available and have anecdotal value in the treatment of headache. Most of these drugs, such as metaxalone (Skelaxin), have central actions that may be the mechanism by which they could reduce head pain, symptomatically and preventively.

See standard references for additional untoward reactions, guidelines, contraindications, and warnings.

6. Caffeine sodium benzoate

Caffeine sodium benzoate may be of value in the treatment of low cerebrospinal fluid (CSF) pressure headache, such as following a spinal tap or in spontaneous low-pressure syndromes (see Chapter 15). A dose of 0.5 g (500 mg) is given intravenously in one of several regimens:

- An ampule (500 mg) may be added to D_5W lactated Ringer's solution (500–1000 ml) and administered over several hours or longer; and
- An ampule (500 mg) administered via a syringe containing 25 mg of normal saline by "slow push."

Careful monitoring for palpitations and other effects of caffeine is required.

See standard references for additional untoward reactions, guidelines, contraindications, and warnings.

7. Capsaicin

Capsaicin, the active ingredient of hot peppers, selectively diminishes sensations of heat pain and neurogenic vasodilation by desensitizing unmyelinated/C-fiber nociceptors. It may be effective in controlling the pain of diabetic neuropathy, postherpetic neuralgia, causalgia, reflex sympathetic dystrophy, and other disorders of the peripheral nerve. Concentrations of 0.025% and 0.075% are available. Capsaicin has been reported useful in the treatment of cluster headache via intranasal application (Fusco, 1994).

8. Sustained use of opioids for intractable headache

In the last several years, several reports have suggested the efficacy and general safety of chronically administered, maintenance opioids in the treatment of refractory headache. Currently a long-term trial of efficacy and safety is underway (J.R.S., B.H.), employing strict entry criteria, monthly monitoring, and psychological and pain assessments over the course of 5 years (Saper, 1997). At this time, however, the use of maintenance opioids in the treatment of chronic headache cannot be advised until long-term safety and efficacy can be established. Preliminary data suggest that approximately 25% of patients entered into the long-term study appear to benefit in a measurable way after 2 years, and in this selected population, risks of diversion and excessive use were minimal. The long-term risks cannot currently be judged. Clearly most authorities recognize that in patients with severe and intractable headache who fail to respond to standard treatments, more aggressive therapy may be necessary. However, this treatment cannot be recommended at this time because of the risks of inappropriate patient selection, long-term hazards, and other complications.

9. Lidocaine nasal spray (4% solution)

The use of lidocaine was popularized by wide U.S. press coverage of an article purporting its value (Maizels, 1996). A previous study by Kudrow (1995) also suggested its value. Criticism of the study design and other related issues have challenged the study results, which appear to have been largely misinterpreted by the lay press. Although the value of lidocaine in both cluster and migraine headaches may be defined by future study, its use is worth considering in selected cases. Improper techniques may have reduced the potential value in some patients.

TABLE 6.21.   SELECTED DRUGS USED IN THE PHARMACOTHERAPY OF HEAD, NECK, AND FACE PAIN[a]

Drug Name	Mg/Dose	Standard Daily Admin	Notes
SYMPTOMATIC DRUGS			
ANALGESICS			
Excedrin[b]	—	varies	Avoid more than 2 days/week of use
NSAIDs			Avoid more than 2 days/week of use
naproxen sodium[b] (p.o.)	275–550	bid-tid	Avoid extended, daily use
indomethacin (p.o.)	25–50	bid-tid	"
indocin SR	75	1 q day or bid	"
indomethacin (p.r.)	50	bid-tid	"
meclofenamate (p.o.)	50–200	bid	"
ibuprofen[b] (p.o.)	600–800	bid-tid	"
ketorolac (p.o.)	10	qid	"
ketorolac (IM)	30	tid	Appears particularly valuable when ergot derivatives & narcotics must be avoided and parenteral therapy is necessary. No more than occasional, short-term use is advisable because of renal toxicity, most likely in predisposed patients
SPECIAL MIGRAINE DRUGS			
isometheptene combinations (Midrin[b] etc.)	—	2 caps at onset; 1–2 q 30–60 min	Max 5–6 caps/day; 2 days/week
ergotamine tartrate[b] (ET) oral (Cafergot, Wigraine, etc.)	1 mg ET, 100 mg caffeine	2 tabs at onset; 1–2 q 30–60 min	Max 4–6/day; 2 days/week
suppositories (Cafergot, Wigraine)	2 mg ET, 100 mg	1/3–1 at onset; may repeat in 60 min	Max 2/day; 2 days/week

sublingual (Ergomar, Ergostat)	2 mg ET	1 at onset; may repeat after 15 min	Max 2/day; 2 days/week
dihydroergotamine (DHE) IM/IV	0.25–1 mg	0.25–1 mg SC, IM, IV tid	Can be used 2–3 times/day in conjunction with antinauseant, analgesic, etc. IM more effective than SC. Fig. 5.1, Table 5.6.
DHE nasal spray[b]	1 mg	See protocols in text, Chapters 16 and 19	Use no more than 2–3 times/week, on separate days
		1 spray each nostril (1/2 mg/spray), repeat in 15 minutes (4 sprays = 2 mg)	
sumatriptan[b] (parenteral)	6 mg SC	May repeat in 1 hour	Cannot be used within 24 hours of ergotamine-related meds or other triptans; should not be used in presence of cardiovascular and/or cerebrovascular disease, severe hypertension, Prinzmetal angina, or peripheral vascular disorders. No more than 2 doses in 24 hours. Limit 2 days/week usage
sumatriptan[b] (oral)	25–50 mg	Take at HA onset; may repeat at 2 hours; max 100 mg/day	"
sumatriptan[b] (nasal spray)	5 or 20 mg	1 spray in 1 nostril only may repeat in 2 hours; max 40 mg/24 hours	"
zolmitriptan[b] (oral)	2.5–5 mg	1 at onset; may repeat in 2 hours; max 10 mg/24 hours	"
naratriptan[b] (oral)	2.5 mg	1 at onset; may repeat in 4 hours; max 5 mg/24 hrs	"

continued

TABLE 6.21. SELECTED DRUGS USED IN THE PHARMACOTHERAPY OF HEAD, NECK, AND FACE PAIN[a]

Drug Name	Mg/Dose	Standard Daily Admin	Notes
rizatriptan[b] (oral)	10–20 mg	1–2 at onset; may repeat in 2 hours; max 40 mg/24 hours	" "
ANTINAUSEANTS/ NEUROLEPTICS			
chlorpromazine (p.o.)	25–100	bid-tid	Limit 3 days/week, expect for persistent nausea; avoid extended use. Monitor for hypotension
(supp)	25–100	bid-tid	" "
(IM)	25–100	bid-tid	" "
(IV)	7.5–15 mg	bid-tid	see Chapters 6–9
metoclopramide (p.o. - tablet & syrup)	10–20	tid	Limit 3 days/wk, except for persistent nausea; avoid extended use. Monitor for hypotension
(parenteral)	10	tid	" "
promethazine			
(p.o.)	25–75	tid	" "
(IM)	25–75	tid	" "
perphenazine			
(p.o.)	4–8	bid-tid	" "
(IM)	5	bid	" "
droperidol			
(IM)	1.25–5	bid-tid	" "
(IV)	1.25–5	bid-tid	" "
ANTIHISTAMINES			
hydroxyzine (p.o., IM)	25–75	bid-tid or at hs	Can be used as symptomatic or preventive treatment
cyproheptadine (p.o.)	2–4	tid-qid	"
STEROIDS			
prednisone	40–60	in 1 or divided doses	4–10 day program. Avoid repeated use

PREVENTIVE DRUGS
(avoid sustained use for more
than 6 months w/o trial reduction)

**TRICYCLIC
ANTIDEPRESSANTS**

amitriptyline	10–150	Divided doses or hs	Bedtime dose aids sleep disturbance
nortriptyline	10–100	" "	" "
doxepin	10–150	" "	" "

OTHER ANTIDEPRESSANTS

fluoxetine	20	20–80 mg/day in divided dose	Actual efficacy for HA uncertain. Administer fluoxetine with care to patients using lipophilic beta blockers (propranolol, metoprolol, etc.) or switch to hydrophilic beta blockers such as nadolol. Value for HA of numerous other antidepressants under investigation

others (SSRIs, etc.)

MAO INHIBITORS

phenelzine	15–30	15–90 mg/day in divided dose	Dietary & medication restrictions mandatory

**BETA ADRENERGIC
BLOCKERS**

propranolol[b,c]*	20–50	tid–qid (standard dose)	Monitor cardiac function, BP, pulse, lipids
Inderal LA[b,c]*	80–160	bid	" "
atenolol	50–100	bid	" "
timolol[b]	10–20	bid	" "
metoprolol[c]*	50–100	bid	" "
nadolol	20–120	bid	Monitor cardiac function, BP, pulse, lipids eliminated by kidneys

continued

TABLE 6.21.   SELECTED DRUGS USED IN THE PHARMACOTHERAPY OF HEAD, NECK, AND FACE PAIN[a]

Drug Name	Mg/Dose	Standard Daily Admin	Notes
CALCIUM CHANNEL ANTAGONISTS			
verapamil	80–160	tid-qid	Monitor cardiac function, BP, pulse
nimodipine	30–60	tid	" " "
diltiazem	30–90	tid	" " "
ERGOTAMINE DERIVATIVES			
methysergide[b]	1–2	tid-5 times per day	After 6 months of tx, review cardiac, pulmonary, & retroperitoneal regions for fibrotic changes. Carefully observe contraindications
methylergonovine	0.2–0.4	tid-qid	" "
ANTICONVULSANTS			
valproate[b]	125–500	1–2 g/day in divided doses	Monitor hepatic & metabolic parameters carefully. Consider dose reduction when used w/ antidepressants, lithium, verapamil, phenothiazines benzodiazepines, other anticonvulsants. Observe warnings carefully. Avoid using with barbiturates
carbamazepine	100–200	300–1200 mg/day in divided doses	Monitor hepatic & metabolic parameters carefully. Consider dose reduction when used w/ anticonvulsants, lithium, verapamil, phenothiazines. Observe warnings carefully. *Reduces oral contraceptive efficacy.*

gabapentin	100–400	1800–3600 mg/day	Actual value for HA uncertain. May cause agitation & other CNS AEs
OTHERS			
baclofen	10–20	tid-qid	Increase and decrease dose slowly, allow tolerance to develop; taper when discontinuing
lithium	150–300	bid-tid	Reduce dose in conjunction with verapamil, other calcium channel antagonists, and NSAIDS. Monitor metabolic parameters
oxygen inhalation	100% O_2 with mask	7 liters/min for 10–15 min	Must be used at onset of attack of cluster headache; avoid around extreme heat or flame, such as cigarettes.
Stadol Nasal Spray (butorphanol)[b]	1 mg/spray; max use 2 dose days/week		Useful for acute migraine but important side effects. Dependency and addictive potential significant. Avoid in patients with addictive or obsessive drug-taking patterns or history of drug overdose. Avoid in patients with daily or almost daily HA. Withdrawal symptoms can be severe.

[a]Only a few of the medications listed in this table are either approved specifically for headache or have been shown by controlled studies to be effective for headache. Others are included, because they have been recommended by various sources as possibly useful for the treatment of some cases of headache.
[b]Drugs that have been approved by the FDA for the treatment of migraine, cluster headache, or tension-type headache.
[c]Usage w/fluoxetine requires dose reduction. *Fluoxetine use requires dose reduction.

TABLE 6.22. **SELECTED SYMPTOMATIC MEDICATION GROUPS FOR HEADACHE AND FACIAL PAIN BY ROUTE OF ADMINISTRATIVE**

Oral	Rectal	Parental	Nasal Spray
Analgesics	Ergotamine tartrate	Analgesics	DHE
Over the-Counter	Neuroleptics	Narcotic	Sumatriptan
NSAIDs	Chlorpromazine	Agonist-antagonist	Butorphanol
Naproxen sodium	Prochlorperazine	DHE	
Indomethacin	Indomethacin	Ketorolac	
Meclofenamate	Morphine sulfate	Neuroleptics	
Mixed analgesics		Hydroxyzine	
Fiorinal		Steroids	
Fiorinal w/codeine		(hydrocortisone)	
Fioricet		Sumatriptan	
Tylenol w/codeine		Butyrophenones	
Vicodin (hydrocodone)			
Percocet (oxycodone)			
Specific Migraine			
Drugs			
Ergotamine tartrate			
Isometheptene			
Triptans			
Phenothiazines/			
antihistamines			
Chlorpromazine			
Perphenazine			
Hydroxyzine			
Steroids			
Prednisone			

TABLE 6.23. **SELECTED WARNINGS ON INTERACTIONS OF COMMONLY USED HEADACHE MEDICATION COMBINATIONS**

Drugs	Warnings
Lithium and verapamil/CCA[a]	Lithium toxicity potentiated
Valproate and TCA, fluoxetine	Enhanced valproate effects, potential liver toxicity
Valproate and barbiturate (? benzodiazepine)	Idiosyncratic sedation/coma
Anticonvulsant (except valproate) and oral contraceptives	Reduced efficacy of oral contraceptives
MAOI with most TCAs	Serotonin syndrome/hypertensive crisis
MAOI and isometheptene	Hypertensive crisis
MAOI and meperidine	Stimulant reaction, sudden death, serotonin syndrome
MAOI and fluoxetine	Serotonin syndrome, sudden death
MAOI and carbamazepine	Hypertensive crisis
MAOI and sumatriptan, rizatriptan, zolmitriptan	Enhanced vasoconstrictive effects
Fluoxetine and phenothiazine	Enhanced extrapyramidal effects
Fluoxetine and MAOI	Serotonin syndrome/sudden death
Fluoxetine and lithium	Potentiates lithium toxicity
CCA[a] and anticonvulsants	Enhanced anticonvulsant effect
CCA[a] and lithium	Potentiates lithium toxicity
Propranolol/metoprolol and fluoxetine	Increased beta blocker blood levels

[a]Calcium channel antagonists.

References

Aloisi P, Marrelli A, Porto C, et al. Visual evoked potentials and serum magnesium levels in juvenile migraine patients. *Headache,* 37:383–385, 1997.

Ayd FJ Jr. Guides for safe and effective use of combined tricyclic MAOI therapy. *International Drug Therapeutic Newsletter.* Pg 14, 1979.

Ballenger JC, Post RM. Carbamazepine in alcohol withdrawal syndromes and schizophrenic psychoses. *Pharmacol Bull,* 20:572–574, 1984.

Bartlik BD, Kaplan P, Kaplan HS. Psychostimulants appear to reverse sexual dysfunction secondary to selective serotonin reuptake inhibitors. *J Sex Marital Ther* (in press).

Bernstein JE, Korman NJ, Bickers DR, et al. Topical capsaicin treatment of postherpetic neuralgia. *J Am Acad Dermatol,* 21:265–270, 1989.

Beutefisch CM, Gutierrez A, Gutmann L. Choreoathetotic movements: Possible side effects of gabapentin. *Neurology,* 46:851–852, 1996.

Boehnert MT, Lovejoy FH. The value of the QR restoration vs. the serum drug level in predicting seizures and ventricular arrhythmias after an acute overdose of tricyclic antidepressants. *N Engl J Med,* 313:474–479, 1985.

Brown TM, Skop BP, Mareth TR. Pathophysiology and management of the serotonin syndrome. *Ann Pharmacother,* 30:527–533, 1996.

Brubache JR. Treating serotonin syndrome. *J Clin Toxicol,* 35:213–214, 1997.

Bucci JA, Manoharan A. Methysergide-induced retroperitoneal fibrosis: Successful outcome and two new laboratory features. *Mayo Clin Proc,* 72:1148–1150, 1997.

Buckoms AJ, Litman RE. Clonazepam in the treatment of neuralgic pain syndromes. *Psychosomatics,* 26:933–936, 1985.

Buzzi MG, Moskowitz MA. The antimigraine drug sumatriptan (GR43175) selectively blocks neurogenic plasma extravasation from blood vessels in dura mater. *Br J Pharmacol,* 99:202–206, 1990.

Callaham MM, Raskin NH. A controlled study of dihydroergotamine in the treatment of acute migraine headache. *Headache,* 26:168–171, 1986.

The Capsaicin Study Group. Treatment of painful diabetic neuropathy with topical capsaicin. *Arch Internal Med,* 151:2225–2229, 1991.

Clary C, Schweitzer E. The treatment of MAOI hypertensive crisis with sublingual nifedipine. *Clin Psychiatry,* 48:249–250, 1987.

Davis CP, Torre BR, William C, et al. Ketorolac vs. meperidine—plus—promethazine treatment of migraine headache: Evaluations by patients. *Am J Emerg Med,* 13:146–150, 1995.

Diamond S, Dalessio DG. *The Practicing Physician's Approach to Headache.* 5th Edition. Baltimore, Williams & Wilkins, 1991.

Dihydroergotamine Nasal Spray Multicenter Investigators. Efficacy, safety, and tolerability of dihydroergotamine nasal spray as monotherapy in the treatment of acute migraine. *Headache,* 35:177–184, 1995.

Duarte C, Dunaway F, Turner L, et al. Ketorolac vs. meperidine and hydroxyzine in the treatment of acute migraine headache: A randomized, prospective, double-blind trial. *Ann Emerg Med,* 21:1116–1121, 1992.

Dunbar SA, Katz NP. Chronic opioid therapy for non-malignant pain in patients with a history of substance abuse: Report of 20 cases. *J Pain Symptom Manage,* 11:163–171, 1996.

Facchinetti F. Magnesium prophylaxis of menstrual migraine: Effects on intracellular magnesium. *Headache,* 31:298–301, 1991.

Facchinetti F, Borella P, Sances G, et al. Oral magnesium successfully relieves premenstrual mood changes. *Obstet Gynecol,* 78:177–181, 1991.

Facchinetti F, Montorsi S, Borella P, et al. Magnesium prevention of premenstrual migraine: A placebo-controlled study. (In) *New Advances in Headache Research* (2nd edition). RC Rose (Ed). London, Smith-Gordon, 1991.

Ferrari MD, Haan J. Drug treatment of migraine attacks. (In) *Headache.* PJ Goadsby, SD Silberstein (Eds). Pgs 117–129, Boston, Butterworth-Heinemeann, 1997.

Folks DG. Monoamine oxidase inhibitors: Re-appraisal of dietary considerations. *J Clin Pharmacol,* 3:246–252, 1983.

Fromm GH, Terrence CF, Chattha AS. Baclofen in the treatment of trigeminal neuralgia: Double- blind study and long-term follow-up. *Ann Neurol,* 15:240–244, 1984.

Fusco BM, Marabine S, Maggi CA, et al. Preventive effective repeated nasal applications of capsaicin in cluster headache. *Pain,* 59:321–325, 1994.

Gallagher RM. Acute treatment of migraine with dihydroergotamine nasal spray. *Arch Neurol,* 53:1285–1291, 1996.

Gigsman HJ, Ferrari MD. Dihydroergotamine nasal spray. *Neurology,* 45:397, 1995.

Gitlin NJ. Effects of depression and antidepressants on sexual function. *Bull Menninger Clin,* 59:232–248, 1995.

Goadsby PJ, Gundlach AL. Localization of ^{3}H-dihydroergotamine binding sites in the cat's central nervous system: Relevance to migraine. *Ann Neurol,* 29:91–94, 1991.

Goldstein J. Ergot pharmacology in alternative delivery systems for ergotamine derivatives. *Neurology,* 42 (supp 2):45–46, 1992.

Harrison WM, McGrath PJ, Stewart JW,et al. MAOIs and hypertensive crisis: The role of OTC drugs. *J Clin Psychiatry,* 50:64–65, 1989.

Hering R, Kuritzky A. Sodium valproate in the treatment of cluster headache: An open clinical trial. *Cephalalgia,* 9:195, 1989.

Hering R, Kuritzky A. Sodium valproate in the prophylactic treatment of migraine: A double- blind study vs. placebo. *Cephalalgia,* 12:81–84, 1992.

Horn AC, Jarret SW. Ibuprofen-induced aseptic meningitis in rheumatoid arthritis. *Ann Pharmacother,* 31:1009–1011, 1997.

Hoshi K, Ma T, Ho IK. Precipitated kappa-opioid receptor agonist withdrawal increases glutamate in rat locus coeruleus. *Eur J Pharmacol,* 314:301–306, 1996.

Jabbari B, Bryan GE, Marsh EE, et al. Incidence of seizures with tricyclic and tetracyclic antidepressants. *Arch Neurol,* 42:480–481, 1985.

Jensen R, Brinck T, Olesen J. Sodium valproate has a prophylactic effect in migraine without aura: A triple-blind, placebo-controlled, crossover study. *Neurology,* 44:647–651, 1994.

Ketorolac tromethamine. *The Medical Letter.* 32:79–81, 1990.

King SA, Strange AJ. Benzodiazepine use by chronic pain patients. *Clin J Pain,* 6:147, 1990.

Koch M, Dez I, Ferrario F, et al. Prevention of nonsteroidal anti-inflammatory drug-induced gastrointestinal mucosal injury. Metanalyses, randomized, controlled clinical trials. *Arch Intern Med,* 11:2321–2332, 1996.

Kudrow L, et al. Rapid and sustained relief of migraine attacks with intranasal lidocaine. *Headache,* 35:79–82, 1995.

Lance JW. Preventive treatment in migraine. (In) *Headache,* PJ Goadsby, SD Silberstein (Eds). Pgs. 131–141, Boston, Butterworth-Heinemeann, 1997.

Larkin GL, Prescott JE. A randomized, double-blind trial, comparative study of the efficacy of ketorolac tromethamine vs. meperidine in the treatment of severe migraine. *Ann Emerg Med,* 21:919–924, 1992.

Lassen LH, Thomsen LL, Kruse C, et al. Histamine-$_1$ receptor blockade does not prevent nitroglycerine-induced migraine. Support for the NO hypothesis of migraine. *Ur J Clin Pharmacol,* 49:335–339, 1996.

Lechin F, Vanderdigs B, Lechin ME, et al. Pimozide therapy for trigeminal neuralgia. *Arch Neurol,* 9:960–964, 1989.

Leone M, Attanasio A, Gratzzi L, et al. Transdermal clonidine in the prophylaxis of episodic cluster headache: An open study. *Headache,* 36:559–560, 1997.

Levenson ML, Lipsy RJ, Fuller DK. Adverse effects and drug interactions associated with fluoxetine therapy. *Ann Pharmacother,* 25:657–661, 1991.

Lewis CT, Molland EA, Marshall VR, et al. Analgesic abuse, uteric obstruction, and retroperitoneal fibrosis. *BMJ,* 2:76, 1975.

Lipton RL, Stewart WF, Ryan RE, et al. Efficacy and safety of acetaminophen, aspirin and caffeine in alleviating migraine headache pain through double-blind, randomized, placebo-controlled trials. *Arch Neurol,* 55:210–217, 1998.

Lodi R, Montagna P, Soriani S, et al. Deficit of brain and skeletal muscle bioenergetics and low brain magnesium in juvenile migraine: An in-vivo 31P magnetic resonance spectroscopy interictal study. *Pediatr Res,* 42:866–871, 1997.

Luckins A. A review of combined tricyclic and MAOI therapy. *Compr Psychiatry,* 18:221–230, 1977.

MacPhee GJA. Verapamil potentiates carbamazepine toxicity: A clinically important inhibitory interaction. *Lancet,* 1:700–703, 1986.

Maizels M, Scott B, Coehn W, et al. Intranasal lidocaine for the treatment of migraine: A randomized, double-blind, controlled study. *JAMA,* 276:319–21, 1996.

Martin PG. Serotonin syndrome. *Ann Emerg Med,* 28:520–526, 1996.

Mathew NT, Ali S. Valproate in the treatment of persistent chronic daily headache. An open-label study. *Headache,* 31:71–74, 1991.

Mathew NT, Saper JR, Silberstein DS, et al. Migraine prophylaxis with divalproex. *Arch Neurol,* 52:281–6, 1995.

Mathew NT, Teitjen GE, Lucker C. Serotonin syndrome complicating migraine pharmacotherapy. *Cephalalgia,* 16:323–327, 1996.

Mathew RJ, Wilson WH. Caffeine-induced changes in cerebral circulation. *Stroke,* 16:814–817, 1985.

Mauskop A, Altura BT, Cracco RQ, et al. Intravenous magnesium sulfate rapidly alleviates headache of various types. *Headache,* 36:154–160, 1996.

Mazzotta G, Sarchielli P, Alberti A, et al. Electromyographical ischemic chest and intracellular and extracellular magnesium concentration in migraine and tension-type headache. *Headache,* 36:357–561, 1996.

McQuay HJ, Carroll D, Watts PG, et al. Codeine 20 mg. increases pain relief from ibuprofen 400 mg. after third molar surgery. A repeat dosing comparison of ibuprofen in an ibuprofen-codeine combination. *Pain,* 37:7–13, 1989.

Merikangas KR, Merikangas JR. Combination monoamine oxidase inhibitor and beta blocker treatment of migraine with anxiety and depression. *Biol Psychiatry,* 38:603–610, 1995.

Mills JC. Serotonin syndrome. A clinical update. *Crit Care Clin,* 13:763–783, 1997.

Mishima K, Takeshima T, Shimomura J, et al. Platelet ionized magnesium, cyclic AMP, and cyclic GMP levels in migraine and tension-type headache. *Headache,* 37:561–564, 1997.

Molaie M, Molaie MD. Serotonin syndrome presenting with migraine-like stroke. *Headache,* 37:519–521, 1997.

The multinational oral sumatriptan and Cafergot comparative study group. A randomized, double- blind comparison of Cafergot and sumatriptan in the treatment of migraine. *Eur Neurol*, 31:314–322. 1991.

Murphy JJ, Heptinstall S, Mitchell JRA. Randomized, double-blind, placebo-controlled trial of feverfew in migraine prevention. *Lancet*, 2:189–192. 1988.

The oral sumatriptan dose-defining study group. Sumatriptan—an oral dose-defining study. *Eur Neurol*, 31:300–305, 1991.

The oral sumatriptan multiple-dose study group. Evaluation of a multiple-dose regimen of oral sumatriptan for the acute treatment of migraine. *Eur Neurol*, 31:306–313. 1991.

Pearce CJ, Gonzalez FM, Wallin JD. Renal failure and hyperkalemia associated with ketorolac tromethamine. *Arch Intern Med*, 153:1000–1002, 1993.

Peikert A, Wilimzig C, Kohne-Vollard R. Prophylaxis of migraine and oral magnesium: Results from a prospective, multicenter, placebo-controlled, double-blind, randomized study. *Cephalalgia*, 16:257–263, 1996.

Peroutka SJ. The pharmacology of current antimigraine drugs. *Headache*, 30 (supp 1):5, 1990.

Peroutka SJ. 5-hydroxytryptamine receptor subtypes in the pharmacology of migraine. *Neurology*, 43(supp 3):S34–38, 1993.

Pfaffenrath V, Oestreich W, Haase W. Flunarizine (10–20 mg.) IV vs. placebo in the treatment of acute migraine attacks: A multicenter, double-blind study. *Cephalalgia*, 10:77–81, 1990.

Pfaffenrath V, Wissely P, Meyer C, et al. Magnesium in the prophylaxis of migraine : A double-blind, placebo-controlled study. *Cephalalgia*, 16:436–440, 1996.

Portenoy RK. Chronic opioid therapy in non-malignant pain. *J Pain Symptom Manage*, 5(supp):46–61, 1990.

Ramadan NM, Halvorson H, Vande-Linde A, et al. Low brain magnesium in migraine. *Headache*, 29:416, 590–593, 1989.

Ramadan NM. Selective occipital cortex magnesium deficiency reduction and familial hemiplegic migraine may reflect an ion channel disorder. Presented at the 1996 American Academy of Neurology meeting, San Francisco, CA, March 1996.

Raskin NH. Repetitive intravenous dihydroergotamine as therapy for intractable migraine. *Neurology*, 36:995–997, 1986.

Reeves SE, Sharbrough FW, Crahn LE. Movement disorders associated with the use of gabapentin. *Epilepsy*, 37:988–990, 1996.

Ries RK, Roy-Byrne PP, Ward NG, et al. Carbamazepine treatment for benzodiazepine withdrawal. *Am J Psychiatry*, 146:536–537, 1989.

Rumor MM, Schlichting DA. Clinical efficacy of antihistaminics as analgesics. *Pain*, 25:7–22, 1986.

Saadah HA. Abortive headache therapy in the office with intravenous dihydroergotamine in the treatment of acute migraine headache. *Headache*, 32:143–146, 1992.

Sandler D, Smith JC, Weinberg CR, et al. Analgesic use in chronic renal disease. *N Engl J Med* 320:1238–1243, 1989.

Saper JR. Drug treatment of headache: Changing concepts and treatment strategies. *Semin Neurol*, 7:178–191, 1987.

Saper JR. Ergotamine dependency: A review. *Headache*, 27:435–458, 1987.

Saper JR. Daily chronic headache—Tension headaches, migraine, and combined headaches: The transformation concept. (In) *Drug-Induced Headache,* HC Diener and M Wilkinson (Eds). Pgs 5–7, Berlin, Springer-Verlag, 1988.

Saper JR. Chronic headache syndromes. *Neurol Clin,* 7:387–412, 1989.

Saper JR, Hamel RL, Lake AE III, et al. Structured opioid maintenance therapy for refractory chronic headache (abstract). *Headache,* 37:329, 1997.

Saper JR, Sheftell F. Headache in the abuse-prone individual. (In) *The Headaches, 2nd Edition,* J Olesen, P Tfelt-Hansen, KMA Welch (Eds). New York, Lippincott Williams & Wilkins, in press.

Schoenen J, Jacquy J, Lenaerts M. Effectiveness of high dose riboflavin in migraine prophylaxis. A randomized, controlled trial. *Neurology,* 50:466–470, 1998.

Sechzer PG, Abel L. Post-spinal anesthesia headache treated with caffeine: Evaluation with demand method. Part I. *Curr Ther Res,* 24:307–312, 1978.

Shrestha M, Singh R, Moreden J, et al. Ketorolac vs. chlorpromazine in the treatment of acute migraine without aura. *Arch Internal Med,* 156:1725–1728, 1996.

Silberstein SD, Shulman EA, Hopkins MM. Repetitive intravenous DHE in the treatment of refractory headache. *Headache,* 30:334–339, 1990.

Simone DA, Ochoa J. Early and late effects of prolonged topical capsaicin on cutaneous sensibility of neurogenic vasodilation in humans. *Pain,* 47:285–294, 1991.

Solomon GD. Verapamil and migraine prophylaxis: A five-year review. *Headache,* 29:425–427, 1989.

Sorensen KV. Valproate: A new drug in migraine prophylaxis. *Acta Neurol Scand,* 78:346–348, 1988.

Soyka D, Taneri Z, Oestreich W, et al. Flunarizine IV in the acute treatment of common or classical migraine attacks: A placebo-controlled, double-blind trial. *Headache,* 29:21–27, 1989.

Strom BL, Berlin JA, Kinman JL, et al. Parenteral ketorolac and risk of gastrointestinal and operative site bleeding. *JAMA,* 275:376–382, 1996.

Subcutaneous sumatriptan international study group. Treatment of migraine attacks with sumatriptan. *N Engl J Med* 5:316–321, 1991.

Tallian JB, Nahata MC, Lo W, et al. Gabapentin associated with aggressive behavior in pediatric patients with seizures. *Epilepsy,* 37:501–502, 1996.

Tfelt-Hansen P, Johnson ES. Ergotamine. (In) *The Headaches.* J Olesen, P Tfelt-Hansen, KMA Welch (Eds). Pgs 313–322, New York, Raven Press, 1993.

Tfelt-Hansen P, Lipton RB. Dihydroergotamine. (In) *The Headaches.* J Olesen, P Tfelt-Hansen, KMA Welch (Eds). Pgs 323–3327, New York, Raven Press, 1993.

Tandan R, Lewis GA, Krvinski PB. Topical capsaicin in painful diabetic polyneuropathy: Controlled study with long-term follow-up. *Diabetes Care,* 15:8–14, 1992.

Topics in Pain Management. JR Saper (Ed). Volume 12, No. 6, Pgs 21–22, Baltimore, Williams & Wilkins, January 1997.

Van Gerpen JA, Shuster EA. A report of NSAID-induced leptomeningeal enhancement not associated with aseptic meningitis (abstract). At the American Academy of Neurology Meeting, April, 1998.

Wang SJ, Silberstein SD, Young WB. Droperidol treatment of status migrainosis and refractory migraine. *Headache,* 37:377–382, 1997.

Ward N, Whitney C, Avery D, et al. The analgesic effects of caffeine in headache. *Pain,* 44:151–155, 1991.

Watson CPN, Evans RJ, Watt VR. Post-herpetic neuralgia and topical capsaicin. *Pain,* 33:333–340, 1988.

Weiller C, May A, Limmroth V, et al. Brainstem activation in human migraine attacks. *Nat Med,* 1:858–860, 1995.

Welch KMA. Naproxen sodium in the treatment of migraine. *Cephalalgia,* 6(supp 4):85, 1986.

Welch KMA. Drug therapy of migraine. *N Engl J Med,* 329:1476–1483, 1993.

Westbrook L, Cicalar S, Wright H. The effectiveness of alprazolam in the treatment of chronic pain: Results of a preliminary study. *Clin J Pain,* 6:32–36, 1990.

White K, Simpson G. Combined use of MAOIs and tricyclics. *J Clin Psychiatry,* 45:67–69, 1984.

Winner P, Ricalde O, LeForce B, et al. A double blind study of subcutaneous dihydroergotamine vs. subcutaneous sumatriptan in the treatment of acute migraine. *Arch Neurol,* 53:180–184, 1996.

Wolf SM, Shinnar S, Kang H, et al. Gabapentin toxicity in children manifesting as behavioral changes. *Epilepsy,* 36:1203–1205, 1995.

Ziegler D, Ford R, Kriegler J, et al. Dihydroergotamine nasal spray for the acute treatment of migraine. *Neurology,* 44:447, 1994.

Ziegler DK, Hurwitz A, Preskorn S, et al. Propranolol and amitriptyline in the prophylaxis of migraine. *Arch Neurol,* 50:825–830, 1993.

6 Supplement

Drug Interactions:
The Cytochrome P-450 Enzyme System

This supplement to Chapter 6 describes the P-450 enzyme system and its effect on many of the medications used to treat headache and pain. Tables S6.1 and S6.2 can be used to guide the selection of medications and their doses.

The treatment of difficult pain disorders often requires the simultaneous use of several medications; thus, the risk of drug-drug interaction is increased. A number of factors affect the potential for an adverse drug interaction, including genetic characteristics, nutritional status, renal function, gender, age, environmental factors, and the presence of liver disease. Drug interactions are caused by increases or decreases in absorption, protein binding displacement, distribution, presystemic elimination, hepatic drug metabolism, and renal excretion.

Metabolites are important in the consideration of drug interactions. Water-soluble agents can be readily excreted unchanged in the urine or other body secretions. Lipid-soluble compounds require transformation into more water-soluble metabolites, which are then excreted. Some metabolites are not readily recognized by drug receptors, which leads to decreased pharmacological activity. Other metabolites have a high binding affinity to the receptor and thus lead to increased activity and potential toxicity, particularly if the metabolite accumulates because of a long half-life or decreased elimination. This is the case with meperidine (Demerol). *The metabolite of meperidine is normeperidine, which has central nervous system stimulant properties and a longer half-life than the parent product; thus, it accumulates with repetitive use. This accumulation can lead to seizures, particularly in patients who simultaneously use other drugs that lower their seizure threshold. In this and other cases, the metabolite, rather than the parent product, occasionally interacts adversely with other agents.*

One of the most important factors determining drug interaction and the risk of combined therapy is metabolism within the liver through oxidation and/or conjugation reactions. Oxidative, or phase I pathway, metabolism involves oxidation, reduction, and hydrolysis. The oxidative reactions are accomplished by the cytochrome P-450 systems of enzymes, which are also known as "mixed function oxidase" or "mono-oxygenases." The mammalian cytochrome P-450 is divided into two major classes: the mitochondrial P-450s, which primarily involve steroid synthesis, and the microsomal P-450s, which are involved in drug metabolism.

The P-450 system is further divided into families, subfamilies, and individual P-450s. Families are designated by a Roman numeral, subfamilies by capital letters, and individual P-450s by Arabic numbers (e.g., P-450 II D 6).

Conjugation, or the phase II pathway, is the second metabolizing enzyme system. The drug or metabolite from phase II pathway metabolism is coupled to an endogenous substance, which forms water-soluble polar metabolites that are more readily excreted. Conjugation reactions are accomplished by such enzymes as glucuronyl transferases, acetyltransferases, and sulfotransferases. Conjugation reactions other than with glucuronic acid may be catalyzed by nonmicrosomal enzymes. The route of drug degradation occurs mainly in the liver but may also take place in the plasma and other tissue sites, including the white blood cells, skin, and lung.

Genetic variations involving the P-450 system result in differences in the patient's ability to metabolize certain drugs. Some individuals cannot metabolize specific agents at all. Polymorphism is a prominent feature of cytochrome P isoenzymes. For example, approximately 10% of Japanese individuals, 90% of Middle Eastern individuals, and 72% of the United States population are labeled as slow acetylators and cannot efficiently metabolize the drug isoniazid. Other agents possibly affected by genetic factors include procainamide, clonazepam, phenelzine, and caffeine. The ultimate effect is a decrease in metabolism, which makes the patient more vulnerable to the side effects of the drug.

Of particular concern here is what may occur when drugs that require metabolism by the identical enzyme system compete for binding to and metabolism by that particular enzyme system. The activity and efficiency of the P-450 liver enzymes may be induced or inhibited by certain drugs (Table S6.1). Some medications may do both. Oral contraceptives can increase the metabolism of some drugs and reduce that of others. Similarly, when ingested acutely, ethanol inhibits the P-450–mediated oxidation of certain drugs; however, when ingested chronically, ethanol is a potent inducer, thus increasing the metabolism of (and reducing the effect of) certain drugs.

To reduce the possibility of significant untoward consequences, it is best to avoid (when possible) agents that significantly alter the metabolic pathways of other drugs being used concurrently. Both unwanted increases and decreases in availability pose risks. If the use of an alternate agent is not possible, careful follow-up for signs of toxicity, lack of efficacy, and therapeutic drug monitoring is warranted. A dose adjustment is often necessary.

TABLE S6.1. **DRUGS THAT INFLUENCE THE P-450 ENZYME SYSTEM**

CYP enzyme	Inhibitor	Inducer	Substrate	
1a2	Fluvoxamine Mexiletine	Cigarette smoke Omeprazole Rifampin	Acetaminophen Amitriptyline Caffeine Clozapine Clomipramine	Imipramine Olanzapine Phenacetin Testosterone Theophylline TCAs (demethylation)
2C8-10	Cimetidine Fluoxetine (suspected) Fluvoxamine Omeprazole Sertraline (suspected)	Phenobarbital Rifampin	Benzphetamine (2C8) Diclofenac (2C8) Diazepam (2C8) Hexobarbital (2C9) Ibuprofen (2C9)	Mephenytoin (2C9) Mephobarbital (2C9) Phenytoin Tolbutamide (2C9) (S)-Warfarin (2C9)
2 C18/19			Diazepam Mephenytoin Naproxen	Propanolol Retinoic acid Tolbutamide
2D 6	Amiodarone Cimetidine Chloroquine Fluoxetine Fluphenazine Fluvoxamine Haloperidol Norfluvoxamine Paroxetine Primaquine Quinidine Sertraline (suspected)	Not induced by common inducers	Amitriptyline Chloroquine (possible) Chlorpromazine Clomipramine Clozapine Codeine Debrisoquine Desipramine Dextromethorphan Encainide Flecainide Fluoxetine	Nortriptyline Oxamniquine Oxycodone Paroxetine Perphenazine Phenformin Primaquine (possible) Promazine Propafenone Propoxyphene Propanolol (minor) Risperidone

continued

TABLE S6.1S. DRUGS THAT INFLUENCE THE P-450 ENZYME SYSTEM

CYP enzyme	Inhibitor	Inducer	Substrate	
2 E1	Disulfiram	Ethanol	Acetaminophen	Ethanol (minor)
3A3	Cimetidine	Isoniazid	Chlorzoxazone	Halothane
	Nefazodone		Erythromycin	Midazolam
	Ranitidine			
3A4	Clarithromycin	Barbiturates	Amitriptyline	Hydrocortisone
	Erythromycin	Carbamazepine	Alfentanil	Imipramine
	Fluconazole	Glucocorticoids	Alprazolam	Ketoconazole
	Fluoxetine	Phenylbutazone	Amiodarone	Miconazole
	Fluvoxamine	Phenytoin	Astemizole	Midazolam
	Grapefruit juice	Rifampin	Azithromycin	Nifedipine
	Ketoconazole		Carbamazepine	Progesterone
	Nefazodone		Cisapride	Quetiapine
	Sertraline		Clarithromycin	Quinidine
	Troleandomycin		Clomipramine	Tacrolimus
			Cyclosporine	Tamoxifen
			Dapsone	TCA (demethylation)
			Diltiazem	Terfenadine
			Erythromycin	Testosterone
			Ethinyle estradiol	Triazolam
3A5			Lidocaine	Nifedipine
			Lovastatin	Troleandomycin
3 A7			Midazolam	Testosterone
			Progesterone	Triazolam

(Substrate column for 2 E1 top entries: Haloperidol, Hydrocodone, Imipramine, Metoprolol, Mexiletine; with TCAs (hydroxylation), Thioridazine, Timolol, Venlafaxine)

Table S6.1 lists many drugs and other agents that frequently are used concurrently (not necessarily by intent) in patients with pain and headache and that influence the P-450 enzyme system. The reader should use Table S6.1 in the following manner:

- Determine what medications a patient is taking, together with any additional medicines being considered for administration.
- Determine whether any of these medications are listed as inhibitors, inducers, or substrates.
- Determine whether any of these medications inhibit or induce the enzyme system with respect to other medications the patient is taking in the same CYP enzyme category (horizontal row across).
- Either adjust dosage or find alternate treatment.

Table S6.2 lists some drug combinations frequently encountered in the treatment of pain. Certain drugs are identified that have a potential effect on certain other agents with particular results.

TABLE S6.2. **SELECTED "PAIN" DRUG INTERACTIONS**

Drug	Effect on P-450	Medication Affected	Result
Phenytoin Carbamazepine Barbiturate	Induces	Oral contraceptives	Reduces oral contraceptive efficacy
Fluvoxamine Fluoxetine Paroxetine Sertraline?	Inhibits	Lipophilic beta-blockers (propranolol metoprolol, timolol)	Increases beta-blockade (bradycardia, heart block, hypotension, etc.)
Fluvoxamine Fluoxetine Paroxetine Sertraline? Nefazodone	Inhibits	Certain TCAs Some benzodiaz-epines (not clonazepam)	Increase blood level and thus anticholinergic effects (hypotension, bradycardia, seizures) Increase sedation, somnolence
Fluoxetine Nefazodone	Inhibits	Terfenadine Astemizole Cisapride	Increases blood level, inducing potential toxic reactions, Torsades de Pointes

7

Serotonin Syndrome

I. Introduction

Serotonin syndrome (SS) is a potentially serious, drug-related complication that arises from the use of serotoninergic agents or disease states that increase serotonin (see Table 7.1). Medications that cause SS increase CNS serotonin neurotransmission. Though many cases are mild, SS may progress to cardiac arrest, coma, seizures, or multiple organ failure with disseminated intravascular coagulation. While most patients with SS improve with supportive care, some patients require specific drug therapy. Because the syndrome may manifest with selected symptoms rather than a full range of neuropsychiatric, autonomic, and neuromuscular events, it is likely that many cases go undetected or are incorrectly assigned to other causes.

Mathew and colleagues (1996) reported six patients with migraine who developed symptoms suggestive of SS. Five of the patients were taking one or more serotonergic agents for migraine prophylaxis. These **included** sertraline, paroxetine, lithium, imipramine, or amitriptyline. The syndrome appeared to develop in close temporal proximity to the administration of a symptomatic agent that had serotoninergic receptor agonist properties. In three instances the agent involved was sumatriptan, given subcutaneously, and in another three instances it was dihydroergotamine, given intravenously. The symptoms were transient, and full recovery occurred.

II. Clinical Symptomatology and Diagnosis
A. Symptoms

SS is expressed through a wide range of symptoms involving neuropsychiatric, autonomic, and neuromuscular manifestations. Signs and symptoms may vary greatly in form and intensity and often begin within hours after an additional serotonergic agent is added to a treatment program. A high index of suspicion is required in patients with **relevant** symptomatology, particularly those who are taking any one of the many medications, or combinations, that increase CNS serotonin transmission. The use of these agents, together with symptoms consistent with SS, should alert to the possibility of this disorder.

SS does not have a gender preference; however, populations at greatest risk (probably from medication requirements) include those with unipolar or bipolar depression, obsessive-compulsive

TABLE 7.1.   **DRUGS ASSOCIATED WITH SEROTONIN SYNDROME**

MAOIs
TCAs (clomipramine, imipramine, etc.)
SSRIs
L-tryptophan
LSD
Lithium
L-dopa
Buspirone
Imitrex
"Ecstasy"
Dextromethorphan
Meperidine
Pentazocine
Dextromethorphan
Trazodone
Cocaine
Fenfluramine

disease, eating disorders with depression, and Parkinson's disease. It has been reported in those under ten and over eighty years of age. SS is idiosyncratic, thus not appearing to **predictably** result from dose or duration of use. The syndrome may occur in those who are at or below therapeutic dose and may not occur in those who have taken significant overdoses. It can occur in patients taking monotherapy but is more likely with combination treatments. Because certain drugs, such as fluoxetine, sertraline, paroxetine, MAOIs, and others, may remain in the system for weeks following discontinuance, combination therapy may inadvertently occur when a new drug is administered weeks after discontinuation of one of these agents. Table 7.2 identifies selected drug combinations implicated in reported serotonin syndrome cases.

Three categories of symptoms are recognized: neuromuscular, autonomic, and cognitive and behavioral (neuropsychiatric) (see Table 7.3). Symptoms from one or two of the categories may be dominant, and onset and severity of symptoms are variable.

1. Neuromuscular symptoms

Symptoms of neuromuscular dysfunction are frequently reported and include myoclonus and hyperreflexia (in over 50% of reported cases). The patient may complain of cramping or muscle rigidity that may be limited to the lower extremities. Severe responses, such as opisthotonos and trismus, have been reported. Rhabdomyolysis can result from prolonged, severe muscle reactions. Shivering occurs in up to 25% of cases. Teeth

TABLE 7.2. **SELECTED COMBINATIONS CAUSING SS**

L-tryptophan and MAOI
MAOI and TCA
MAOI and SSRI
Meperidine and MAOI
fluoxetine and L-tryptophan
fenfluramine and SSRI
dexfenfluramine and sumatriptan
dextromethorphan and non-selective MAOI
fluoxetine and pentazocine
buspirone and trazodone
antidepressant and sumatriptan or DHE

TABLE 7.3. **SYMPTOMS OF SEROTONIN SYNDROME**

Neuromuscular
    Myoclonus
    Hyperreflexia/extensor plantar response (Babinski sign)
    Muscle rigidity
    Tremor
    Ataxia/incoordination
    Shivering/chills
    Nystagmus/ocular oscillation
    Teeth chattering
    Opisthotonos
    Trismus
    Oculogyric crises
    Rhabdomyolysis
Autonomic dysfunction
    Hyperthermia
    Diaphoresis
    Sinus trachycardia
    Hypertension
    Tachypnea
    Dilated pupils (mydriasis)
    Unreactive pupils
    Flushed skin
    Hypotension
    Diarrhea
    Abdominal cramps
    Salivation
Neuropsychiatric
    Confusion/disorientation
    Dizziness
    Agitation
    Anxiety
    Hypomania
    Drowsiness/lethargy
    Seizures
    Insomnia
    Hallucinations
    Autism
    Delirium
    Coma/unresponsiveness

chattering, facial twitching, nystagmus, and Babinski signs have been reported. The symptoms are usually bilateral. Neuromuscular irritability and restlessness may represent mild expressions of the disorder, as can extremity tremor and incoordination.

2. **Autonomic symptoms**

    Autonomic symptoms are most common. Diaphoresis is one of the primary symptoms of SS. Also common are hyperthermia, hypertension, asymptomatic sinus tachycardia (100–180), tachypnea, hypotension, dilated pupils (mydriasis), flushing, salivation, abdominal pain, and diarrhea. Hypotension may be a sign of poor prognosis.

3. **Cognitive and behavioral symptoms**

    The most commonly encountered neuropsychiatric symptoms are agitation and confusion. These are often subtle and unrecognized. Anxiety and hypomania may be misinterpreted as reflective of an underlying psychiatric disorder, withdrawal, or simple drug side effect. Seizures occur in up to 14% of reported cases and are generally major motor in nature. Other symptoms include insomnia, headache, hallucinations (usually visual), and dizziness. Coma may occur.

B. **Diagnostic Testing**

    The diagnosis is established by the presence of characteristic symptoms and the exclusion of other disorders (see Differential Diagnosis section). Most laboratory studies are normal, but occasionally electrolyte disturbances, elevated liver enzymes, and hyperammonemia are present. Leukocytosis may occur. ECGs may demonstrate sinus tachycardia. Elevated creatinine kinase levels of noncardiac origin are the result of muscle activity. Organ failure, metabolic acidosis, hypoxia, and disseminating intravascular coagulation are seen in advanced cases.

III. Treatment

Treatment consists of the following: discontinuance of all medications that enhance serotonin transmission, supportive care, and administration of antidotal therapy, if necessary (see Table 7.4).

With supportive care and discontinuance of the offending agent(s), most patients show improvement within the first 12–24 hours. Symptoms may last longer in instances in which significant complications occur, such as organ failure, or when drugs with prolonged action (such as fluoxetine or MAOIs) are involved.

Patients with hyperpyrexia can be cooled through the use of mist fans or by other measures, but antipyretics are generally ineffective. Seizures are treated with benzodiazepines or barbiturates.

TABLE 7.4.   PRINCIPLES OF TREATMENT OF THE SEROTONIN SYNDROME

Discontinue offending agent(s)
Supportive care
   Cooling
   Fluids
   Vital sign support
Antidotal treatment
   Cyproheptadine
   Benzodiazepines
   Propranolol
   Methysergide
   Others
Intensive care (fulminant symptoms)
   Reverse major autonomic disturbances, including hypertension
   Address organ failure, including respiratory distress, arrhythmias, disseminated
     intravascular coagulation (DIC)
   Treat seizures
   Etc.

Benzodiazepines are the first choice of treatment for neuromuscular symptomatology and for treatment of seizures. Nondepolarizing paralyzing agents are also of benefit in some instances. Dantroline has also been used.

Many of the symptoms of serotonin syndrome respond to drugs that block 5-HT_{1A} and 5-HT_2 receptors. Among these are cyproheptadine (blocks 5-HT_1 and 5-HT_2), methysergide (blocks 5-HT_2), and propranolol (p.o. or IV) (blocks 5-HT_{1a}). Of the available agents, cyproheptadine is the most consistently effective "antiserotinergic" agent. It has antimuscarinic, antihistaminic, and antiserotonin effects. Dosing should begin at 4 to 8 mg and can be repeated every couple of hours until therapeutic response is achieved. Maximum daily dose is 12 mg in children and 32 mg in adults.

The 5-HT_3 antagonists ondansetron (Zofran) and granisetron (Kytril) do not induce the syndrome and can be used for control of nausea.

IV. Differential Diagnosis

SS is most frequently confused with simple anxiety, hypertensive crisis, withdrawal symptoms, simple adverse reactions, muscle cramps, or the neuroleptic malignant syndrome (NMS). NMS generally occurs following the use of dopamine antagonists. The symptoms resemble those of SS and also include hyperthermia, dehydration, and increased liver enzymes. According to Mills (1997), the two disorders may represent two different pathways to the same clinical phenomenon. Adverse effects associated with the SSRIs include extrapyramidal symptoms, such as dystonia, akathisia, and Parkinsonism. In addition to the above, SS may be confused with **excessive dosing** from agents that

have stimulant actions, such as cocaine, amphetamine, methylphenidate, nicotine, lithium, antimuscarinic (anticholinergic) agents, and Ecstasy (3–4 methylenedioxymethamphetamine).

V. Conclusion

Many of the agents used alone or in combination for the treatment of headache can cause SS. Thus, caution must be applied in assessing adverse effects in patients using one or more of these agents. Personal experience suggests that partial expression of SS may go underdiagnosed or diagnosed incorrectly.

References

Ames D, Wirshing WC. Ecstasy: The serotonin syndrome and neuroleptic malignant syndrome: A possible link. *JAMA,* 269:869–870, 1993.

Baetz M, Malcolm D. Serotonin syndrome from fluvoxamine and buspirone. *Can J Psychiatry,* 40:428–429, 1995.

Bodner RA, Lynch T, Lewis L, et al. Serotonin syndrome. *Neurology,* 45:219–223, 1995.

Bostwick JM, Brown TM. A toxic reaction from combining fluoxetine and phentermine. *J Clin Psychopharmacol,* 16:189–190, 1996.

Brown TM, Scop BP. Pathophysiology and management of the serotonin syndrome. *Ann Pharmacother,* 30:527–533, 1996.

Demirkiran M, Jankovic J, Dean JM. Ecstasy intoxication: An overlap between serotonin syndrome and neuroleptic malignant syndrome. *Clin Neuropharmacol,* 19:157–164, 1996.

Fischer P. Serotonin syndrome in the elderly after antidepressant monotherapy. *J Clin Psychopharmacol,* 15:440–442, 1995.

George TP, Godleski LS. Possible serotonin syndrome with trazodone addition to fluoxetine. *Biol Psychol,* 39:383–386, 1996.

Goldberg RJ, Huk M. Serotonin syndrome from trazodone and buspirone (letter). *Psychosomatics,* 33:235–236, 1992.

Graber MA, Hoehns TB, Perry PJ. Sertraline-phenelzine drug interaction: A serotonin syndrome. *Ann Pharmacother,* 28:732–735, 1994.

Guze BH, Baxter LR. The serotonin syndrome: Case responsive to propranolol. *J Clin Psychopharmacol,* 6:119–120, 1986.

Hansen TE, Dieter K, Keepers GA. Interaction of fluoxetine and pentazocine. *Am J Psychiatry,* 147:949–950, 1990.

Kline SS, Mauro LS, Scala-Barnett DM, et al. Serotonin syndrome vs. neuroleptic malignant syndrome as a cause of death. *Clin Pharmacol,* 8:510–514, 1989.

Kuisma MJ. Fatal serotonin syndrome with trismus. *Ann Emerg Med,* 26:109, 1995.

Lappin RI, Anchincloss EL. Treatment of the serotonin syndrome with cyproheptadine. *Lancet,* 343:475, 1994.

Lenzi A, Raffaelli S, Marazzitti D. Serotonin syndrome-like symptoms in a patient with obsessive-compulsive disorder, following inappropriate increase in fluvoxamine dosage. *Pharmacopsychiatry,* 26:100–101, 1993.

Lieberman JA, Kane JM, Reife R. Neuromuscular effects of monoamine oxidase inhibitors. *Adv Neurol,* 43:231–249, 1986.

Martin TG. Serotonin syndrome. *Ann Emerg Med,* 28:520–526, 1996.

Mathew NT, Teitjen GE, Lucker C. Serotonin syndrome complicating migraine pharmacotherapy. *Cephalalgia,* 16:323–327, 1996.

Miller F, Friedman R, Tanenbaum J, et al. Disseminated intravascular coagulation and acute myoglobinuric renal failure: A consequence of the serotoninergic syndrome. *J Clin Psychopharmacol,* 11:277–279, 1991.

Mills KC. Serotonin toxicity: A comprehensive review for emergency medicine. *Topics Emerg Med,* 15:54–73, 1993.

Mills KC. Serotonin syndrome. *Clin Pharmcol,* 52:1475–1482, 1995.

Mills KC. Serotonin syndrome: A clinical update. *Crit Care Clin,* 13:763–783, 1997.

Miyaoka H, Kamijima K. Encephalopathy during amitriptyline therapy: Are neuroleptic malignant syndrome and serotonin malignant syndrome and serotonin syndrome spectrum disorders? *Int Clin Psychopharmacol,* 10:265–267, 1995.

Muly EC, McDonald W, Stefens D, et al. Serotonin syndrome produced by a combination of fluoxetine and lithium. *Am J Psychiatry,* 150:1565, 1993.

Nierenberg DW, Semprebon M. The central nervous system serotonin syndrome. *Clin Pharmacol Ther,* 53:84–88, 1993.

Power BM, Pinder H, Hackett LP, et al. Fatal serotonin syndrome following a combined overdose of moclobemide, clomipramine, and fluoxetine. *Anaesth Intensive Care,* 23:499–502, 1995.

Reeves RR, Bullen JA. Serotonin syndrome produced by paroxetine and low-dose trazodone. *Psychosomatics,* 36:159–160, 1995.

Rivers N, Horner B. Possible lethal reaction between nardil and dextromethorphan. *Can Med J,* 103:85, 1970.

Rosenberg B, Pearlman CA. NMS-like syndrome with lithium/doxepin combination. *J Clin Psychopharmacol,* 11:75, 1991.

Ruiz F. Fluoxetine and the serotonin syndrome. *Ann Emerg Med,* 24:983–985, 1994.

Sandyk R. L-dopa induced "serotonin syndrome" in a Parkinson patient on bromocriptine (letter). *J Clin Psychopharmacol,* 6:194–195, 1986.

Skop BP, Finkelstein JA, Mareth TR, et al. The serotonin syndrome associated with paroxetine, an over-the-counter cold remedy, and vascular disease. *Am J Emer Med,* 12:642–644, 1994.

Sporer KA. The serotonin syndrome. *Drug Experience,* 13:94–104, 1995.

Tackley RM, Tregaskis B. Fatal disseminated intravascular coagulation following a monoamine oxidase inhibitor/tricyclic interaction. *Anesthesia,* 42:760–763, 1987.

Weiss DM. Serotonin syndrome and Parkinson disease. *J Am Board Fam Pract,* 8:400–402, 1995.

SPECIFIC CONDITIONS
Introduction to Chapters 8-20

The following chapters will profile the primary headache disorders and selected clinical entities, including the neuralgias, atypical facial pain disorders, and several organic/metabolic conditions. The chapters are not meant to provide exhaustive reviews but to highlight practical considerations of each condition, with recommendtions for diagnostic evaluation and treatment.

Details of pharmacotherapy, as recommended under the treatment sections in each chapter, can be found in Chapters 6 and 9. Diagnostic testing is described in Chapter 3.

8

Migraine

I. Introduction

Migraine embodies a large number of clinical presentations, ranging from typical, characteristic attacks to many variant forms. It includes, in our opinion, in some cases what has traditionally been called "ordinary" or minor headaches and so-called episodic "tension-type" headache (see Chapter 10). It may be that some time in the future, the diagnostic criteria for migraine will be broadened to include a variety of other conditions that are now considered separate entities. In practice, what has been called *acute tension headache* and is now called *episodic tension-type headache* is at times indistinguishable symptomatically and therapeutically from mild cases of episodic migraine, particularly in patients with a history of migraine.

In its typical form, migraine is a complex neurophysiological disorder characterized by episodic and, in its progressive form, daily head pain. The headache attacks are often accompanied by neurological, autonomic, and psychophysiological events. Seventy-six percent of women and 57% of men suffer from recurring headache. We believe most suffer from a form of migraine.

Formerly, migraine was divided into two major subgroups: *classic* and *common* migraine. *Classic migraine* is now called (International Headache Society [HIS] classification) *migraine with aura,* and *common migraine* is called *migraine without aura.* (See Table 8.1 and 8.2). Approximately 30% of migraine attacks are "with aura." Many patients have both forms. The aura of migraine may precede, accompany, or follow the actual headache attack.

Since the late 1970s, there has been increasing recognition of migraine's capacity to *transform* from intermittent attacks to daily or almost daily head pain. This "variant" form of migraine, which has been termed *transformational migraine, progressive migraine,* or *pernicious migraine,* represents a progressive form of the illness in which, for uncertain reasons, intermittent migraine attacks increase in frequency, eventually transforming into continuous or almost continuous headache, with periodic attacks of acute migraine superimposed. (See Chapter 4 for a discussion of current concepts of migraine pathogenesis.)

II. Key Clinical Features

Generally, migraine is an inherited disorder. It is most likely that migraine is a syndrome with multiple genetic and environmental im-

TABLE 8.1. **INTERNATIONAL HEADACHE SOCIETY DEFINITION OF MIGRAINE WITHOUT AURA**[a]

1.1 *Migraine without aura*
Previously used terms: common migraine, hemicrania simplex
Diagnostic criteria:
  A. At least five attacks fulfilling B–D
  B. Headache lasting 4 to 72 hours (untreated or unsuccessfully treated)
  C. Headache has at least two of the following characteristics:
    1. Unilateral location
    2. Pulsating quality
    3. Moderate or severe intensity (inhibits or prohibits daily activities)
    4. Aggravation by walking stairs or similar routine physical activity
  D. During headache at least one of the following:
    1. Nausea and/or vomiting
    2. Photophobia and phonophobia
  E. At least one of the following:
    1. History, physical, and neurological examinations do not suggest one of the disorders listed in groups 5–11 (see reference below)
    2. History and/or physical and/or neurological examinations do suggest such disorder, but it is ruled out by appropriate investigations
    3. Such disorder is present, but migraine attacks do not occur for the first time in close temporal relation to the disorder

[a]From Headache Classification Committee of the International Headache Society. Classification and diagnostic criteria for headache disorders, cranial neuralgias, and facial pain. *Cephalagia* 8 (Suppl 7):1–96, 1988.

plications and variations. An autosomal dominant trait with incomplete penetrance has been proposed. Most recently, the gene for familial hemiplegic migraine in association with cerebellar disturbances has been found on chromosome 19 (Joutel, 1993). Gender distribution is approximately equal in childhood; however, in adults, significant migraine affects women in a ratio of approximately 3:1 to men. This dominance likely reflects the aggravating influence of *estrogen* on the migraine mechanism and the generally better prognosis of childhood migraine in males. Most patients develop migraine in the first three decades of life, but migraine can develop for the first time during any decade.

The following phases of migraine are recognized and may occur alone or in combination with any other phase.

A. The Prodrome

The prodrome consists of premonitory phenomena generally occurring hours to days before the headache, and includes mental, nonspecific neurological, constitutional, or autonomic symptoms. Neurological phenomena, such as photophobia and phonophobia (increased sensitivity to light and sound, respectively) and hyperosmia (increased sensitivity to smells), are common. Table 8.3 lists selected prodromal features of migraine. The presence of stiff neck as part of the prodrome has led many to consider erro-

TABLE 8.2. **NEW INTERNATIONAL HEADACHE SOCIETY DEFINITION OF MIGRAINE WITH AURA**[a]

1.2 *Migraine with aura*
Previously used terms: classic migraine, classical migraine, ophthalmic, hemiparesthetic, hemiplegic, or aphasic migraine
Diagnostic criteria:
A. At least two attacks fulfilling B
B. At least three of the following four characteristics:
    1. One or more fully reversible aura symptoms indicating focal cerebral cortical and/or brainstem dysfunction
    2. At least one aura symptom develops gradually over more than 4 minutes, or two or more symptoms occur in succession
    3. No aura symptom lasts more than 60 minutes. If more than one aura symptom is present, accepted duration is proportionally increased
    4. Headache follows aura with a free interval of less than 60 minutes. (It may also begin before or simultaneously with the aura.)
C. At least one of the following:
    1. History, physical, and neurological examinations do not suggest one of the disorders listed in groups 5–11 (see reference below)
    2. History and/or physical and/or neurological examinations do suggest such disorder, but it is ruled out by appropriate investigations
    3. Such disorder is present, but migraine attacks do not occur for the first time in close temporal relation to the disorder
1.2.1 *Migraine with typical aura*
Diagnostic Criteria:
A. Fulfills criteria for 1.2 including all four criteria under B
B. One or more aura symptoms of the following types:
    1. Homonymous visual disturbance
    2. Unilateral paresthesias and/or numbness
    3. Unilateral weakness
    4. Aphasia or unclassifiable speech difficulty

[a]From Headache Classification Committee of the International Headache Society. Classification and Diagnostic criteria for headache disorders, cranial neuralgias, and facial pains. *Cephalalgia* 8 (Suppl 7):1–96, 1988.

neously "tension headache" or cervical pathology as the origin of the complaint.

B. The Aura

The *aura* is composed of focal neurological symptoms that usually precede the headache and evolve over 5–20 minutes, usually lasting less than 60 minutes. Occasionally, the aura may begin simultaneously with the headache phase or after it has begun. The aura may occur alone, not accompanied or followed by a subsequent headache. If the aura is prolonged, it may meet the criteria established for *migraine with prolonged aura* (*complicated migraine* or *hemiplegic migraine*). In this instance, the aura lasts more than 60 minutes, but full recovery occurs within 3 weeks. Occasionally, patients have only this form. Rarely, patients with *migraine with aura* may experience neurological deficits lasting 3 or more weeks. The exact nature and relationship of these symp-

TABLE 8.3. **SELECTED PRODROMAL FEATURES OF MIGRAINE**

Mental and mood changes (depression, anger, euphoria, hypomania, etc.)
Stiff neck
A chilled feeling, peripheral vasoconstriction
Sluggishness/fatigue/excessive tiredness/yawning
Increased frequency of urination
Anorexia
Constipation or diarrhea
Fluid retention
Flood cravings

toms to migraine are not known. Oral contraceptives, smoking, and other risk factors that may be important should be controlled when possible in patients with moderate to severe migraine with aura, particularly if symptoms other than visual aura are present.

The most common symptoms of the aura are visual, particularly *fortification spectra,* which are zigzag or scintillating images. Table 8.4 lists selected features of the aura.

C. The Headache

The headache of migraine may be unilateral or bilateral and located anywhere about the head or neck. Forty percent of headaches are bilateral; 60% are unilateral. It may be mild or severe, with a throbbing, pulsating quality, though these characteristic features are not always present. The headache may last hours to days but rarely less than 4 hours in duration. Some attacks can last weeks. Severe, debilitating, prolonged attacks are referred to as *status migrainosis* or *intractable migraine.*

A small percentage of migraine attacks occur without head pain. Examples include childhood migraine with "*migraine equivalents*" only (see page 162), and in the adult, *late onset migraine (transient migraine accompaniments)* (see page 158). Other adult forms unassociated with headache also occur. The diagnosis is established by the presence of typical features and by ruling out other paroxysmal conditions, such as seizure disorders, transient ischemic attacks (TIA), pheochromocytoma, etc.

Table 8.5 lists many of the symptoms that can accompany the pain. They overlap the symptoms of the aura. In fact, any neurological, constitutional, autonomic, or emotional symptom may occur as part of the aura or as an accompanying symptom to the headache.

D. The Postdrome

After a severe attack of migraine, patients often feel tired, "washed out," irritable, and listless, with impaired concentration and general fatigue. Muscle weakness and aching, anorexia, or food craving are common. A feeling of euphoria or hypomania may follow or precede the attack.

TABLE 8.4. **SELECTED FEATURES OF THE AURA**

Visual	Motor	Sensory	Brainstem Disturbances
Scotomata (formed or unformed figures[a])	Hemiparesis Aphasia	Hypersensitivity to feel and touch	Ataxia Loss or change in
Fortification scotomata (zigzag or scintillating figures)	(See brainstem disturbances)	Paresthesiae Reduced sensation (hypesthesia)	level of consciousness Diplopia Tinnitus or hearing
Light sensitivity		(See brainstem disturbances)	loss Vertigo
Photopsia (unformed flashes of light)			Dysarthria Bilateral motor or
Distortions in shape and size			sensory symptoms

[a]In "retinal migraine," these occur unilaterally rather than bilaterally.

TABLE 8.5. **SELECTED FEATURES ACCOMPANYING THE HEADACHE OF MIGRAINE**

Gastrointestinal
   Anorexia
   Nausea and vomiting
   Diarrhea
Visual disturbances
   Blurring
   Light sensitivity (photophobia)
Other
   Fatigue/depression/irritability/anger
   Mental dullness/hypomania/confusion
Motor disturbances
Sensory disturbances
   Dysesthesiae/hyperesthesiae
   Phonophobia/hyperacusis
   Pain throughout the body
Brainstem features
   Vertigo
   Ataxia
   Loss of consciousness
   Diplopia
   Other
Fluid retention/polyuria
Autonomic disturbances
   Hypertension
   Hypotension
   Tachycardia/bradycardia
   Nasal congestion
   Peripheral vasoconstriction

III. Variant Forms of Migraine With Aura and Without Aura
A. Late-Life Migraine

As described by Fisher in 1980, *late-life migraine,* also called *transient migraine accompaniments,* represents attacks of episodic neurological events after the age of 45, occurring in the absence of headache, and believed to result from migraine pathophysiology. The attacks last up to 72 hours and are frequently characterized by scintillating scotoma, with migrating episodic neurological symptoms that include paresthesiae, aphasia, and other sensory and motor symptoms.

Patients may or may not have previously experienced migraine. The diagnosis can be established only after ischemic cerebrovascular disease (TIAs, giant cell arteritis, etc.) and other organic causes of episodic neurological symptoms, including cardiogenic disease, have been ruled out. Generally, the transient nature of these symptoms, their migraine quality, and the buildup over 20–30 minutes distinguish these from other more serious ailments. The workup should include studies for risk factors for stroke, including clotting disorders (antiphospholipid antibody syndrome, etc.) and computed tomography (CT), magnetic resonance imaging (MRI), magnetic resonance angiogram (MRA), and contrast arteriography, if necessary (see Table 3.6, Chapter 3). Regarding treatment, some authorities recommend aspirin or ticlopidine 250 mg twice daily. Anticonvulsants such as divalproex may also be tried, since neurogenic origin to symptoms is possible. Calcium channel blockers may also have a role in treatment.

B. Basilar (Brainstem) Migraine

Basilar migraine, also called *basilar artery migraine, vertebrobasilar migraine,* or the *Bickerstaff syndrome,* was first believed to result from spasm of the basilar artery, and subsequent ischemia. Many authorities now believe that neuronal dysfunction, with or without ischemia, underlies the neurological events. The condition frequently affects young people (most often females) and belongs to the subgroup *migraine with aura.*

The aura reflects involvement of the basilar or brainstem region, and symptoms include:

- Visual field disturbances;
- Dizziness/vertigo;
- Diplopia;
- Ataxia;
- Dysarthria;
- Tinnitus/hearing loss;
- Bilateral sensory and motor disturbances; and
- Changes in the level of consciousness, including loss of consciousness.

A dramatic form of *basilar migraine* is *stuporous migraine* or *confusional migraine.* Symptoms include the subacute onset of stupor, confusion, and/or severe tiredness, often in association with imbalance and other brainstem signs. Obscene utterances and obstreperous behavior are also noted. The EEG is frequently markedly slowed, which can be a striking feature. The condition is often diagnosed erroneously as "hysterical in origin" or due to drug-induced states. Spontaneous improvement occurs in days to a week.

C. Ophthalmoplegic Migraine

This variant of migraine is characterized by repeated acute attacks of headache associated with diplopia due to paresis of one or more extraocular muscles and often associated with a dilated pupil. Other cranial nerves may be involved. Diagnostic considerations include:

- Diabetic cranial neuropathy;
- Intracranial aneurysm/tumor;
- Tolosa-Hunt syndrome (painful ophthalmoplegia);
- Acute glaucoma;
- Ocular pseudotumor; and
- CNS infiltrative or infectious disease.

D. Hemiplegic Migraine

Hemiplegic migraine occurs in both sporadic and familial forms. It begins in childhood, sometimes as early as 1–2 years, and generally ceases in later life. The hemiplegia, usually part of the aura, can last 30–60 minutes, or longer. Other neurological events may also occur. Severe attacks may last days or weeks. The headache, often throbbing, follows the hemiplegia or may occur with it. A male predominance appears to exist. CSF pleocytosis may be present.

In 1993, Joutel and colleagues identified a region of DNA on human chromosome 19 that appeared genetically linked to the clinical diagnosis of familial hemiplegic migraine (FHM). Other chromosomal linkages, other than chromosome 19, are possible. Cerebellar dysfunction may also occur, particularly in those cases linked to chromosome 19. An abnormality in a neuronal P/Q calcium channel has also been proposed.

E. Retinal Migraine

Retinal migraine is characterized by repeated attacks of headache, preceded or accompanied by visual impairment or blindness involving one eye. The visual impairment lasts less than 1 hour. Headache usually follows the attacks but can be simultaneous or absent. Ischemic phenomena, including embolic disease and ischemic optic atrophy, and other organic causes must be ruled out. Carotid ultrasound studies and CT scan/MRI are recommended.

F. Migraine and Vestibular Dysfunction

Migraineurs, compared to nonmigraineurs, have a significantly higher prevalence of central and combined central and peripheral vestibular dysfunction, including hearing loss (Buchholz, 1996; Savundra, 1997). Migraine is associated with both specific vestibular disorders and nonspecific ones, including benign paroxysmal vertigo of childhood and benign recurring vertigo in adults. In a recent review in *Headache,* Baloh (1997) noted that motion sensitivity with bouts of motion sickness occur in about two-thirds of patients with migraine, and episodes of vertigo occur in about one-fourth of patients. Vertigo may actually represent a "migraine equivalent" in some. Migraine may mimic Meniere's disease.

Benign paroxysmal vertigo of childhood, as well as benign paroxysmal torticollis of infancy (a familial self-limited disorder characterized by recurring episodes of head tilt, pallor, and vomiting) both appear to evolve over time to migraine in some individuals. A family history of migraine is common. Benign paroxysmal vertigo generally affects infants and preschool children, but older children are not spared. Attacks of vertigo, inability to sit without being maintained, and pallor, together with nausea and abdominal pain, are often noted. The attacks may last seconds to minutes but may continue for hours. A relationship to basilar migraine is suspected (Davidoff, 1998).

In a study of 100 patients with a diagnosis of migraine-related vestibulopathy (Cass, 1997), dominant clinical features included chronic movement-associated disequilibrium, unsteadiness, space and motion discomfort, and episodic vertigo, which could manifest as the aura prior to a migraine attack.

Testing abnormalities can be found and may include directional preponderance on rotational testing, unilateral reduced caloric responsiveness, and vestibular system dysfunction on posturography.

Baloh (1997) notes that the recent recognition of a brain calcium-channel gene in families with hemiplegic migraine and in families with episodic vertigo and ataxia suggests a possible mechanism for the neurotologic symptoms in patients with the more common forms of migraine. A calcium-channel defect, expressed in the brain and/or inner ear, could lead to reversible hair cell depolarization and the auditory and vestibular symptoms.

Treatment of the vestibular symptoms associated with migraine generally requires the use of anti-migrainous therapy (Bikhazi, 1997). Other treatments include vestibular sedatives, (promethazine, benzodiazepines, and meclizine), vestibular rehabilitation, and therapies directed at anxiety.

G. Progressive Migraine (Transformational Migraine)

The authors of this book consider *progressive migraine,* also referred to as *pernicious migraine* and *transformational migraine,* to be a variant of migraine. It is covered in detail in Chapter 11.

H. Carotodynia

Carotodynia is sometimes described as a variant of migraine. See Chapter 14.

I. Icepick Pain

Icepick-like, jabbing head pain is frequently encountered in migraine patients, occurring during and independent of actual migraine attacks. The phenomenon is also seen in exertional headache syndromes and *hemicrania continua* (see Chapter 15). The brief, painful paroxysms are not serious but are often frightening. The pain may occur in the temple, face, or external ear. The mechanism is not understood. Indomethacin and perhaps other NSAIDs may be specifically helpful.

J. Exertional Migraine (See Chapter 15)

IV. Migraine in Childhood

Approximately 39–70% of children experience at least occasional headache. Some authors believe that most childhood headaches are forms of migraine. Migraine in children is often similar to adult migraine, but attacks are usually of shorter duration. Gastrointestinal (GI) complaints, mental changes, and abdominal discomfort are more common in children and may be characteristic features of the childhood attacks.

In children, episodic symptoms of disequilibrium, anxiety, nausea and vomiting, nystagmus, or other symptoms can occur in the absence of headache. These symptoms may represent precursors to more typical migraine attacks in later years. The symptoms are sometimes referred to as *migraine equivalents* and include:

- Dizziness/vertigo/disequilibrium;
- Nausea and vomiting/abdominal pain;
- Sudden irritability;
- Anorexia;
- Sensitivity to light and sound;
- Cyclic vomiting;
- Diarrhea;
- Personality change; and
- Periodic attacks of limb and joint pain.

Children with migraine are often treated effectively with biofeedback and behavioral, cognitive therapies. Medicines should be avoided if possible, but pharmacotherapy, if appropriate, should not be withheld. See Chapter 11 for further discussion on biofeedback, relaxation, and psychotherapy. Also see discussion of non-medicinal therapy in later sections of this chapter. Dietary restrictions can also be very useful in children (see Chapter 3).

V. Migraine and Its Comorbidities

Comorbidity refers to the greater than coincidental association of two conditions in the same individual. In recent years migraine has been recognized to be comorbid with a number of neurological and neuropsychiatric disorders. These include stroke, epilepsy, depression, and anxiety disorders, among other conditions (see below). The occurrence of comorbidity has diagnostic and treatment implications, as well as epidemiological and etiological ones. This section will emphasize two of the most important *neurologically* significant comorbid conditions associated with migraine—stroke and epilepsy. However, from a practical consideration, the neuropsychiatric comorbid conditions are much more prevalent and important in the day-to-day treatment of patients with migraine.

Recent population-based studies demonstrate an association between migraine and major depression, as well as between migraine and neuroticism. Other neuropsychiatric conditions, in which the odds ratio was elevated for an association with migraine, include bipolar spectrum disorders, generalized anxiety disorders, panic disorders, simple phobia, and social phobia. Depression and anxiety disorders often occur together with migraine (Breslau, 1991, 1995, 1994; Lipton, 1997; Merikangas, 1993, 1997). For further discussion, see Chapter 5 in *Headache* by Lipton and Stewart (Goadsby and Silberstein, 1997), and Merikangas and Stevens, 1997, in *Neurologic Clinics* (February, 1997).

A. Migraine and Stroke

The association between migraine and stroke is complex. Several points should be emphasized. Headache is common with stroke, regardless of stroke form. Migraine appears to be a modest risk factor for ischemic stroke in young woman, particularly those who smoke and use high estrogen-containing oral contraceptives. Though there is an increased incidence of stroke in migraine, overall it is relatively rare. Genetic implications may have an important influence on migraine-related cerebral infarction.

Welch (1994) recognizes four categories of relationship between migraine and stroke. These include: coexistent stroke and migraine; stroke with clinical features of migraine; migraine-induced stroke; and uncertain cases. In the category of *coexistent stroke and migraine,* there exists a clearly defined stroke syndrome, but this occurs remotely in time from a typical migraine attack. Some cases may be coincidentally related or related by mutual underlying risk factors, such as mitral valve prolapse or an antiphospholipid antibody syndrome (see below).

In the category of *stroke with clinical features of migraine,* there exists a structural lesion that is unrelated to migraine pathogenesis, but which presents with clinical features of a migraine attack. One subtype is referred to as *symptomatic,* and the other as *migraine mimics.* In the *symptomatic* form, the structural disease causes episodes of typical migraine with aura, an example of which might be an AV malformation. In the *migraine mimics* subtype, stroke is accompanied by headache and neurological events that resemble or mimic migraine.

In the classification of *migraine-induced stroke,* a neurological deficit of stroke is identical to the neurological symptoms of prior migraine attacks, and the stroke occurs in the course of a typical migraine attack. Other causes of stroke are excluded.

In the final classification between migraine and stroke, *uncertain cases,* a causal link is difficult. Intrinsic and extrinsic factors may be influential, such as excessive use of vasoconstrictive medications, the presence of systemic vasculitis, the antiphospholipid antibody syndrome, mitochondrial encephalopathies, oral contraceptive use, and others.

Thus, the relationship between migraine and stroke remains an enigma. Migraine is a risk factor for stroke but is difficult to assess statistically. Case-controlled and population-based studies suggest that the strongest association between migraine and stroke is found in women under 45, mostly in those with migraine and aura, and especially in those who smoke or use oral contraceptives. It is likely to be a rare occurrence.

Various external factors may contribute to the risks in patients with migraine. These include hemoconcentration, hypercoagulability, use of oral contraceptives, cigarette smoking, and other causes of endothelial damage, including those related to smoking, diabetes, hypertension, elevated cholesterol, and others. Low-estrogen oral contraceptive preparations do not appear likely to increase the risk of stroke (Petitti, 1996).

The *antiphospholipid antibody syndrome* is a constellation of symptoms that include headache, recurring ischemic neurological events, left-sided heart failure, neuropsychological disturbances, recurring thrombotic events (cerebral or otherwise), livedo reticularis, and miscarriages. Patients with elevated circulating antibodies are thought to be at particular risk for occlusive vascular disease. By way of background, antiphospholipid antibodies are circulating immunoglobulins, including anticardiolipin antibody and lupus anticoagulant. Antibodies to cardiolipin, a serologically active phospholipid, first isolated from beef heart, bind to cause a positive or false-positive venereal disease research laboratories (VDRL) test, because cardiolipin is one of the antigens in the VDRL assay. Patients with long-standing false-positive VDRL have a high prevalence of autoimmune diseases, including systemic lupus erythematosus (SLE) and hemolytic anemia.

The role of antiphospholipid antibody (aPl) in migraine is controversial. Exposure of phospholipids in damaged endothelial membranes to blood may lead to formation of aPl, a documented risk factor for ischemic stroke. Migraineurs with aPl have neuroimaging abnormalities consistent with ischemic stroke more often than the non-migraineurs. Conflicting studies have been published regarding the frequency of aPl in migraine-induced infarction. Transient focal neurological events and headache are often associated with the antiphospholipid syndrome. Treatment guidelines remain uncertain, with some advocates recommending aspirin and others recommending anticoagulation for patients with high risk or actual stroke.

Other migraine and stroke risk factors include immunological disturbances and genetic-based migraine-related stroke. In this latter category is the CADASIL (Cerebral Autosomal Dominant Arteriopathy with Subcortical Infarcts and Leukoencephalopathy) syndrome. This acronym, for what was earlier described as hereditary multi-infarct dementia, includes recurring subcortical infarcts with eventual dementia and pseudobulbar palsy. Early in its course, migraine with aura may play a prominent role. The CADASIL locus has been found on chromosome 19q12.

B. Migraine and Epilepsy

Significant evidence suggests that migraine and epilepsy are comorbid (Ottman, 1994), with a reported median prevalence of 5.9%, which exceeds prevalence of epilepsy in the general population (approximately 0.5%). The prevalence of migraine in those with epilepsy is in a range of 8–23%.

Speculation on the basis of this comorbidity remains unsettled. Both illnesses may share common EEG patterns, including posterior slowing and episodic, paroxysmal features. Some seizure patients experience migraine-like headaches before (aura to seizure), during, or following the seizure. Some with severe migraine experience loss of consciousness similar to that seen in certain forms of epilepsy. Moreover, the aura for epilepsy and that of migraine may be similar, or in some cases the same, leading to a seizure on one occasion and to a headache attack on another. Patients with overlapping symptoms or substantially altered EEGs may benefit from the use of both or either antimigraine and antiseizure medications.

Regardless of the etiology, the comorbid association between migraine and epilepsy is significant, both diagnostically and therapeutically. Drugs that lower seizure threshold should be used with caution in patients with both conditions. Among these are the tricyclic antidepressants, SSRIs, neuroleptics, and meperidine. Using treatments that might control both conditions, such as divalproex sodium, has particular advantage in these circumstances. (For further discussion, see Lipton and Stewart, Chapter 5, in *Headache* [Goadsby and Silberstein, 1997].)

VII. Migraine-Provoking Influences

Migraine is an illness in which genetic or acquired factors predispose patients to attacks. A variety of external or internal events appear likely to provoke an attack. *Internalized, cyclic rhythms reflecting the chronobiological mechanisms of the hypothalamus may be the key factor determining the specific, temporal vulnerability toward a headache.* During this period, other internal as well as external factors may further lower the migraine threshold. Table 8.6 lists a number of factors considered likely to induce/provoke a migraine (see also Tables 3.2 and 3.3 in Chapter 3). Reliability of any of these factors is variable, thus explaining the failure of any one to consistently precipitate an attack.

Certain mental states, food craving, excessive tiredness, light and sound sensitivity (perception of bright light or sound), and food taken during the craving are not "provoking factors," as some people have misinterpreted them to be. Actually, they reflect events of the prodrome or aura. By the time these symptoms occur, the attack is already underway!

Hormonal changes represent one of the more important internal activating factors. The most predictable time for migraine is around the *menstrual period*. Migraine may also worsen in the first phases of *pregnancy*. Migraine may change its frequency and quality around the time of *menopause,* worsening or improving.

Oral contraceptives frequently, but not necessarily, aggravate migraine. Rarely do they relieve migraine. Moreover, the use of *supplemental estrogens* at or around the time of menopause may worsen the condition. Exceptions are common, since estrogen deficiency

TABLE 8.6.   **SELECTED POTENTIAL PROVOKING FACTORS OF MIGRAINE**

Stress/anger
Missing meals
Sleep (too much or too little)
Certain foods (see Table 3.3, Chapter 3)
Weather changes
Hormonal changes
   Oral contraceptives
   Menstrual periods
   Pregnancy
Certain medicines
Scintillating, flashing, or bright light
Alcohol
Emotional "letdown"
Exhilaration/anticipation
General metabolic or infectious conditions
Localized cranial disturbances
Smoking/ambient smoke
Strong perfume/odors (paint, cleaning solutions, exhaust fumes, etc.)

may also provoke migraine. Based on anecdotal data, it is believed by some that the use of synthetic estrogens, such as estradiol (Estrace, Estraderm) or estropipate (Ogen) are less likely to incite migraine than conjugated forms, such as Premarin.

VIII. Specific Diagnostic Testing

The neurological examination in patients with migraine is usually normal, except in the presence of migraine with aura or complicated migraine. Occasionally, "soft" sensory findings are present. No routine diagnostic test establishes the presence of migraine (PET scanning is still impractical, except for research protocols). *The clinician must exclude other conditions that may mimic or overlap symptoms of migraine, or coexist with it* (see Chapters 3 and 5).

Clinically, provocation by specific instigating factors is a relatively reliable clue. The association of the following factors with migraine gives support for the diagnosis:

1. Headache occurring within minutes to an hour or two after the ingestion of red wine;
2. Headache occurring exclusively at or around the time of a menstrual period;
3. Headache occurring after emotional "letdown";
4. Headache associated with sleeping later than usual; and
5. Headache provoked by weather changes.

The presence of a family history and characteristic clinical features similarly support the diagnosis but cannot be used to categorically eliminate the need for testing. Migraine may be imitated by organic disease (see Chapter 5) and aggravated by coexistent disease. A thorough evaluation is recommended except in typical, intermittent cases with absolutely characteristic clinical and provocative features, as noted above. Testing for variant and progressive forms include CT scan or MRI and perhaps EEG (in cases which fulfill testing guidelines) (see Chapter 3). Electrocardiogram (ECG) and metabolic studies assist to rule out certain disorders that can cause headache and also to establish a safety baseline for pharmacotherapy, many drugs of which possess cardiac, liver, or renal implications.

IX. Principles of Treatment

As in all headache disorders, the most fundamental principle of treatment is establishing the correct diagnosis. A detailed compilation of information regarding the character of the attacks, provoking and relieving factors, and accompaniments is essential. In approaching migraine therapeutically, there are two strategies of treatment:

- Treating the individual attack (acute, symptomatic, abortive, reversal therapy); and
- Preventing an attack (prophylactic therapy).

Symptomatic and preventive measures are available in both pharmacological and nonpharmacological forms.

A. Nonmedicinal Therapy

There are relatively few useful, self-administered means of symptomatically reversing a migraine attack without medication. Actions that can be taken include:

- Applying ice;
- Taking refuge in a cool, quiet dark environment;
- Practicing biofeedback and relaxation techniques; and
- Inducing sleep (perhaps the best treatment).

Avoiding provoking factors and utilizing biofeedback and behavioral and stress management techniques, along with improvement in general health, can be helpful preventitively. Biofeedback and cognitive/behavioral treatment can be extremely useful and aid in avoiding medicines in some cases. See Chapter 11 for a discussion of biofeedback and behavioral treatment for headaches.

The following are some additional recommendations:

1. Discontinue smoking;
2. Exercise regularly;
3. Keep day-to-day activities the same, as much as possible; and
4. Avoid foods and circumstances that may provoke headache.

Migraine patients appear vulnerable to changes in regular patterns. Weekend and holiday changes in the patterns of living, for example, may provoke an attack. Attempting to stabilize activities such as eating times and patterns, sleeping (retiring and awakening), stress, and pleasure activities may bring benefit to some patients with headache. Many migraine patients regulate their schedules compulsively as a result of this phenomenon.

B. The Pharmacotherapy of Migraine

Details of proper dosing and medication administration were discussed in Chapter 6 and are further elaborated upon in Chapter 9. This section provides a summary of pharmacotherapy of migraine.

1. Symptomatic vs. preventive approaches

Both a symptomatic and a preventive approach can be used (see Chapter 6). Employing both approaches is required when attack frequency warrants preventive measures and breakthrough headaches require symptomatic treatment. Even under the best preventive circumstances, acute attacks may occur. The symptomatic and preventive approaches can be described as follows:

a. *Symptomatic therapy*—To reverse or control the headache and accompaniments once the attack has begun; and

b. *Preventive therapy*—To minimize the frequency and intensity of expected attacks.

2. Criteria for symptomatic treatment alone (see Chapter 6)

a. When acute attacks occur no more than two times per week; and

b. When use of the symptomatic treatment is effective and not contraindicated by other health factors.

The headache frequency may satisfy the criteria for preventive measures, but certain patients do very well with symptomatic treatments alone and do not exceed safety guidelines for their use.

3. Criteria for preventive treatment (see Chapter 6)

a. When attacks of migraine occur at a frequency greater than 4–8 attacks/month*;

b. When despite the infrequency of attacks, the devastating nature of the condition justifies the use of daily (preventive) medication; and

c. When symptomatic medications are contraindicated or ineffective. Most patients on preventive treatment will require acute treatment for breakthrough attacks;

Some authorities suggest preventive treatment for patients with more than two headache attacks per month. However, many patients with up to 4–8 attacks per month do well with symptomatic treatment alone. Individual consideration is essential. Preventive treatment imposes risks, some very serious, and should be recommended only in those patients in whom these risks are worth imposing. Alternately, menstrual migraine, occurring once per month, may require preventive treatment only at or around the time of menses (to be discussed later in this chapter).

4. Principles of treatment

a. Provide sufficient but not excessive symptomatic treatment, perhaps with back-up alternatives for moderate and severe attacks, and firm limits on frequency and usage per week and;

b. Use oral, rectal, or nasal spray preparations initially;

c. Use nasal, rectal, or parenteral forms of medication when attacks are accompanied by significant nausea or vomiting or when there is evidence of delayed GI absorption (gastroparesis) (often present in even mild to moderate headache attacks);

d. Use adjunctive oral metoclopramide to reverse gastroparesis and improve absorption from the GI tract during severe attacks when oral symptomatic drugs are administered;

e. Administer nasal, rectal, or parenteral forms of symptomatic medication (DHE [parenteral and nasal], sumatriptan [nasal or parenteral], indomethacin suppositories, etc.) for attacks that are not responsive to oral medication;

f. Employ preventive treatment when criteria are met, and provide symptomatic treatment for breakthrough attacks;

g. Develop a program of symptomatic and preventive medication, often in combination, to establish the most beneficial treatment;

h. Administer preventive medication for several months, if effective, and then reconsider alternate treatment or impose a "drug holiday" when possible;

i. Provide patients with a range of treatment options for breakthrough attacks. Encourage the avoidance of emergency department treatment except when all means of "at home" therapy have proven ineffective. *Do not deny patients the*

*use of emergency department treatment for acute, resistant
headache. In cases of recurring or inappropriate emergency service utilization, consider hospitalization, since rebound or other confounding factors are often present* (see
Chapter 9);

j. Consider hospitalization treatment prior to the development of complications and/or addiction/dependency syndromes for patients with severe attacks who overuse treatment or whose treatments are clearly ineffective; and

k. Clinician availability for advice for acute attacks not responsive to "at home" treatment is an essential component of an
effective therapeutic relationship and patient compliance.

X. Specific Treatment Approaches
A. Symptomatic Treatment
1. The aura

The aura rarely requires treatment, and it is uncertain
whether medications provide any meaningful benefit. The
anecdotal use of sublingual nifedipine (10 mg) to reverse focal neurological disturbances has been recommended but is
generally unnecessary, since the symptoms usually reverse
spontaneously within 10–20 minutes. For particularly severe
attacks with recurrent neurologically significant aura, aspirin
therapy, symptomatically or preventively, may have value,
though this has not been established as protective in migraine.

2. The headache

The following groups of medications are useful for the acute
headache attack. The reader should refer to Chapters 6 and 9
for tables and descriptions of each of these medications and the
method of administration, side effects, and contraindications.

a. Mild to moderate attacks

1) Simple OTC analgesics, mixed (barbiturate-containing)
analgesics, hydroxyzine (has analgesic effects), etc.
2) Nonsteroidal anti-inflammatory agents
3) Oral or nasal antimigraine medications (ergotamine
tartrate, DHE nasal spray, Midrin, oral or nasal sumatriptan, rizatriptan, naratriptan, zolmitriptan, etc.)

b. Moderate to severe attacks

1) Rectal NSAIDs (indomethacin)
2) Mixed (barbiturate-containing) analgesics
3) Specific antimigraine medications (DHE nasal spray,

sumatriptan [nasal, oral], rizatriptan, zolmitriptan, naratriptan, Midrin, etc.)

4) Mixed analgesic/narcotic preparations (containing codeine, oxycodone, hydrocodone, etc.)

c. Severe attacks

1) Sumatriptan (parenteral or nasal)
2) DHE (parenteral or nasal)
3) Oral rizatriptan, zolmitriptan, naratriptan
4) Butorphanol nasal spray
5) Parenteral ketorolac
6) Rectal/parenteral neuroleptics
7) Rectal barbiturate
8) Rectal or parenteral opioid

d. Treatment of nausea, vomiting, and diarrhea

1) Rectal/parenteral neuroleptics, ondansetron
2) Oral antidiarrheic agents

B. Preventive Medications for Migraine
1. Categories of medication

The following categories of medication are useful in the prevention of migraine:

a. β-adrenergic blockers;

b. Calcium channel blockers;

c. Antidepressants (TCA, MAOIs); (SSRIs have not yet been established as convincingly helpful in migraine prevention)

d. Anticonvulsants (divalproex); (gabapentin, clonazepam, and carbamazepine are not yet accepted generally as effective in migraine prevention);

e. Ergot derivatives (methysergide*, methylergonovine*); and

f. Nonsteroidal anti-inflammatory drugs.

Both methysergide and methylergonovine cause fibrotic reactions. Careful monitoring and drug holidays are recommended (see Chapter 6).

2. Principles of preventive medication use

a. Select appropriate initial agent—first-line drugs include beta adrenergic blockers, TCAs, and divalproex, because of its hepatic and other adverse effects, should be used as a first-line agent when others cannot be used or are ineffective, or where comorbid illness, such as seizures or bipolar disease, makes this choice appropriate;

b. Increase dose at a reasonable pace, carefully monitoring for adverse effects, blood pressure, pulse rate, etc.

c. If treatment is ineffective at therapeutic levels, add a complementary treatment or discontinue and begin another preventive agent. Some agents require several weeks or perhaps months of therapy at therapeutic levels before effectiveness can be judged; and

d. Combined preventive treatment (strategic co-therapy) is necessary in some difficult-to-control conditions but must be used cautiously.

3. Combination preventive treatment (strategic co-therapy)

Strategic co-therapy may be used for difficult-to-manage cases when risk considerations support combined usage. Combination therapy should be avoided except in intractable cases when monotherapy is ineffective. Currently, evidence does not exist to support widespread use of combined therapy, although anecdotal experience suggests the usefulness in intractable cases. Careful monitoring and screening for cardiac, liver, and renal abnormalities, as well as blood pressure and pulse abnormalities are mandatory. Be aware of additive effects of the combined drugs, such as anticholinergic influence (constipation, urine retention, cardiac effects), vasoconstriction, liver toxicity, the *serotonin syndrome,* etc. A detailed description of the *serotonin syndrome,* which results from single or coadministration of agents that exert a serotonergic effect, can be found in Chapter 7.

Combination treatment should be used with careful and regular monitoring, including regular office visits and metabolic testing. Liver function should be carefully watched, as should renal, hematological, and other parameters. In addition to the risks listed earlier, combination therapies raise concern regarding influence on P-450 isoenzyme system. This influence may result in excessive or low blood levels. Generally speaking, combination therapies should be avoided except when clearly necessary and when administered by clinicians with experience in combination therapies (see Chapter 6 for further discussion of P-450 isoenzyme system and headache-related drugs, and Chapter 7 for the serotonin syndrome).

C. Rebound or Toxic Headache Syndromes

The excessive use of symptomatic medications, including analgesics, ergot agents, sumatriptan (and other triptans?), and perhaps high-dose NSAIDs, can result in a headache/medication cycle referred to as *rebound headache* or "analgesic rebound headache" (see Chapters 6, 9, and 11).

The *rebound syndrome* is a self-sustaining clinical phenomenon, rendering preventive medications ineffective until discontinuance and withdrawal occur. Withdrawal may require hospitalization and time to stabilize physiological systems until preventive medication can reduce the frequency of attacks and alternate forms of symptomatic treatment, at restricted intervals, can be employed. The key features of this syndrome include:

- Insidious increase of headache frequency;
- Dependable and irresistible use of increasing amounts of offending agents at regular, predictable intervals;
- Failure of alternate medications or preventive medications to control headache attacks;
- Development of psychological and/or physiological dependency;
- Predictable onset of headache within hours to days following the last dose of symptomatic treatment; and
- Awakening with or experiencing a headache at the same time each day when this has not previously been a feature of past headache patterns.

Effective termination of *rebound* can of itself reduce the frequency of headaches. If attempts to reduce the medications result in severe intensification of pain and accompaniments, hospitalization is required (see Chapter 9).

D. Guidelines for Treating Menstrual Migraine

Patients with menstrual migraine often require aggressive and innovative treatment that combines preventive and symptomatic approaches. The following considerations are recommended.

1. Symptomatic treatment

    a. NSAIDs, Midrin;

    b. DHE (nasal or parenteral);

    c. Sumatriptan (parenteral, nasal, oral), oral rizatriptan, naratriptan, or zolmitriptan; and

    d. Opioid or related analgesics (oral, rectal, or nasal spray);

2. Preventive treatment

    a. Standard preventive agents, including NSAIDs and ergot derivatives (methylergonovine, methysergide);

    b. 3-day use of DHE nasal spray, sumatriptan (oral or nasal

spray), rizatriptan, zolmitriptan, naratriptan, oral ergotamine tartrate (usage of these agents in this way should only
be carried out when their use is limited throughout the remainder of the month);

c. Hormonal manipulation (i.e., estrogen patch applied prior
to headache onset) (see Silberstein, 1991), to prevent precipitous drop of estrogen, which is thought to incite the
headache event; and

d. The preventive use of magnesium supplementation (not
yet established as effective in menstrual migraine) (see
Chapter 6).

Often, a combined preventive/symptomatic program is necessary. Preventive treatment can be started several days before
predictable onset of headache vulnerability and discontinued
2–4 days after menses begins. Menstrual migraine is believed
to result from the premenstrual drop of estrogen.

E. Migraine and Pregnancy

Approximately 70% of active migraineurs improve during pregnancy. However, worsening during the first trimester is common.
Generally, though not always, improvement occurs in the second
and third trimesters. Diagnostic testing should be avoided whenever
possible, but sometimes cannot. The EEG is safe during pregnancy
but is rarely useful except when suspected seizures, encephalopathy, loss of consciousness, or transient neurological events are present. CT imaging is generally avoided, and currently the same is true
of MRI. In rare instances, these tests have been performed.

It is best to avoid medications during pregnancy, if at all possible. Biofeedback may have value and should be considered in
appropriate cases. The authors of this text prefer the use of acetaminophen or opioids or combinations of these. Nausea and emesis can be treated with metoclopramide, trimethopenzamide,
chlorpromazine, prochlorperazine, and promethazine. Preventive
medications are generally avoided, but beta adrenergic blockers
have been used, as have tricyclic antidepressants.

A full discussion and disclosure of medical options during
pregnancy, if deemed necessary, should occur between physician,
patient, and spouse. For a more complete discussion of this topic,
see Silberstein, 1997.

F. Severe Dietary Limitations

Patients with migraine headaches rarely benefit from severe dietary limitation. Implementation of an elimination diet has been
recommended for some of these cases, with good results anecdo-

tally, at least temporarily. Patients should be referred to a dietary consultant for implementation.

References

Abramowicz M (Ed). Transdermal estrogen. *Med Lett Drugs Ther,* 28:119–120, 1986.

Airing CD. Late-life migraine. *Arch Neurol,* 48:1174–1177, 1991.

Andermann F. Clinical features of migraine-epilepsy syndrome. (In) *Migraine and Epilepsy.* F Andermann, E Lugeresi (Eds). Boston, Butterworth, Pgs 3–30, 1987.

Baloh RW. Neurotology of migraine. *Headache,* 37:615–621, 1997.

Basser LS. The relation of migraine and epilepsy. *Brain,* 92:285–300, 1969.

Bickerstaff ER. The basilar artery and the migraine-epilepsy syndrome. *Royal Society Medical Proceedings,* 55:167–169, 1962.

Bickerstaff ER. Ophthalmoplegic migraine. *Rev Neurol,* 110:582–588, 1964.

Bickerstaff ER. Basilar artery migraine. (In) *Handbook of Clinical Neurology,* Vol. 48. FC Rose (Ed). Amsterdam, Elsevier Science Publishing, Pgs 135–140, 1986.

Bikhazi, Jackson C, Ruckenstein, MJ. Efficacy of anti-migrainous therapy in the treatment of migraine-associated dizziness. *Am J Otol,* 18:350–354, 1997.

Bradshaw P, Parsons M. Hemiplegic migraine: A clinical study. *QJM,* 34:65–85, 1965.

Breslau N, Andreski P. Migraine: personality and psychiatric comorbidity. *Headache,* 35:382–386, 1995.

Breslau N, Davis GC. Migraine, major depression, and panic disorder: A prospective epidemiological study of young adults. *Cephalalgia,* 12:85, 1992.

Breslau N, Davis GC, Andreski P. Migraine, psychiatric disorders, and suicide attempts: An epidemiological study of young adults. *Psychiatry Res,* 37:11–23, 1991.

Breslau N, Davis GC, Schultz LR, et al. Migraine and major depression: A longitudinal study. *Headache,* 7:387, 1994.

Breslau N, Merikangas KR, Bowen CL. Comorbidity of migraine and major affective disorders. *Neurology,* 44(supp 7):S17–S22, 1994.

Bruyn GW. Complicated migraine. (In) *Handbook of Clinical Neurology,* Vol. 5. PJ Vincan, GW Bruyn (Eds). New York, John Wiley and Sons, Pgs 59–95, 1968.

Bruyn GW. Migraine equivalents. (In) *Handbook of Clinical Neurology,* Vol. 48. FC Rose (Ed). Amsterdam, Elsevier Science Publishers, Pgs 155–171, 1986.

Callahan N. The migraine syndrome in pregnancy. *Neurology,* 18:197–199, 1968.

Caplan L. Intracerebral hemorrhage revisited. *Neurology,* 38:624–627, 1988.

Caplan L, Chedru F, Lheramitte F, et al. Transient global amnesia and migraine. *Neurology,* 31:1167–1170, 1981.

Carolei A, Marini C, DeMatteis G, et al. History of migraine and risk of cerebral ischemia in young adults. *Lancet,* 347:1503–1506, 1996.

Cass SP, Furman JM, Ankersjernek, et al. Migraine-related vestibulopathy. *Ann Otol Rhinol Laryngol,* 106:182–189, 1997.

Cole AJ, Aube M. Migraine with vasospasm and delayed intracerebral hemorrhage. *Arch Neurol,* 47:53–56, 1990.

Cull RE. Investigation of late-onset migraine. *Scott Med J,* 40(2):50–52, 1995.

Davidoff R. *Benign Paroxysmal Vertigo of Childhood in Neurobase.* 2nd Edition. S Gillman, GW Goldstein, SG Waxman (Eds). San Diego, Arbor Publishing Company, 1998.

Dexter JD, Weitzman ED. The relationship of nocturnal headaches to sleep stage patterns. *Neurology,* 20:513–517, 1970.

Diener HC, Dichgans J, Scholz E, et al. Analgesic-induced chronic headache. Long-term results of withdrawal therapy. *J Neurol,* 236:9–14, 1989.

Ehyai A, Fenichel GM. The natural history of acute confusional migraine. *Arch Neurol,* 35:368–369, 1978.

Elliott MA, Parudka SJ, Welch S, et al. Familial hemiplegic migraine, nystagmus, and cerebellar atrophy: Clinical description of chromosome localization. *Ann Neurol,* 39:100, 1996.

Emery ES. Acute confusional state in migraine with children. *Pediatrics,* 60:110–114, 1977.

Fenichel GM. Migraine as a cause of benign paroxysmal vertigo of childhood. *J Pediatr,* 71:114–115, 1967.

Fenichel GM. *Clinical Pediatric Neurology: A Signs and Symptoms Approach.* Philadephia, WB Saunders, 1993.

Fisher CM, Adams RD. Transient global amnesia. *Acta Neurol Scand,* 40 (supp 9):1–83, 1964.

Fisher CM. Late life migraine accompaniments as a cause of unexplained transient ischemic attacks. *Can J Neurol Sci,* 7:9–17, 1980.

Fisher CM. Transient global amnesia: Precipitating activities and other observations. *Arch Neurol,* 39:605–608, 1982.

Fisher CM. Late life migraine accompaniments—further experience. *Stroke,* 17:1033–1042, 1986.

Gallucci M, Feliciani M, Martucci N, et al. Complicated migraine: An NMR and CT comparison. *Cephalalgia,* 5 (supp 3):376–377, 1985.

Gascon G, Barlow C. Juvenile migraine presenting as an acute confusional state. *Pediatrics,* 45:628–635, 1970.

Golden GS, French JS. Basilar artery migraine in young children. *Pediatrics,* 56:722–726, 1975.

Goldensohn ES. Paroxysmal and other features of the electroencephalogram in migraine. *Res Clin Stud Headache,* 4:118–128, 1976.

Harrison MJG. Hemiplegic migraine. *J Neurol Neurosurg Psychiatry,* 44:652–653, 1981.

Holroyd KA, Andrasik F. A cognitive-behavioral approach to recurrent tension and migraine headache. (In) *Advances in Cognitive-Behavioral Research and Therapy.* PC Kendell (Ed). New York, Academic, Pgs 275–320, 1982.

Iniguez C, Pascual C, Pardo A, et al. Antiphospholipid antibodies in migraine. *Headache,* 31:666–668, 1991.

Jacome DE. EEG features in basilar artery migraine. *Headache,* 27:80–83, 1987.

Jensen TS, Olivarius B, Kraft M, et al. Familial hemiplegic migraine: A reappraisal on a long-term follow-up study. *Cephalalgia,* 1:33–39, 1981.

Joutel A, Bousser M, Biousse V, et al. A gene for familial hemiplegic migraine maps to chromosome 19. *Nat Genet,* 5:40–45, 1993.

Kuritzky A, Ziegler DK, Hassanein R. Vertigo motion sickness and migraine. *Headache,* 21:227–231, 1981.

Lance JW, Anthony M. Some clinical aspects of migraine. A prospective survey of 500 patients. *Arch Neurol,* 15:356–361, 1966.

Lanzi G, Balottin U, Ottolini A, et al. Cyclic vomiting and recurrent abdominal pains as migraine or epileptic equivalents. *Cephalalgia,* 3:115–118, 1983.

Lauritzen M, Trojaborg W, Olesen J. The eeg in common and classic migraine attacks. (In) *Advances in Migraine Research and Therapy.* FC Rose (Ed). New York, Raven Press, Pgs 79–84, 1982.

Lee CH, Lance JW. Migraine stupor. *Headache,* 17:32–38, 1977.

Levine SR, Brey RL. Antiphospholipid antibodies and ischemic cerebrovascular disease. *Semina Neurol,* 11:329–338, 1991.

Lipton RB, Stewart WF. Epidemiology and comorbidity of migraine. (In) *Headache: The Blue Book of Practical Neurology.* PJ Goadsby, SD Silberstein (Eds). Boston, Butterworth-Heinemeann, 1997.

Merikangas KR, Angst J, Isler H. Migraine and psychopathology: Results of the Zurich cohort study of young adults. *Arch Gen Psychiatry,* 47:849, 1990.

Merikangas KR, Merikangas JR, Angst J. Headache syndromes and psychiatric disorders: Association and familial transmission. *J Psychiatr Res,* 27:197–210, 1993.

Merikangas KR, Stevens DE, Angst J. Headache and personality: Results of the community sample of young adults. *J Psychiatr Res,* 27:187, 1993.

Merikangas KR, Stevens DE. Comorbidity of migraine and psychiatric disorders. *Neurol Clin,* 15:1–13, 1997.

Meyer JS, Konno S, Akiyama H, et al. Late-life migraine accompaniments. (In) *Neurobase,* 3rd Edition. S Gilman, GW Goldstein, SG Waxman (Eds). Arbor Publishing Company, 1997.

Neurologic Clinics: Advances in Headache. NT Mathew (Ed). Saunders, February, 1997.

Olesen J. Some clinical features of the acute migraine attack. An analysis of 750 patients. *Headache,* 18:268–271, 1978.

Ottman R, Lipton RB. Comorbidity of migraine and epilepsy. *Neurology,* 44:2105, 1994.

Parrish RM, Stevens H. Familial hemiplegic migraine. *Minn Med,* 60:709–715, 1977.

Peatfield RC, Fozard JR, Rose FC. Drug treatment of migraine. (In) *Handbook of Clinical Neurology,* Vol. 48. FC Rose (Ed). Amsterdam, Elsevier Science Publishers, Pgs 173–216, 1986.

Petitti DB, Sidney S, Bernstein A, et al. Stroke in users of low-dose oral contraceptives. *N Engl J Med,* 335:8–15, 1996.

Pfaffenrath V, Kommissari I, Pollmann W, et al. Cerebrovascular risk factors in migraine with prolonged aura and without aura. *Cephalalgia,* 11:257–161, 1991.

Rapoport A, Weeks R, Sheftell F, et al. Analgesic rebound headache: Theoretical and practical implications. *Cephalalgia,* 5 (supp 3):448–450, 1985.

Raskin NH, Schwartz RK. Icepick-like pain. *Neurology,* 30:203–205, 1980.

Savundra PA, Carroll JD, Davies RA, et al. Migraine-associated vertigo. *Cephalalgia,* 17:505–510, 1997.

Shulman EA, Silberstein SD. Symptomatic and prophylactic treatment of migraine and tension-type headache. *Neurology,* 42 (supp 2):16–21, 1992.

Silberstein SD. Twenty questions about headaches in children and adolescents. *Headache,* 30:716–724, 1990.

Silberstein SD, Merriam GR. Estrogens, progestins, and headache. *Neurology,* 41:786–793, 1991.

Silberstein SD, Merriam GR. Estrogens, progestins, and headache. *Neurology,* 41:786–793, 1991.

Silberstein SD. The role of sex hormones in headache. *Neurology,* 42 (supp 2):37–42, 1992.

Solomon GD, Spaccavento LJ. Lateral medullary syndrome after basilar migraine. *Headache,* 22:171–172, 1982.

Somerville BW. The role of estradiol withdrawal in the etiology of menstrual migraine. *Neurology,* 22:355–365, 1972.

Somerville BW. Estrogen withdrawal migraine I and II. *Neurology,* 25:239–244, 245–250, 1975.

Stewart WF, Linet MS, Celentano DD. Migraine headaches and panic attacks. *Psychosom Med,* 51:559, 1989.

Sulkava R, Kovanen J. Locked-in syndrome with rapid recovery: A manifestation of basilar artery migraine? *Headache,* 23:238–239, 1983.

Teitjen GE. Migraine and antiphospholipid antibodies. *Cephalalgia,* 12:69–74, 1992.

Teitjen GE, Day M, Norris L, et al. The role of anticardiolipin antibodies in young persons with migraine and transient focal neurological events: A prospective, frequency-matched study. *Neurology* (in press).

Tinuper P, Cortelli P, Sacquengna T, et al. Classic migraine attack complicated by confusional state: EEG and CT study. *Cephalalgia,* 5:63–68, 1985.

Tomsak RL, Jergens PB. Benign recurrent transient monocular blindness: A possible variant of acephalgic migraine. *Headache,* 27:66–69, 1987.

Tzourio C, Iglesias S, Hubert JB, et al. Migraine and risk of ischemic stroke: A case-controlled study. *Br Med J,* 307:289–292, 1993.

Watson P, Steele JC. Paroxysmal disequilibrium in the migraine syndrome of childhood. *Arch Otolaryngol* 99:177–179, 1974.

Welch KMA, Darnley D, Simpkins RJ. The role of estrogen in migraine: A review and hypothesis. *Cephalalgia,* 4:227–236, 1984.

Whitty CWM. Familial hemiplegic migraine. (In) *Handbook of Clinical Neurology,* Vol. 48. FC Rose (Ed). Amsterdam, Elsevier Science Publishers, Pgs 141–153, 1986.

9

Treatment of Intractable, Severe Migraine: Parenteral Treatment Protocols, Hospitalization, and Referral Guidelines

I. Introduction, Definition, and Overview

Episodic migraine is defined as a severe migraine headache that is usually self-limited (less than 72 hours) if untreated. Although generally responsive to self-administered treatments, occasionally the attack is either unresponsive to self-treatment and/or accompanied by such intense pain, nausea, and vomiting that acute care intervention is mandatory.

Intractable (persistent, protracted, progressive) migraine is defined as a sustained (persistent, not self-limited), severe migraine and accompaniments that are not effectively terminated (sustained control) by standard outpatient interventions. This condition generally requires continuing acute therapeutic treatments over a day or longer, sometimes as much as 8–10 days. The illness is similar (or the same as) that which has been historically referred to as *status migrainosis*. Patients can be severely incapacitated and at risk if the condition is protracted. Also, attacks may evolve to a chronic and continuing form, similar to daily chronic headache.

A. Clinical Features of *Acute, Intractable Migraine*

1. **Continuing, persistent, severe head, neck, or face pain**
2. **Progressive physical and emotional accompaniments that may include:**
   a. Nausea, vomiting, and diarrhea;
   b. Dehydration;
   c. Despair/depression;
   d. Alteration of normal sleeping, eating, and activities of daily living; and
   e. Additional migraine accompaniments: Photo- and phono-sensitivity, malaise, focal neurological symptoms, etc.

3. **Toxicity and/or withdrawal symptoms from excessive use of symptomatic medication, with or without a history of dependency/addiction**

B. Treatment Overview

Treatment of *intractable (persistent, disabling) migraine* departs markedly from the treatment of more ordinary or self-limited headache events. *The principal challenge to effective treatment is to match the intensity of treatment to the severity of illness.* Patients with these severe states of pain require aggressive intervention, which usually mandates one or more of the following:

1. Parenteral pain therapy;
2. Rehydration;
3. Control of nausea and vomiting;
4. Removal of provoking factors, including medications;
5. Support (psychological and physiological); and
6. Monitoring in an acute care setting.

C. Other Considerations

Patients with *intractable migraine syndromes* suffer the often escalating consequences of head pain *plus* accompaniments, some of which are more serious and debilitating than the headache itself. In the presence of toxic medication effects or "rebound" dependency (see below), withdrawal symptomatology is likely when excessively used, symptomatic medications are withdrawn. If present, dehydration may result from a combination of factors, including reduced fluid intake over days or weeks, increased fluid and electrolyte loss through emesis, diarrhea, and polyuria, and diaphoresis.

II. Contributing Factors to Acute, Intractable Migraine

The following are considered factors that might contribute to the intractable headache status.

A. Drug-related Causes

The *rebound phenomenon,* as described in Chapters 6, 8, and 11, is a self-sustaining condition characterized by a persisting and recurring headache against a background of chronic and regular use of centrally-acting analgesics, ergotamine tartrate, and perhaps certain triptans that are capable of producing this medication/headache cycle. Generally, patients will undergo weeks, months, or even years of excessive use of centrally-acting analgesics or ergotamine tartrate (and probably short-acting triptans) prior to the presentation. Attempts to withdraw or discontinue the overused medications may result in a dramatic escalation of pain that often understandably but unwisely prompts the physician to readminister the medication, or for the patient to seek other sources of medication for self-administration.

In addition to the "rebound effect," which reflects both physiological and psychological dependence, toxic symptoms (including headache) can result from excessive use of certain drugs (caffeine, ergot preparations, opiates, acetaminophen, etc.), thereby further contributing to the intractable state.

Removal of the offending agent(s) is critical to establishing effective treatment. Patients are refractory to standard treatments during active phases of the rebound phenomenon. Successful discontinuance of the offending agent may itself result in a substantial reduction in the frequency of headache, although initially a marked increase in headache intensity may occur (the rebound effect) before response to treatment or spontaneous improvement occurs.

B. Endocrine Disturbances

Endocrine factors, including estrogen replacement or the use of oral contraceptives, for example, may contribute to prolonged, protracted migraine. Similarly, progesterone products, including the "depo" (sustained release) forms, appear likely to aggravate migraine conditions.

C. The Presence of Disease (see Chapter 5)

The presence of comorbid intracranial, cranial, cervical, or systemic disease, particularly if the peripheral pathways of the trigeminal system or the occipitocervical junction are involved, can be a major factor contributing to acute, intractable headache. Table 9.1 lists selected disorders that can manifest as persisting or acute headache, at times mimicking persistent, intractable migraine (see Chapter 5 for discussion of the differential diagnosis of headache).

D. Head Injury

See Chapter 13 for discussion on post-traumatic headache.

E. Severe, Intense Psychological Duress

F. *Intractable Migraine* without Apparent Cause

Intractable migraine occasionally develops without apparent aggravating influence and probably reflects intrinsic physiological mechanisms.

III. Choosing the Proper Setting for Treatment

Patients with *acute, intractable migraine* may sometimes benefit from aggressive outpatient services, including emergency department therapy, but frequently require hospitalization for acute treatment. The decision to treat patients through the emergency department vs. hospitalization is based on several variables.

A. Clinical Variables That Determine Treatment Setting

While there is pressure to treat patients on an outpatient rather than an inpatient basis, it must be emphasized that unless pain is

TABLE 9.1.   **SELECTED CONDITIONS THAT MIMIC MIGRAINE OR INDUCE PERSISTENT HEADACHE**

Sphenoid sinusitis
Arnold Chiari malformation
Internal carotid dissection
Temporal arteritis
Intracranial hypertension
Intracranial hypotension
Cerebral venous occlusion
CNS infection, infiltrative disease
Toxic/metabolic disturbances
Facet joint syndrome
Hormonal disturbances
Occult dental disorders
Glaucoma
Connective tissue disorders

responsibly controlled, continued high-cost utilization and recurring use of offending medication are likely to result in even higher costs. Thus, the sooner effective care can be administered in any setting, the greater the long-term savings will be. The following clinical variables and conditions can be used to determine the most appropriate setting for care:

1. The intensity and duration of pain;
2. The presence and intensity of toxicity, "rebound," or dependency (physiological and/or psychological);
3. The "addiction" potential of excessively used drugs (predicts the difficulty of discontinuance and likelihood of withdrawal symptoms);
4. The patient's drug dependency profile;
5. Capacity of the patient to cope with pain on an outpatient basis as treatment trials are undertaken;
6. Anticipated difficulty of establishing a preventive program;
7. Need for supportive measures
   a. Fluids
   b. Repetitive parenteral pain control treatment
   c. Treatment of withdrawal symptoms (nausea and vomiting, seizures from barbiturate withdrawal, muscle cramps, diarrhea, and abdominal pain from narcotic withdrawal, etc.);
8. The presence of complicating medical problems, including
   a. Moderate to severe cardiac disease
   b. CNS disorders, including seizures and others listed in Table 9.1
   c. Severe hypertension/hypotension

d. Severe peripheral vascular disorders
e. Serotonin syndrome (see Chapter 7)
f. Others; and

9. Moderate to severe psychological and behavioral health disorders confounding treatment on an outpatient basis.

B. Emergency Department Treatment

Emergency department service is appropriate in the following circumstances:

1. To treat moderate to severe headache that is *unaccompanied* by drug toxicity, dependency, or rebound, since these conditions, if present, will continue to provoke subsequent attacks until treated more specifically;
2. To rapidly rule out accompanying severe neurological or medical illness (subarachnoid hemorrhage, acute sphenoid sinusitis, etc.); and,
3. When headaches are associated with a suicidal potential (suicidal risk evaluation is necessary).

Emergency department treatment is less suitable when headaches are accompanied by:

1. Dehydration, electrolyte depletion, and/or hypotension, which require prolonged therapy or sustained monitoring;
2. Toxic/rebound or dependency states, requiring days to weeks to resolve (patients with intense rebound syndromes or drug dependency patterns can rarely be detoxified or effectively treated on an outpatient basis due to the intensification of headache during the process of withdrawal);
3. Intractable nausea, vomiting, or diarrhea, requiring many hours or days to treat and that may recur;
4. Concurrent medical illness influencing or limiting the sustained effective treatment of headache;
5. The likelihood of delayed withdrawal phenomena, with potential for marked increase in pain, seizures, diarrhea, leg and abdominal cramps, etc.;
6. A pattern of multiple emergency department treatments; and
7. The likelihood that emergency services will not be able to address the headache patient's needs promptly and effectively.

Although emergency department treatment for acute headache is improving, historically it has been suboptimal. Cynical treatment and delay in treatment still characterize the experience of many headache patients in emergency departments, no matter how ill they are. While narcotic administration may be appropriate in certain circumstances, it is not appropriate in others. In fact, a pattern of repetitive use of certain opioid treatments, particularly meperidine, even when no more frequent than approximately *once a week*, can induce a pattern of *delayed "rebound,"* in which the continued administration of the meperidine results in the "rebound" syndrome. Unfortunately, emergency department physicians are often distracted by "more serious" problems and resort to short-term palliation and by so doing inadvertently sustain confounding factors. Although in some circumstances it is necessary to administer opioid medications for the treatment of acute headache, the availability of more appropriate and effective agents, such as dihydroergotamine, injectable sumatriptan, parenteral neuroleptics, parenteral ketorolac, and others, make these alternatives far more appropriate in most, but not all, instances.

C. Hospitalization (also see Chapter 11)

The following are among the criteria justifying admission to the hospital or a similar acute care setting. Some patients require but a few days to "break" the cycle and correct the treatable disturbances. Intermittent headaches generally follow. Other patients, however, require a more lengthy stay. These patients generally have a long history of sustained severe daily headache, usually suffer from severely confounding comorbid disease, and will, for a variety of reasons, fail to respond to short-term interventions. Because of the severity of their symptoms, outpatient treatment is generally unsuitable, and without sufficient controls, patients will resort to the re-use of offending treatments and other desperate actions. Long-term success and effective outcome results (see Chapter 2) require sustained headache reduction, appropriate confrontation of behavioral and related phenomena, and implementation of suitable headache relief methods. Currently under development is a 3-phase treatment concept, whereby after a short acute care stay, the patient is "stepped down" to subacute level care and subsequently to a day care treatment concept. This may provide the most cost-effective means to effectively treat extreme cases of intractable headache. Outcome results from tertiary care headache programs are discussed in Chapter 2 and demonstrate the likely cost effectiveness and potential long-term savings that can result from appropriate treatment of this complex population.

The criteria for hospitalization include the following:

1. The presence of moderate to severe, intractable headache that fails to respond to appropriate and aggressive outpatient or

emergency department measures and requires repetitive, sustained parenteral treatment (e.g., DHE, etc.);

2. The presence of continuing nausea, vomiting, or diarrhea;
3. The need to detoxify and treat toxicity, dependency, or rebound phenomena and/or monitor protectively against withdrawal symptoms, including seizures, in cases in which this cannot be achieved effectively or safely on an outpatient basis;
4. The presence of dehydration, electrolyte imbalance, and prostration that requires monitoring and intravenous fluids;
5. The presence of unstable vital signs;
6. The presence of repeated, previous emergency department treatments;
7. The likely presence of serious disease (e.g., SAH, intracranial infection, cerebral ischemia, severe hypertension, etc.);
8. The need to rapidly develop both immediate pain reduction and an effective pharmacological prophylaxis in order to sustain improvement achieved by parenteral therapy (aggressive daily drug manipulation, requiring careful monitoring and drug level evaluation);
9. The necessity to urgently address other comorbid conditions contributing to or accompanying the headache, including medical and/or psychological illness; and
10. The presence of concurrent medical and/or psychological illnesses requiring careful monitoring in high- risk situations.

IV. Protocols for Managing Acute, Intractable Migraine
A. General Measures

1. Assess vital signs;
2. Rule out organic disease;
3. Monitor;
4. Carefully assess for the presence of dehydration and replace fluids and electrolytes as necessary;
5. Treat nausea, vomiting, and diarrhea; control blood pressure if necessary;
6. Discontinue offending medications (if withdrawal is likely, appropriate measures should be undertaken);
7. Implement acute parenteral pain management (to be discussed);
8. When appropriate, gradually implement preventive measures to achieve pain control after acute care is terminated;
9. Identify appropriate outpatient symptomatic (abortive, acute) treatments for use after discharge to assure compliance and reduce anxiety and recidivism when periodic attacks occur;

10. When appropriate, refer for psychological and behavioral evaluation and treatment, family counseling, drug overuse treatment, etc. Address obsessive drug-taking patterns when present; and

11. Instruct patient and family in the use of treatments and self-help measures to avoid future hospitalizations.

B. Parenteral Protocols
1. General measures

a. Inform patient of procedure, risks, and advantages;
b. Establish baseline vital signs;
c. Perform and review baseline electrocardiogram;
d. Establish peripheral IV access;
e. Consider administering "piggy-back" or have available IV fluids for emergency needs;
f. Following administration, monitor vital signs during the first hour and as appropriate thereafter; and
g. Establish availability of emergency equipment and personnel.

2. Choose from among the following parenteral protocols:

a. General measures: vital signs, rule out comorbid disease, ECG, etc.
b. Parenteral treatments

1) Intramuscular or intravenous DHE (see protocol)
2) Intramuscular ketorolac
3) Subcutaneous sumatriptan
4) Intravenous neuroleptics/antiemetics
5) Parenteral opioids
6) Intravenous steroids
   (Please see Chapter 6 for further details on these protocols.)

3. Specific protocols (see Chapter 6 for additional details):

a. Intravenous DHE (see Figure 9.1, Table 9.2)
b. Intravenous neuroleptics (must monitor carefully for orthostatic hypotension and other adverse effects for several hours post-administration; administer IV diphenhydramine if *acute dystonic reactions occur*)

1) Chlorpromazine
   i. 7.5–20 mg chlorpromazine (Thorazine)

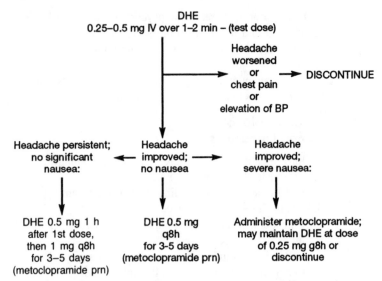

Figure 9.1. Algorithm for IV DHE administration

TABLE 9.2. **INTRAVENOUS PROTOCOL FOR DIHYDROERGOTAMINE ADMINISTRATION**

A. Protocol
   1. 0.25–0.5 mg IV "push" (test dose), over 2 minutes via heparin lock apparatus. (Do not administer in presence of moderate or greater hypertension.)
   2. If tolerated, DHE 0.5–1 mg IV "push" q 8 hours.
   3. Administer 10 mg metoclopramide (IV[a] or IM) before DHE administration, if nausea occurs.
   4. Maintain for 3–5 days, if tolerated. May repeat program one time.
B. Guidelines for Use
   1. Administer metoclopramide before or with DHE administration if necessary to control nausea. Discontinue if not necessary.
   2. DHE to be administered via 1–2 minute slow "push."
   3. Most patients stabilize at end of day 3, but extension of program for 2–3 more days may be necessary.
   4. Discontinue DHE via a 1–3 day gradual reduction program if patient is pain-free for 2 days.
   5. Hospitalization is most appropriate for sustained therapy, during which careful monitoring for blood pressure elevation, chest pain, severe nausea, etc. can be carried out and necessary concurrent therapies can be administered, including establishment of an effective preventive program.
   6. Discontinue or substantially reduce dose if significant elevation of blood pressure, severe nausea, chest pain, severe leg cramps, or other significant adverse reactions occur.

[a]10 mg slow "IV push" or in 50 cc 5% dextrose in water (D5W) over 20–30 minutes.

      ii. In 25–50 cc saline "drip" or slow "push" (over 2 minutes)

     iii. b.i.d.–t.i.d.; administer as needed

  2) Prochlorperazine (Compazine)

      i. 10 mg prochlorperazine (Compazine)

     ii. In 25–50 cc saline "drip" or slow "push" (over 2 minutes)

    iii. b.i.d.–t.i.d.; administer as needed

c. Parenteral ketorolac

  1) 30 mg IM t.i.d.

  2) 3-day regimen for intractable headache

Ketorolac therapy imposes a risk to renal function and should not be used in those with significant renal risk factors, including those with severe dehydration, renovascular disease, diabetes, or in the elderly. Restrict use to a 3-day regimen.

d. Hydrocortisone

  1) 100 mg hydrocortisone intravenous "push" (2 cc)

  2) q 6 hr for 24 hr

  3) q 8 hr for 24 hr

  4) q 12 hr for 24 hr

This drug should be used restrictively because of potential adverse events, including avascular necrosis of bone. The clinical need, total amount of steroids previously administered, and frequency of use are important considerations in determining usage and length of administration. Carefully review for the presence of infection and other contraindications.

C. Other Measures

Treatment of severe nausea and vomiting is performed via the standard use of antinauseants (see Chapter 6).

D. Referral to Tertiary (Quaternary) Centers

While many patients with straightforward and even complex headache conditions will respond to primary care outpatient therapy utilizing appropriate interventions, many patients with severely intractable conditions require more advanced and sustained outpatient and/or inpatient intervention. The following are recommended criteria for referral to tertiary centers of care for headache (see Chapter 2 for concepts regarding the stratification of headache care):

a. Intractable cases failing to respond to standard treatments provided at primary and secondary levels of care;
b. Patients unable to refrain from the excessive use of symptomatic medications that contribute to persisting pain (rebound);
c. Patients with medical illnesses (comorbid disease) that confound and/or complicate the treatment of headache;
d. Patients in whom behavioral and psychological factors are interwoven and enmeshed with the headache disorder, such that standard primary and secondary treatment interventions are not alone likely to produce beneficial results;
e. Patients who require a combination of detoxification, headache interruption, and the development of preventive programming such that standard primary and secondary treatment is unlikely to provide the adequate pace or intensity of treatment necessary to achieve maximal results;
f. Cases of headache that require comprehensive, team-oriented, coordinated, interdisciplinary intervention; and,
g. Persistent headache that requires advanced diagnostic and treatment services not generally found at primary and secondary levels of care.

E. Conclusion

The effective and safe treatment of intractable headache requires commitment and experience. Patients are often physiologically at risk and emotionally distraught. The appropriate setting of care for the case at hand must be determined using reasonable criteria. The implementation of treatment must occur in an inpatient setting when outpatient or emergency department services are either inadequate or unlikely to address complicating and confounding factors that are present. Referral to tertiary centers of care is required in selected cases.

The reader is referred to Chapters 2 and 11 for further discussion of hospitalization, criteria for hospitalization, comprehensive care concepts, treatment of medication overuse, and the treatment of daily chronic headache (Chapter 11).

References

Baumgartner CP, Wesseley P, Bingol C, et al. Long-term prognosis of analgesic withdrawal in patients with drug-induced headache. *Headache,* 29:510–514, 1989.

Belegrade MJ, Ling LJ, Schleevogt MB, et al. Comparison of single dose meperidine, butorphanol, and dihydroergotamine in treatment of vascular headache. *Neurology,* 39:590–592, 1989.

Bell R, Montoya D, Shuaib A, et al. A comparative trial of three agents in the treatment of acute migraine headache. *Am J Emerg Med,* 19:1079–1082, 1990.

Callaham M, Raskin NH. A controlled study of dihydroergotamine in the treatment of acute migraine headache. *Headache,* 26:168–171, 1986.

Diener HC, Dichgans J, Scholz E, et al. Analgesic-induced chronic headache: Long-term results of withdrawal therapy. *J Neurol,* 236:9–14, 1989.

Diener HC, Tfelt-Hansen P. Headache associated with chronic use of substances. (In) *The Headaches.* J Olesen, P Tfelt-Hansen, KMA Welch (Eds). Pg 721, New York, Raven Press, 1993.

Edmeads J. Emergency management of headache. *Headache,* 28:675–679, 1988.

Hering R, Steiner TJ. Abrupt outpatient withdrawal from medication in analgesic-abusing migraineurs. *Lancet,* 337:1442, 1991.

Jones J, Sklar D, Dogherty J, et al. Randomized double-blind trial of intravenous prochlorperazine for the treatment of acute headache. *JAMA,* 261:1174–1176, 1989.

Lake AE, Saper JR, et al. Inpatient treatment for chronic daily headache: A prospective long-term outcome study. *Headache,* 30:299, 1990.

Lipton RB, Lowenkopf T, Bajwa ZH, et al. Cardiac cephalgia: A treatable form of exertional headache. *Neurology,* 49:813–816, 1997.

Mathew NT, Stubbits E, Nigam MR. Transformation of episodic migraine into daily headache: Analysis of factors. *Headache,* 22:66, 1982.

Neuman M, Demarez JP, Harmer JR, et al. Prevention of migraine attacks through use of dihydroergotamine. *Int J Clin Pharmacol Res,* 6:11–13, 1986.

Rapoport A, Weeks R, Sheftell F, et al. Analgesic rebound headache: Theoretical and practical implications. *Cephalalgia,* 5(supp 3):448–450, 1985.

Rapoport AM, Weeks RE, Sheftell FD, et al. The "analgesic washout period": A critical variability in the evaluation of headache treatment efficacy. *Neurology,* 36(suppl 1):100, 1986.

Rapoport AM, Silberstein SD. Emergency treatment of headache. *Neurology,* 42(3 suppl 2):43–44, 1992.

Raskin NH. Repetitive intravenous dihydroergotamine as therapy for intractable migraine. *Neurology,* 36:995–997, 1986.

Saper JR, Jones JM. Ergotamine tartrate dependency: Features and possible mechanisms. *Clin Neuropharmacol,* 9:244–256, 1986.

Schnider P, Aull S, Baumgartner C, et al. Long-term outcome of patients with headache and drug abuse after inpatient withdrawal: 5-year follow-up. *Cephalalgia,* 16:481–485, 1996.

Silberstein SD, Schulman EA, Hopkins MM. Repetitive intravenous DHE in the treatment of refractory headache. *Headache,* 30:334–339, 1990.

Silberstein SD, Silberstein JR. Analgesic/ergotamine rebound headache: Prognosis following detoxification and treatment with repetitive IV DHE. *Headache,* 32:352, 1992.

10

Episodic Tension-Type Headache

I. Introduction

In the past, *tension headache* was a poorly defined disorder that was attributed to muscle contraction and various degrees of psychopathology. It was not clearly distinguished from migraine. Both conditions may be associated with bilateral pain and occasionally accompanied by the same clinical features, such as nausea, vomiting, and photosensitivity; aggravated and provoked by many of the same stimuli; have the same male to female ratio and hereditary pattern; and are treated effectively by many of the same medications.

Moreover, epidemiological studies have failed to identify features that could distinguish "tension headache" from migraine on clinical or physiological grounds. The inability to clearly differentiate these two headache types on clinical, epidemiological, therapeutic, and diagnostic grounds has led some authorities to believe that indeed they may reflect the same pathophysiological disturbance and should not be considered separately. Some authorities have suggested that they may simply represent different points on a broad clinical continuum with migraine at one end and tension or tension-like headache at the other (Raskin, 1988).

After considerable debate and controversy, the International Headache Society's (IHS) classification employed the term *tension-type headache* (TTH) for what was previously called *tension headache, muscle contraction headache, stress headache,* and *ordinary headache* (see Table 10.1.) Moreover, the IHS classification has subdivided TTH into episodic and chronic forms. It has also subdivided the entity into whether or not attacks are associated with tenderness of pericranial musculature, and also separated the entity according to provocative factors. The IHS effort underscores the absence of recognized etiology and precisely defined manifestations.

Because of the significant uncertainty regarding most aspects of this disorder and the strong differences of opinion that prevail, the authors of this book have decided against a detailed review of this entity. The reader is encouraged to review more detailed considerations of this topic. This chapter mainly addresses the episodic form of TTH. The chronic form will be discussed in Chapter 11.

Episodic TTH is distinguished from the chronic form primarily by frequency of attacks. The episodic form occurs no more than 15 days per month, while the chronic form occurs more than 15 days per

TABLE 10.1. **NEW INTERNATIONAL HEADACHE SOCIETY DEFINITION OF TENSION-TYPE HEADACHE**[a]

2.1 *Episodic tension-type headache*
Previously used terms: tension headache, muscle contraction headache, psychomyogenic headache, stress headache, ordinary headache, essential headache, idiopathic headache, and psychogenic headache
Diagnostic criteria:
  A. At least 10 previous headache episodes fulfilling criteria B–D listed below. Number of days with such headache < 180/year (< 15/month)
  B. Headache lasting from 30 minutes to 7 days
  C. At least two of the following pain characteristics:
    1. Pressing/tightening (non-pulsating) quality
    2. Mild or moderate intensity (may inhibit, but does not prohibit activities)
    3. Bilateral location
    4. No aggravation by walking stairs or similar routine physical activity
  D. Both of the following:
    1. No nausea or vomiting (anorexia may occur)
    2. Photophobia and phonophobia are absent, or one but not the other is present
  E. At least one of the following:
    1. History, physical, and neurological examinations do not suggest one of the disorders listed in group 5–11
    2. History and/or physical and/or neurological examinations do suggest such disorder, but it is ruled out by appropriate investigations
    3. Such disorder is present, but tension-type headache does not occur for the first time in close temporal relation to the disorder

2.1.1 *Episodic tension-type headache associated with disorder of pericranial muscles*
Previously used terms: muscle contraction headache
Diagnostic criteria:
  A. Fulfills criteria for 2.1
  B. At least one of the following:
    1. Increased tenderness of pericranial muscles demonstrated by manual palpation of pressure algomater
    2. Increased EMG level of pericranial muscles at rest or during physiological tests

2.1.2 *Episodic tension-type headache unassociated with disorder of pericranial muscles*
Previously used terms: idiopathic headache, essential headache, psychogenic headache
Diagnosis criteria:
  A. Fulfills criteria for 2.1
  B. No increased tenderness of pericranial muscles, if studied; EMG of pericranial muscles shows normal levels of activity

2.2 *Chronic tension-type headache*
Previously used terms: chronic daily headache
Diagnostic criteria:
  A. Average headache frequency 15 days/month (180 days/year) for 6 months fulfilling criteria B–D
  B. At least two of the following pain characteristics:
    1. Pressing/tightening quality
    2. Mild or moderate severity (may inhibit but does not prohibit activities)
    3. Bilateral locations
    4. No aggravations by walking stairs or similar routine physical activity
  C. Both of the following:
    1. No vomiting
    2. No more than one of the following: Nausea, photophobia, or phonophobia

continued

TABLE 10.1. **NEW INTERNATIONAL HEADACHE SOCIETY DEFINITION OF TENSION-TYPE HEADACHE**[a]

D. At least one of the following:
 1. History, physical, and neurological examinations do not suggest one of the disorders listed in groups 5–11
 2. History and/or physical and/or neurological examinations do suggest such disorder, but it is ruled out by appropriate investigations
 3. Such disorder is present, but tension-type headache does not occur for the first time in close temporal relation to the disorder

2.2.1 *Chronic tension-type headache associated with disorder of pericranial muscles*

2.2.2 *Chronic tension type headache unassociated with disorder of pericranial muscles*

[a]From Headache Classification Committee of the International Headache Society. Classification and diagnostic criteria for headache disorders, cranial neuralgias, and facial pain. *Cephalalgia* 1988, 8 (Suppl 7):1–96, 1988.

month. The chronic form may be associated with nausea as an isolated associate symptom, further blurring the distinctions between TTH and migraine.

According to some authors, episodic TTH may be two distinct disorders. When it occurs in patients who also suffer migraine, it is often migrainous-like, having some migraine features. It may be nothing more than a mild case of migraine. When episodic TTH occurs in patients without migraine, it may have less migrainous features and may be more easily distinguished. The "spectrum" concept may be best applied as a concept that applies to the range of headache of a given individual, rather than as a range of inter-related headaches. These distinctions will eventually be delineated more definitively as more research and diagnostic detail emerge.

II. Symptom Overview

Episodic TTH has neither a prodrome nor aura. The pain is usually dull and band-like, mild to moderate in severity, and nonpulsatile. Pain intensity often increases with attack frequency. Most patients have bilateral pain, but unilateral headache occurs in up to 20% of patients. Episodic TTH does not usually interfere with daily activities, and physical activity usually has no influence on the headache. Some patients feel soreness in their neck or cranial musculature, but studies of muscle do not reliably demonstrate increased muscle contraction, as has been assumed historically.

Episodic TTH usually responds to treatments appropriate for migraine, both pharmacological and nonpharmacological. Specific antimigraine medication, such as DHE and the triptans, may effectively treat the condition.

The possible relationship between fibromyalgia and TTH is a curious one. Further study may provide the basis for a better understanding of each of these two entities and any linkages, as well as shed light on the relationship between fibromyalgia and temporomandibular disorders.

In the next chapter, Chapter 11, transformational migraine, chronic TTH, and chronic daily headache will be reviewed. The reader is referred to a scholarly review of the topic of TTH by Schoenen and Wang, in *Headache* (Goadsby and Silberstein, 1997).

References

Drummond PD. Scalp tenderness and sensitivity to pain in migraine and tension headache. *Headache,* 27:45–50, 1987.

Goebel H, Weigle L, Kropp P, et al. Pain sensitivity and pain reactivity of pericranial muscles in migraine and tension-type headache. *Cephalalgia,* 12:142–151, 1992.

Hatch JP, Moore PJ, Cyr-Provost M, et al. The use of electromyography and muscle palpation in the diagnosis of tension-type headache with and without pericranial muscle involvement. *Pain,* 49:175–178, 1992.

Iversen HK, Langemark M, Andersson PG, et al. Clinical characteristics of migraine and tension-type headache in relationship to new and old diagnostic criteria. *Headache,* 30:514–519, 1990.

Jensen R, Paiva T. Episodic tension-type headache. (In) *The Headaches.* J Olesen, P Tfelt-Hansen, KMA Welch (Eds). Pgs 497–502, New York, Raven Press Ltd., 1993.

Jensen R, Rasmussen BK, Olesen J. Cephalic muscle tenderness and pain threshold in headache: A population study. *Pain,* 52:193–199, 1993.

Raskin NH. Tension headache. (In) *Headache.* 2nd edition. Pgs 215–228, New York, Churchill-Livingstone, 1988.

Rasmussen BK. Migraine and tension-type headache in a general population: Precipitating factors, female hormones, sleep pattern, and relation to lifestyle. *Pain,* 53:65–72, 1993.

Schoenen J, Wang W. Tension-type headache. (In) *Headache.* PJ Goadsby, SD Silberstein (Eds). Pgs 177–200, Boston, Butterworth-Heinemeann, 1997.

11

Daily Chronic Headache: Transformational Migraine and Others

I. Introduction

This chapter focuses on headaches that occur in a daily or almost daily pattern *and* that the authors believe most often reflect the clinical manifestations and variations of migraine or migraine-like headaches. Many cases of daily or almost daily headache will have progressed from periodic, acute migraine patterns. Others will have begun with this persistent pattern (new-onset daily headache).

Admittedly, the term *daily chronic headache* (DCH) is seriously inadequate and confusing. Taken literally, the term would include *any* headache, from whatever origin, that occurs daily or almost daily. Thus, it could be used to describe *organic* headache disorders, as well as a variety of other headache syndromes that produce daily head, neck, or face pain.

The classification of chronic daily headache is still controversial. To the authors of this text, the term refers to a *primary headache syndrome* (organic causes of daily headache must be excluded). The condition occurs more frequently than 15 days a month and lasts longer than 4 hours a day (to exclude chronic cluster headache). The International Headache Society (IHS) classification (see Chapter 10, Table 10.1) suggests that the term *chronic tension-type headache* be substituted for *daily chronic headache*. DCH can be arbitrarily subdivided into the following categories:

1. Transformed migraine (TM), with or without medication overuse;
2. Chronic tension-type headache (chronic TTH), with or without medication overuse;
3. New daily, persistent headache (NDPH), with or without medication overuse; and,
4. Hemicrania continua (HC), with or without medication overuse (see Chapter 15).

Daily headaches associated with organic disease or of traumatic origin will be discussed elsewhere in this text. HC will be discussed in Chapter 15. This chapter will focus on migraine and its progression to DCH.

II. Transformational Migraine (progressive migraine, etc.)
A. Definition of Transformational Migraine

Transformational migraine specifically refers to the presence of periodic, acute migraine that over time "transforms" or progresses to a more frequent and then continuous or almost continuous pattern, with superimposed acute attacks. Graham (1968) made the original observation that migraine could progress from intermittent to daily, prompted sometimes by dependency on ergotamine tartrate.

While drug provocation (rebound) is often present and likely to influence or prompt the progression to almost daily headache, drug-induced factors are not always to blame, sometimes being a secondary phenomenon. The transformation of migraine may reflect a variety of other physiological influences, including genetic, psychological, internal or external physiological events (i.e., hormonal), or traumatic mechanisms, among others. Transformation (progression) may be the natural pattern of the illness, not necessarily induced by external, controllable factors.

The term "transformational migraine" is credited to Mathew (1982), although other authors, including Graham (1968) and Saper (1982), had observed the evolutive nature of migraine prior to that time.

B. Clinical Features of Transformational Migraine

The clinical features of transformational migraine are listed in Table 11.1. In general, most patients begin their headache years with intermittent, occasional attacks of migraine or migraine-like headaches. Generally, after an interim period of 5–10 years and between the ages of 25 and 40, individuals will begin to experience an increase in headache frequency. The headaches will become daily or almost daily, and will generally be mild to moder-

---

TABLE 11.1.   **CLINICAL FEATURES OF TRANSFORMATIONAL MIGRAINE**

Intermittent migraine by age 20–30 years
Between ages 25 and 40, gradual increase in headache frequency
Daily or almost daily mild to moderate head, neck, or face pain
Periodic acute severe attacks of migraine, at varying frequency
Frequently occurring accompaniments:
• Sleep disturbance
• Overuse of analgesics or ergotamine tartrate
• Anxiety/depressive states
• Reduction of quality of life and activities of daily living
• A family history of headaches
• A family history of substance overuse, anxiety, or depressive states

ate in severity. Head, neck, or face pain may dominate. A sense of tight neck muscles and tenderness in the trapezii are common. Periodically, acute, severe attacks of migraine will occur at varying frequencies ranging from two or more per week to monthly or less. In addition, frequently accompanying comorbid illness is present. Sleep disturbance, overuse of analgesics or ergotamine tartrate, anxiety and depressive states, and general deterioration in the quality of life are common. An ever-increasing effort to obtain sufficient medication to control symptoms and a progressive sense of desperation are common features.

Early studies (Saper, 1982) suggest that two-thirds of patients with daily chronic headache that had progressed from intermittent migraine were depressed, had sleep disturbances, overused medication, and often had a similar family history. Since that time, additional studies have established the presence of these and other comorbid conditions, which appear more likely than by chance alone to accompany migraine. In Chapter 8, an additional discussion of the comorbidities associated with migraine and its variants can be found. Although uncertain, it seems that these comorbidities, particularly depression, anxiety disorders, and other neuropsychiatric conditions, are more likely in those patients with DCH of transformational migraine than with episodic migraine alone. As with migraine, a female predominance exists.

III. Diagnostic Studies

There are no diagnostic studies to establish the diagnosis of DCH as a form of migraine. Because of the daily pattern, however, it is imperative to rule out head and neck organic pathology, including intracranial obstructive disease, dental disease, sphenoid sinusitis, CNS ischemia, vasculitis, intracranial infection, cervical pathology, systemic disease, and many others (see Chapters 5 and 13–19).

IV. Principles of Treatment

The principles of treatment for DCH can be found in Table 11.2.

V. Specifics of Treatment
A. Nonmedical Treatment
1. Introduction

Nonmedical treatment begins by identifying and removing any external factor that can provoke or aggravate headaches and implementing appropriate adjustments. Biofeedback, stress management, cognitive therapy, family therapy, substance overuse counseling, life-style changes, exercise, and

TABLE 11.2. **PRINCIPLES OF TREATMENT OF DAILY CHRONIC HEADACHE (PROGRESSIVE MIGRAINE)**

Proper diagnosis (rule out structural, organic disease and treat accordingly, if found)
Reduction of aggravating factors
Reduction of analgesics, the triptans, or ergotamine tartrate overuse
Implementation of nonpharmacological treatment (see below).
• Lifestyle changes
• Discontinue smoking
• Regular eating and sleeping patterns
• Exercise
• Etc.
Implementation of pharmacotherapy (preventive and sumptomatic)
Treatment of neuropsychiatric, comorbid, and behavioral disturbances that occur as a
  consequence or coexist, and aggravate the condition or inhibit improvement
Assessment of life-style changes, family dynamics, and other factors that might have
  occurred as a consequence or coexist, and aggravate the condition or inhibit
  improvement
Education of patients and family regarding the chronic nature of this entity, establishing
  reasonable expectations and limitations

other health-related adjustments are important and perhaps essential interventions that can be critically helpful in some individuals.

2. Psychotherapy, biofeedback, cognitive, and behavioral treatments

If nothing else, patients with frequent pain need support, understanding, and sometimes expressive behavioral or other psychotherapeutic interventions. However, within the population of headache sufferers there are those individuals with clearly evident psychiatric, stressful, and/or behavioral disturbances that markedly contribute to, occur as a response to, or represent psychobiological, comorbid accompaniments to the primary headache problem. The comorbid accompaniments may be disturbances that share or are related to the same fundamental pathogenetic mechanisms common to the primary headaches of a migraine or transformed migraine type. Whatever their origin, the presence of these psychiatric, psychosocial, and behavioral disturbances requires proper evaluation and treatment, and successful therapy of these problems may be key to headache control.

Psychotherapy and behavioral treatment alone are rarely adequate to control troublesome headaches and should be undertaken within the framework of a broad, comprehensive therapeutic approach that includes pharmacotherapy. Many patients with severe headaches improve psychologically when proper treatment for headaches is achieved. Others cannot gain control over their headaches *until* psychological and behavioral factors are effectively addressed. Although occasionally patients with severe headaches benefit from psychotherapy alone, most often a combined and comprehensive pharmacological and nonpharmacological approach is required.

Biofeedback, stress management, and behavioral/cognitive therapies do help many patients with headache, including those without psychological problems or evident distress, and do provide primary, effective intervention. These therapies also serve as adjunctive interventions in patients with frequent headaches who require medicines. Use of these therapies is recommended whenever the clinical need is present. They should be administered by well-trained professionals with experience in treating headache disorders.

Among the patients who suffer from DCH are those who also suffer significant neuropsychiatric phenomena beyond those that more typically accompany migraine. It is increasingly apparent that many of the most difficult to manage headache patients experience features of one or more personality disorders or Axis II conditions (Diagnostic and Statistical Manual of Mental Disorders [DSM-IV]). The most troublesome of these is the Borderline Personality Disorder. This condition, and its relationship to headaches, is discussed more completely in Chapter 20.

B. Pharmacotherapy
1. Symptomatic treatment

The treatment of DCH consists of the use of symptomatic medications for acute episodic migraine attacks and preventive migraine therapy for persistent headache (see Chapters 6, 8, and 9).

2. Preventive treatment

Antidepressants. Amitriptyline (Elavil, Endep) and nortriptyline (Pamelor, Aventyl) are currently the most widely used TCAs to treat daily chronic headache. Fluoxetine (Prozac) and other SSRIs are widely used but not well established as effective agents. MAO inhibitors and strategic cotherapy may be required.

β-adrenergic blockers

Calcium channel antagonists

Ergot derivatives (methysergide, methylergonovine)

Anticonvulsants (particularly valproate)

C. Medication Overuse (see Chapters 6, 8, and 9 for further discussion on rebound)

Medication overuse (related to rebound or not) is widespread in the headache population, but this often reflects the absence of adequate, more appropriate therapy and should not be interpreted in and of itself as indicative of a primary addictive disorder.

While many medications can cause physical and psychological dependency, many experts believe that true *addictive disease* is quite rare in the headache population. Addictive disease is best defined as physical and psychological dependency accompanied by severe, devious acts of drug seeking, hoarding, inappropriate use, and use beyond the control of pain or other primary symptoms, illicit activity, and other antisocial behaviors. Overuse or rebound phenomena, even if severe, are alone not indicative of addictive disease in this sense. Many patients who have been inadequately treated will desperately seek effective self-treatment for relief and control of their pain and functional limitations. Many could not perform their duties without these medications, and the overuse and multisourcing may be *adaptive* efforts to maintain some semblance of a normal existence. Physical and psychological dependence can occur, and inappropriate behaviors, which must be addressed clinically, are often present. However, the primary impetus for this is a desperate quest for pain control at any cost. These behaviors must thus be seen in this perspective.

Personality disorders (see Chapter 20) and primary addictive disease are present in some patients with headache. The clinician must distinguish between these cases and those in which *inadequately* treated headaches lead to desperate and inappropriate behavior, including overusage. In this case, the behavior is prompted by the need to control pain or the fear of pain, a term referred to as *cephalgiaphobia*. These individuals require aggressive intervention to address the pain, the behavior, and the complex dynamics that often confound the clinical circumstances. In some ways these individuals are "victims" of the headache disorder and should be treated without needless labeling and harmful prejudice.

Existing terms for drug overuse do not reflect the individual's motivation to overuse medications, which includes the inadequacy of care that may prompt desperate and unreasonable use of medications. The terms *substance overuse* and *substance misuse* may be more appropriate terms for patients who are painful. *Substance overuse* (SO) is nonpejorative and reflects the use of medication which exceeds recommended limits. It implies that the medication is used solely for pain control and that in other ways compliance and behavior are acceptable. With effective pain control, medications are used responsibly. The term *substance misuse* (SM) is likewise motivated by the need to control pain but implies circumstances in which the use of medications is associated with maladaptive and unacceptable behavior. Pain control is still the principal motivator; however, excessive use is confounded by the presence of psychological and behavioral factors which prove troublesome. The distinction between SO and SM is based upon the presence of behavioral disturbances (noncompliance, defiance, multisourcing, obsessive drug-taking, etc.) in SM, whereas these behavioral misadventures and mischief are not present in SO.

In this context, analgesic rebound, for example, could reflect either SO or SM. The distinction would depend upon the presence or absence of attending comorbidities and behaviors. In order for either of the terms to apply, the drug usage *must not* reflect a broader pattern of drug misadventure, nor must it reflect the use of substances beyond the primary purpose of pain control. If the drug usage exceeds these limits, then terms traditionally used to describe substance abuse are more appropriate (see Saper JR and Sheftell F in *The Headaches,* 1998, in press.)

D. Hospitalization

Because of the daily presence of pain, acute episodic attacks, and the frequently associated analgesic or ergotamine overuse patterns in patients with daily headache, hospitalization to address these factors simultaneously may be necessary. Patients are often unwilling or unable to discontinue analgesics in an outpatient setting because of the escalation of pain that predictably follows. Some cannot because of *cephalgiaphobia*. Characteristically, otherwise acceptable treatments are generally ineffective until analgesics, ergotamine tartrate, and sumatriptan (or other triptans) are discontinued and a period of physiological readjustment is established. Excessive drug taking patterns and other aggravating, psychological, and behavioral influences, including disturbed family dynamics, make the simultaneous confrontation of these problems essential for effective management. Admission is justified not simply because of what is done or has to be done, but because of the inability of some patients to withstand the severe pain, which often escalates as adjustment of treatment takes place. This requires aggressive, around-the-clock interventions to speed control, stabilize patients during the withdrawal process, and confront the comorbid and confounding factors that have contributed and at times underlie the intractable nature of the headache process. Outpatient management has already failed in many of these individuals. Moreover, many with complex headache disorders have multifactorial influences aggravating the condition. As it progresses, it becomes more costly to treat and will continue to worsen until aggressive and appropriate services are provided. A rehabilitative model of care is often required to maximize the functional capacity and quality of life potential of these individuals and is available in some tertiary headache centers (see Chapters 2 and 9).

E. Comprehensive Care and Stratification of Care for Headache (see Chapters 2 and 9)

It is increasingly apparent that many patients with chronic headache, of the transformed migraine or other type, are refractory to standard interventions that are provided at a primary or even consulting level. Many of these patients require more advanced and comprehensive services, together with interdisciplinary interventions involving pharmacological, psychological, and rehabilitative models of care. For many patients with difficult and intractable headache conditions, outpatient *and* inpatient services are required, and continuing *maintenance of care* programs are necessary.

The reader is referred to Chapter 9 for a description of criteria, treatment strategies, and hospital management of intractable headache, and further considerations of tertiary care for headache patients.

F. Other Forms of Daily Chronic Headache

This chapter has focused primarily on DCH as it has progressed from intermittent migraine. The reader is reminded that distinguishing between transformational migraine, chronic tension-type headache, and new daily persistent headache is often difficult and arbitrary. Organic disease must be ruled out. Moreover, hemicrania continua, a rare, unilateral, daily headache disorder that uniquely responds to indomethacin (see Chapter 15), also presents with daily headaches.

References

Andrasik F. Psychological and behavioral aspects of chronic headache. (In) *Neurologic Clinics,* NT Mathew (Ed). Pgs 961–976, Saunders, November, 1990.

Baumgartner CP, Wesseley P, Bingol C, et al. Long-term prognosis of analgesic withdrawal in patients with drug-induced headache. *Headache,* 29:510–514, 1989.

Graham JR. Migraine: Clinical aspects. (In) *Handbook of Clinical Neurology,* Volume 5. PJ Vinken, GW Bruyn (Eds). Pgs 45–58, Amsterdam, North Holland Publishing Company, 1968.

Holroyd KA, Andrasik F. A cognitive-behavioral approach to recurrent tension and migraine headache. (In) *Advances in Cognitive-Behavioral Research and Therapy.* PC Kendell (Ed). Pgs 275–320, New York, Academic, 1982.

Kudrow L. Paradoxical effects of frequent analgesic use. *Adv Neurol,* 33:335–341, 1982.

Lake AE III. Relaxation therapy and biofeedback in headache management. (In) *Help for Headaches.* JR Saper (Ed). Pgs 163–182, New York, Warner Books, 1987.

Mathew NT, Reuveni U, Perez F. Transformed or evolutive migraine. *Headache,* 27:102–106, 1987.

Mathew NT. Drug-Induced Headache. (In) *Neurologic Clinics,* NT Mathew (Ed). Pgs 903–912, Philadelphia, WB Saunders, November, 1990.

Mathew NT, Stubits E, Nigam M. Transformation of episodic migraine into daily chronic headache: An analysis of factors. *Headache,* 22:66–68, 1982.

Mathew NT. Transformed migraine, analgesic rebound, and other chronic daily headaches. (In) *Neurologic Clinics,* Volume 15. NT Mathew (Ed). Pgs 167–186, Philadelphia, WB Saunders, 1997.

Rapoport AM, Weeks RE, Sheftell FD, et al. The "analgesic washout period": A critical variable in the evaluation of headache treatment efficacy. *Neurology* (abstract), 36(supp):100–101, 1986.

Saper JR. Changing perspectives in headache treatment. *Clin J Pain,* 2:19–29, 1986.

Saper JR. Ergotamine dependency: A review. *Headache,* 27:435–438, 1987.

Saper JR. Daily chronic headache, tension headache, migraine, and combined headache: The transformation concept. (In) *Drug-Induced Headache.* HC Diener and M Wilkinson (Eds). Berlin, Springer-Verlag, 1988.

Saper JR. Daily chronic headache. *Compr Ther,* 18:6–10, 1992.

Saper JR, Winters M. Chronic "mixed" headaches: Profile and analysis of 100 consecutive patients experiencing daily headache (abstract). *Headache,* 22:145–146, 1982.

Saper JR, Sheftell F. Headache in the abuse-prone individual. (In) *The Headaches, 2nd Edition.* (Eds) J Olesen, P Tfelt-Hansen, KMA Welch. New York: Lippincott-Raven, 1999 (in press).

Solomon S, Lipton RB, Newman LC. Clinical features of chronic daily headache. *Headache,* 32:325–329, 1992.

12

Cluster Headache

I. Introduction

Cluster headache is a devastating, painful affliction. Unlike migraine and daily chronic headache (DCH), this condition primarily affects men. Though each attack is relatively brief (1/2–1 1/2 hours), the pain brings with it fear and desperate behavior in many sufferers.

The term "cluster headache" was originally used to describe the clustering or sequence of bouts of painful attacks that occur from weeks to months at a time and then spontaneously terminate. The headache cycle may return weeks or months later. The interval of quiescence is called the *interim*. It is now recognized that a chronic form of cluster headache exists in which recurring attacks, without interim, occur for years at a time.

The prevalence of cluster headache is reported to be approximately 0.1–0.3% of the population, though some estimates are higher. The attacks can begin at any age, although they usually occur between the ages of 20 and 40 years. A family history of cluster headache is occasionally present (as well as an increased prevalence of migraine).

II. Key Clinical Features

Cluster headache is a periodic (30–90 minute) attack of severe pain, primarily localized to the eye, temple, forehead, or cheek region. Up to 50% of patients may have focal tenderness in the ipsilateral occipitocervical junction.

Cluster headache occurs predominantly in males, compared with the female to male ratio (3:1) of migraine. The frequency of attacks is 1–6 times per day. Alcohol typically provokes an attack. Most (not all) cluster headache patients are heavy smokers and alcohol drinkers. Attacks frequently occur during sleep or napping times. Each attack of cluster headache is usually accompanied by ipsilateral lacrimation and nasal drainage, lid drooping, pupillary change, and conjunctival injection. The clinical features that distinguish cluster from migraine headache are listed in Table 12.1.

In *episodic (classic) cluster headache,* the bouts of headache last 1–4 months, followed by an interim. In *chronic cluster headache,* in which an interim does not occur, bouts of headache occur for years before termination or remission. The *chronic* form may evolve from the *episodic* form or may have a chronic pattern from its onset. During an attack, patients will characteristically pace, cry, scream, or pound their fists.

TABLE 12.1. **CLINICAL FEATURES DISTINGUISHING BETWEEN CLUSTER AND MIGRAINE HEADACHES**[a]

Feature	Cluster	Migraine
Location of Pain	Always unilateral, periorbital; sometimes occipital referral	Unliteral, bilateral
Age at onset (typical)	Onset 20 years or older	10–50 years (can be younger or older)
Sx incidence	Majority male	Majority female
Occurrence of attacks	Multiple daily attacks for several weeks	Usually 2–5 times per month
Time of day	Frequently at night, often the same time each day	Any time
Number of attacks	1–6 per day	1–10 per month
Duration of pain	30–90 min	4–24 hours
Prodromes	None	Often present
Nausea and vomiting	2–5%	85%
Blurring of vision	Infrequent	Frequent
Lacrimation	Frequent	Infrequent
Nasal congestion	70%	Uncommon
Ptosis	30%	1–2%
Polyuria	2%	40%
Family history of vascular headaches	7%	90%
Miosis	50%	Absent
Behavior during attack	Paces, pounds fist	Rests in quiet, dark room

[a]Modified from Diamond S, Dalessio DG. *The Practicing Physician's Approach to Headache.* Fifth edition. Baltimore: Williams & Wilkins, 1992.

III. Proposed Mechanism

Currently, the exact mechanism of cluster headache remains uncertain. The sphenopalatine ganglion and cavernous sinus are among the sites previously considered potentially important for cluster headache pathogenesis. Most recently, PET scanning techniques have revealed the hypothalamic region as important in cluster headache pathogenesis (May, 1998). Critical serotonergic function, which regulates the biological clock, may also be altered (Leone, 1997).

IV. Specific Diagnostic Tests and Differential Diagnoses

The neurological examination of cluster headache is normal, except for changes during the headache that might include ptosis, pupillary change, etc. Soft neurological sensory signs occasionally may be present. There are no specific diagnostic tests for cluster headache, although provocation with alcohol is considered a key and reliable feature.

Among the conditions that must be considered are:

- Chronic paroxysmal hemicrania (to be discussed);
- Disease of the orbit (glaucoma, ocular pseudotumor, etc.);
- Trigeminal neuralgia;

- Tumors of the brainstem or occipitocervical junction;
- Hemicrania continua—episodic;
- Infiltration/infection of brainstem;
- Cavernous sinus disorders (aneurysm, thrombosis, etc.);
- Sphenoid sinusitis (acute);
- Disorders involving the fifth cranial nerve peripheral branches, which may activate central headache mechanisms;
- Carotid artery dissection; and
- SUNCT syndrome (short-lasting unilateral neuralgiform headache attacks with conjunctival injection, tearing, sweating, and rhinorrhea, which may represent either a refinement or a variant of atypical trigeminal neuralgia).

(See Chapters 5, 14, 15, and 16.)

V. Principles of Treatment

The primary treatment strategy is *prevention* of the attacks. Symptomatic treatment is adjunctive. Because of the frequency and brevity of the attacks, symptomatic treatment is not generally the mainstay of therapy. Due to the devastating nature of the condition, patients must be seen by their physicians, whenever appropriate. Visits cannot be postponed when recurring, untreated attacks are occurring.

Patients must be provided effective and aggressive preventive and symptomatic relief measures. Although steroids (to be discussed) are reliably effective, the risks must be weighed against the benefits. Other preventive agents are often more appropriate first-line treatments.

VI. Specific Treatment Approaches (for details see Chapter 6)

A. Symptomatic Treatment

Symptomatic treatment includes:

1. Oxygen inhalation*;
2. Dihydroergotamine (nasal spray or parenteral);
3. Sumatriptan (s.c. and nasal spray) or the other "triptans";
4. Sphenopalatine blockade;
5. Intranasal lidocaine;
6. Intranasal capsaicin;
7. Indomethacin (rectal suppositories, occasionally effective); and
8. Opioids (rectal/Stadol nasal spray; avoid frequent use).

Oxygen (100%) inhalation should be administered via a face mask at 7 liters/min for 10–15 minutes at a time, preferably given at the onset of the attack.

B. Preventive Treatment

The following agents are most appropriate for the prevention of cluster headache:

1. Verapamil is a first-line treatment for prevention of cluster headache, although weeks of therapy may be required before control is established. Verapamil must be administered at relatively high dosages to be effective (120–160 mg t.i.d.–q.i.d). Short-acting forms of verapamil are generally more reliable than long-acting forms due to variations in bioavailability. Thus, long-acting forms often require upward adjustment of dosage.

2. Steroids are reliably effective (80–90%) in preventing attacks during active therapy (see Chapter 6, Tables 6.11 and 6.12). Though not appropriate for prolonged preventive therapy, steroids can be used for:
   a. Difficult-to-treat exacerbations
   b. At the onset of a cycle to allow time for other medications to take effect
   c. As an available "insurance treatment" for breakthrough attacks while traveling or otherwise away from medical care

   The risks of steroids must be carefully explained. Continuous steroid treatment should not be used. Repetitive, interval administration should be considered only in truly resistant cases.

3. Lithium

4. Methysergide/methylergonovine

5. Divalproex sodium

6. Maintenance neuroleptics, such as chlorpromazine, may have a value in rare instances.

7. Transdermal or oral clonidine (possible benefits have recently been reported by D'Andrea, 1995)

8. Daily ergotamine tartrate, daily dihydroergotamine, sumatriptan, or other triptans (The risks of daily use of these agents for prolonged clusters makes this use unacceptable except in the most extreme and debilitating cases. The risks must be weighed against the value, since cluster headache patients, whether they smoke or not, may be at increased risk for cardiovascular disease, and alternate treatments, including hospitalization, are generally effective.)

9. Daily opioids (This must be reserved for extreme cases where all other reasonable treatments have failed or are unacceptable alternatives.)

C. Neural Blockade and Surgery

Sphenopalatine ganglion (SPG) blockade is reported effective in some patients (Saunders, 1997). Though control of an acute attack may be achieved with local application of cocaine or other anesthetic agents, repetitive SPG blockade has not generally achieved acceptance in neurological circles. Various surgical procedures are available, the most popular of which is percutaneous stereotaxic or radiofrequency rhizotomy. Tahu and Tew (1995) reported long-term results of radiofrequency rhizotomy in seven patients with cluster headache. All patients reported relief immediately after surgery. Two patients remained pain-free 5 and 20 years later, respectively. Three patients experienced mild pain recurrence 6–12 months after surgery, and two of these patients were able to control the pain with prescribed medication. The third patient controlled the pain with simple analgesics. Two patients had poor results. Major recurrence was noted in one patient 4 days after surgery and in the other, 2 months after surgery.

According to Mathew (1990), approximately 65–75% of patients had excellent, very good, or good results in his extensive series. Poor results are infrequent, often the consequence of post-surgical difficulties. Repeated surgery is sometimes necessary.

Despite these reports, some authorities believe that surgical success is 50% or less, with significant complications in many. The authors of this text are reluctant to recommend surgery, except in the most extreme cases and when all other options have been explored. Several personally encountered patients have done poorly after surgery. Headaches have recurred, or persistent deafferentation syndromes have emerged.

Recently, Ford and colleagues (1998) reported that gamma knife radiosurgery of the trigeminal nerve provided benefit to five of the six patients treated. The authors suggested that the technique carries negligible short- and long-term risk. The ultimate value of this intervention will await further studies.

Matthew suggests the following criteria for surgery:

1. Chronic cluster headache without pain remission for at least one year in patients who are totally resistant to aggressive medical management for a "reasonable" period of time;
2. Strictly unilateral pain; and
3. Patients who are physiologically stable, not prone to medication overusage, and otherwise medically and mentally healthy.

D. Hospitalization (see Chapter 9 for a detailed description of hospital management; also see Chapters 6 and 11)

Hospitalization for cluster headache patients may be essential during resistant, severe episodes or when patients become desperate. The use of IV fluids, sedation, parenteral DHE, and other parenteral therapies may be required. Patients with cluster headache should generally avoid alcohol, particularly during cluster cycles. Discontinuing smoking may be very important as well, but is quite difficult to achieve, particularly on an outpatient basis. Hospitalization often allows confronting these and other factors, which sometimes are critical. The physician must be firm on these matters. In one author's experience (Saper) and in the published outcome series (Lake, 1993), cluster headache appears to respond better than any of the other primary disorders to the aggressive interventions in a hospital setting.

VII. Other Questionably Related Conditions

A. Cluster Tic Syndrome

The *cluster tic syndrome* features the primary symptoms of cluster headache but with the added component of stabbing, ice-pick neuralgic-like components involving the eye, face, and jaw. The syndrome is found in 10–20% of patients but is often undiagnosed. True *trigeminal neuralgia* may coexist with cluster headache (see Chapter 16).

Alberca and Ochoa (1994) reviewed 37 reported cases of cluster tic syndrome. They noted equal gender representation and found that trigeminal neuralgia usually appeared first. Some attacks appeared to blend both neuralgia and cluster headache symptomatology and could be triggered by touching of the upper lip on the ipsilateral side. Medical treatment was often not effective, although a combination of cluster headache therapy with that for trigeminal neuralgia was sometimes useful.

Several antineuralgic agents are available. These include carbamazepine, phenytoin, baclofen valproate, and clonazepam. Most recently, gabapentin has shown promising results in neuropathic pain disorders. As for surgical interventions, suboccipital surgery (Solomon, 1985) revealed compression of the trigeminal nerve by aberrant vasculature, and following treatment, the neuralgic component resolved.

B. Chronic Paroxysmal Hemicrania (CPH)

Chronic paroxysmal hemicrania (CPH) may be a variant form of cluster headache; it is frequently confused with it and responds quickly to indomethacin. A full description is found in Chapter 15.

C. Hypnic Headache

Hypnic headache is a rare, distinctive nocturnal headache disorder that affects elderly men and women (after age 60). The attacks are usually bilateral, but unilateral pain has been reported (Gould, 1997). The pain is throbbing in quality and occurs 2–4 hours after night-time sleep onset, although attacks after daytime napping are reported (Dodick, 1998). It is usually a short-lived attack with a duration ranging between 15 minutes to 3 hours. Generally, there is an absence of associated autonomic features, although nausea may be present. Hypnic headaches characteristically respond to lithium carbonate (300–600 mg. at h.s.), although caffeine (Dodick, 1998) and indomethacin are also reported to help (Ivanez, 1998). Both genders are affected; however, in Dodick's recent large series, 84% of cases were women. It is generally considered a benign disorder (Gould, 1997; Mosek, 1997; Newman, 1991; Raskin, 1997). At this time, a relationship to cluster headache has not been established. However, the responsiveness to lithium, the periodicity of the attacks, and their nocturnal relationship do raise the question, since these are also features of cluster headache. Raskin (1997) suggests the possibility of disturbances of the "biological clock," which are serotoninergically modulated. Lithium enhances serotoninergic neurotransmission.

D. SUNCT Syndrome

SUNCT syndrome (short-lasting, unilateral, neuralgiform headache with conjunctival injection and tearing) (Sjaastad, 1989) is characterized by the following key clinical features:

1. Short-lasting attacks (30–60 seconds) with neuralgiform features;
2. Autonomic accompaniments;
3. A cyclical pattern of presentation; and,
4. Males more likely than females to be affected.

To date no effective treatment has been identified. The differential diagnosis of SUNCT syndrome includes cluster headache, trigeminal neuralgia, chronic -paroxysmal hemicrania, "ice-pick" headache, organic disease, and sphenoid sinusitis, among others. (See Chapter 15 for further discussion and comparative table.)

References

Alberca R, Ochoa JJ. Cluster tic syndrome. *Neurology,* 44:996–499, 1994.

Caviness VS Jr, O'Brien P. Cluster headache response to chlorpromazine. *Headache,* 20:128–131, 1980.

D'Andrea G, Perini F, Granella F, et al. Efficacy of transdermal clonidine in short-term treatment of cluster headaches. *Cephalalgia,* 15:430–433, 1995.

Diamond S, Dalessio DG. *The Practicing Physician's Approach to Headache.* Fifth edition. Baltimore, Williams & Wilkins, 1992.

Dodick DW, Mosek AC, Campbell JR. The hypnic "alarm clock" headache syndrome. *Cephalalgia,* 18:152–156, 1998.

Ekbom K, Lindgren L, Nilsson BY, et al. Retro-gasserian glycerol injection in the treatment of chronic cluster headache. *Cephalalgia,* 7:21–27, 1987.

Fogan L. Treatment of cluster headache: A double-blind comparison of oxygen vs. air inhalation. *Arch Neurol,* 42:362–363, 1985.

Ford RG, Ford KT, Swaid S, et al. Gamma knife treatment of refractory cluster headache. *Headache,* 38:3–9, 1998.

Fusco BM, Geppetti P, Fancicullaci M, et al. Local application of capsaicin for treatment of cluster headache and idiopathic trigeminal neuralgia. *Cephalalgia,* 11(supp 2):234–245, 1991.

Gabe IJ, Spierings CLH. Prophylactic treatment of cluster headache with verapamil. *Headache,* 29:167–168, 1989.

Gould JD, Silberstein SD. Unilateral hypnic headache: A case study. *Neurology,* 49:1749–1751, 1997.

Herring R, Kuritzky A. Sodium valproate in the treatment of cluster headache: An open label trial. *Cephalalgia,* 9:195–198, 1989.

Ivanez V, Soler R, Barreiro P. Hypnic headache syndrome: A case with good response to indomethacin. *Cephalalgia,* 18:225–226, 1998.

Jammes JJ. The treatment of cluster headache with prednisone. *Diseased Nervous System,* 36:375–376, 1975.

Jotkowitz S. Chronic paroxysmal hemicrania and cluster. *Ann Neurol,* 4:389, 1978.

Kudrow L. *Cluster Headache Mechanisms and Management.* London, Oxford University Press, 1980.

Kudrow L. Response of cluster headache attack to oxygen inhalation. *Headache,* 21:1–4, 1981.

Kudrow L, Kudrow DB. Association of systemic oxyhemoglobin desaturation and onset of cluster headache attacks. *Headache,* 30:474–480, 1990.

Mathew NT. Advances in cluster headache. *Neurol Clin,* 8:867–890, 1990.

Mathew NT. Cluster headache. *Intractable Headache: Inpatient and Outpatient Treatment Strategies.* SD Silberstein (Ed). *Neurology,* 42(supp 2):22–31, 1992.

Mathew NT, Hurt W. Percutaneous radiofrequency trigeminal gangliorhizolysis in intractable cluster headache. *Headache,* 28:328–331, 1988.

Mathew NT, Ruevini U. Cluster-like headache following head trauma. *Headache,* (abstract), 28:307, 1988.

Maxwell RE. Surgical control of chronic migrainous neuralgia by trigeminal gangliorhizolysis. *J Neurol Surg,* 57:459–466, 1982.

May A, Bahra A, Büchel C, et al. Hypothalamic activation in cluster headache attacks. *Lancet,* 352:275–278, 1998.

Morales-Asin F, Mauri JA, Iniquez C. The hypnic headache syndrome: Report of three new cases. *Cephalalgia,* 18:157–158, 1998.

Mosek A, Dodick DW. The hypnic headache syndrome: The Mayo Clinic experience. *Cephalalgia,* 17:312, 1997.

Moskowitz MA. Cluster headache: Evidence for a pathophysiological focus in the superior pericarotid cavernous sinus plexus. *Headache,* 28:584–586, 1988.

Newman LC, Lipton RB, Solomon S. The hypnic headache syndrome. (In) *New*

Advances in Headache Research. FC Rose (Ed). Pgs 31–34, London, Smith-Gordon and Company Ltd., 1991.

Onofrio BM, Campbell JK. Surgical treatment of chronic cluster headache. *Mayo Clin Proc,* 61:537–544, 1986.

Pareja J, Pareja J, Palomo T, et al. SUNCT syndrome: Repetitive and overlapping attacks. *Headache,* 34:114–116, 1994.

Raskin NH. Short-lived head pains. *Neurol Clin,* 15:143–152, 1997.

Saunders M, Zuurmond WWA. Efficacy of sphenopalatine ganglion blockade in 66 patients suffering from cluster headache: A 20–70 month follow-up evaluation. *J Neurosurg,* 87:876–880, 1997.

Sjaastad O. Chronic paroxysmal hemicrania. (In) *Handbook of Clinical Neurology,* Vol. 48. FC Rose (Ed). Pgs 257–266, Amsterdam, Elsevier Science Publishing, 1986.

Sjaastad O. Cluster headache. (In) *Handbook of Clinical Neurology,* Vol. 48. FC Rose (Ed). Pgs 217–246, Amsterdam, Elsevier Science Publishing, 1986.

Sjaastad O, Apfelbaum R, Caskey W, et al. Chronic paroxysmal hemicrania (CPH): The clinical manifestation. A review. *Ups J Med Sci,* (suppl) 31:27–33, 1980.

Sjaastad O, Fredriksen TA, Pfraffenrath V. The cervicogenic headache: Diagnostic criteria. *Headache,* 30:725–726, 1990.

Sjaastad O, Saunte C, Salveen R, et al. Short-lasting unilateral neuralgiform headache attacks with conjunctival injection, tearing, sweating, and rhinorrhea. *Cephalalgia,* 9:147–156, 1989.

Solomon S, Apfelbaum RI, Guglielmo KM. The cluster-tic syndrome and its surgical treatment. *Cephalalgia,* 5:83–89, 1985.

Sweet WH. Surgical treatment of chronic cluster headache. *Headache,* 28:669–670, 1988.

Tahu JM. Long-term results of radiofrequency rhizotomy in the treatment of cluster headache. *Headache,* 35:193–196, 1995.

Watson CPN, Morley TP, Richardson JC, et al. The surgical treatment of chronic cluster headache. *Headache,* 23:289–895, 1985.

Watson P, Evans R. Cluster-tic syndrome. *Headache,* 25:123–126, 1985.

13

Post-Traumatic Headache and Syndrome: Post-Concussion Syndrome, Post-Traumatic Syndrome

"Though no objective signs accompany these complaints, they are so uniform from case to case that the symptoms cannot be regarded as other than genuine."
—*H. Cushing, M.D.*

I. Introduction

The *post-traumatic syndrome* (PTS), previously called *post-concussion syndrome,* is a constellation of symptoms that can follow mild to moderate closed head injury (actual cranial impact). It is also seen following flexion/extension trauma (whiplash) in which no actual cranial contact has occurred (Young, 1997). Eighty-two percent of patients seeking help following whiplash report headache (Balla, 1988). The primary symptoms of PTS, usually strikingly consistent from patient to patient, include one or more of the following:

- Headache, neck, and shoulder pain;
- Sleep disturbance;
- Cognitive abnormalities;
- Mood and personality changes; and
- Dizziness, with or without vertigo.

Long a controversial matter, the prevailing view of most authorities is that the condition is a neurological disorder that may arise *even if frank unconsciousness has not occurred.* Some patients who experience momentary loss of consciousness are not aware that consciousness was lost and report "No" to the ER question, "Did you lose consciousness?" In some cases in which momentary loss of consciousness has occurred, the patient, still in the immediate post-traumatic period, is not yet aware of it, since there may be no frame of reference to allow such recognition if unaccompanied by others who have observed it. Many patients report that they were momentarily dazed but did not lose consciousness. In this perspective, the most appropriate term to describe this condition is *PTS*.

Headache is present in up to 88% of patients with mild head injury, and persists for more than 2 months in 60% of patients, even those with apparently minor trauma. The symptoms do not correlate with the presence or duration of unconsciousness, amnesia, or any identifiable neurodiagnostic finding (Young, 1997). An inverse relationship may exist between the severity of head injury, as determined by the duration of post-traumatic amnesia, and the incidence of headache (Yamaguchi, 1992).

The International Headache Society (IHS), in one of its most controversial sets of criteria, has asserted that the onset of the headache must be within 2 weeks of head injury or of regaining consciousness, if lost. The IHS criteria also distinguish between acute post-traumatic headache, that which lasts less than 8 weeks, and chronic post-traumatic headache, which lasts longer. However, in practice these criteria seem arbitrary and needlessly restrictive. Headaches that occur as a result of trauma may develop well after 2 weeks following the injury (perhaps reflecting progressive central nervous system [CNS] changes) (see *Pathogenesis*). Nonetheless, it is true that from a medico-legal point of view it is not possible to differentiate late post-traumatic headache from that which might occur from another cause during that intervening period of time.

II. Pathophysiology
A. General Considerations

Post-traumatic headache and PTS probably reflect a set of pathophysiological factors that produce a wide-ranging set of symptoms. It is most likely that cognitive, psychological, and behavioral disturbances seen in patients with PTS represent the sequelae of brain injury. Moreover, direct or indirect injury to the neck, jaw, or tissues of the scalp may similarly play a role in the development of many of the headache and other painful symptoms. These acute changes, which may produce pain in the immediate post-traumatic period, may induce delayed and chronic disturbances centrally that involve pain modulation. Peripherally painful injury can induce central pain phenomena, such as *windup* and *sensitization,* that include wide dynamic-range neurons and other recently recognized CNS factors involved in pain. Moreover, the *kindling phenomenon,* seen in experimental epilepsy, could influence the evolution from peripheral injury to chronic, centrally maintained pain, possibly producing a daily persistent headache.

Head injury varies in its cause, pathophysiology, and symptoms. According to Gennarelli (1993), two broad categories of injury can be identified. *Focal injury* is due to direct blows to the head. Examples include contusion, lacerations, and hemorrhage. *Diffuse injuries* are usually caused by sudden movement of the head. Examples of this include concussional injury in which prolonged and delayed events, such as *diffuse axonal injury* (DAI), occur.

Both neural and vascular elements are involved in trauma, and clinical events can be affected by immediate and delayed influences, such as deafferentation, ischemia, cerebral edema, and increased intracranial pressure. Axonal injury, such as that at the Node of Ranvier, can, for example, cause traumatic defects in the axonal membrane. This results in calcium ion accumulation in the intracellular compartment of the axone, a change similar to that which can occur from ischemia and which results in cell damage.

Moreover, the trauma of either head injury or whiplash can produce forces that when applied to the brain, result in DAI, identified histologically. These changes may not require direct impact (Gennarelli, 1993). DAI has been shown most clearly in the corpus callosum, internal capsule, fornices, dorsal lateral midbrain, and pons. DAI has been shown in concussive syndromes (Blumbergs, 1994), but it remains unclear whether it is present in subconcussive compromise. Axones in the upper brainstem, an area important to the production of pain, sleep, and mood control, may be particularly vulnerable as a result of rotational factors that develop between the cerebral hemispheres and cerebellum (Elson, 1994). Hemorrhage in the midbrain, seen on magnetic resonance imaging (MRI), has been reported in a patient with mild head injury (Servadei, 1994).

Moreover, according to the model of Gennarelli (1985), angular acceleration in experimental animals produces many of the features of human head injury, including axonal changes in the brainstem, which is similar to human autopsy cases of mild head injury (Povlishock, 1989). Stretching or compression, in addition to shearing, may cause axonal injury as well, and hydraulic pressure pulse, which lasts only miniseconds, may produce a response similar to that seen in mild or moderate head injury.

Many of the changes seen in closed head injury are not immediately apparent and may evolve over hours to weeks, suggesting that a progressive process may occur for some time following the initial trauma. With respect to the mechanism of this process, a variety of theories have been proposed and include damage mediated through calcium entry, receptor dysfunction, free radical accumulation, and inflammation. Ischemia may also produce injury, as can increased intracranial pressure, seizures, infection, edema, excitotoxicity, and extracranial injury. Cellular changes, disturbances of neurotransmitters, and metabolic disturbances are offered in explanation. Some studies have shown that dopamine receptors are diminished, resulting in excess dopamine in synaptic spaces following trauma. Changes also occur in $5\text{-}HT_2$ and

$5-HT_1$ receptors, as well as in magnesium levels and nitric oxide formation, factors recently gaining attention in theories on the pathogenesis of headache. Changes in receptor density can either be increased or decreased following injury and the reparative process (see references for Chapter 13).

Thus, changes following trauma may include neural, vascular, ionic, neurochemical, and neurotransmitter, deafferentation, and "neuroplastic" dynamics. Also, brain trauma impairs cerebral blood flow autoregulation. Ischemia is associated with a cascade of neural events superimposed upon the original trauma. Glutamate activation and an influx of calcium in the intracellular space result in cytotoxic changes (Gennarelli, 1993)

Other mechanical considerations are relevant as well. These include compression at the level of the foramen magnum, motion at the level of the medulla, injury to the neck, and rotational factors of the cerebral hemispheres and cerebellum. Also important may be the proximity of the brainstem to the skull, tentorial impact (Elson, 1994), and size and structural factors at the occipitocervical junction (as in Arnold Chiari Type I malformation).

The neurocognitive disturbances that are seen in patients with closed head injury may be a reactive response to pain, stress, or loss of normalcy; or, these disturbances may be the direct result of neurobiological changes occurring as a result of the injury. Recent studies have shown a possible neurobiological basis for psychological phenomena following trauma. Single-photon emission computed tomography (SPECT) has been used to study head injury, though not specifically in post-traumatic headache or PTS (Abdel-Dayem, 1994; Gray, 1992; Levin, 1987, 1992). Levin (1992) attempted to correlate neurobehavioral and cognitive deficits with MRI abnormalities. Studies suggest that two types of lesions may be seen on SPECT: circumscribed areas of hypoperfusion, representing contusion, and diffuse occipitotemporal hypoperfusion, which represents multiple small contusions or DAI (Masdeu, 1995).

B. Headache Considerations

The exact mechanism for headache and its accompaniments is not now known. Gross and microscopic abnormalities, including brain hemorrhage, occur in animals following carefully controlled head trauma approximating minor head injury in humans. In addition, the few human autopsy reports that are available, together with animal studies, allow recognition that a variety of pathophysiological mechanisms may be operational to explain the constellation of symptoms seen. Moreover, recognition that trauma to the head and neck produces both biochemical, microscopic, and more gross structural changes offers an opportunity to better explain the myriad of symptoms seen in these conditions.

Soft tissue injury (muscle, tendon, blood vessel, nerve) and direct trauma to the cervical root, spinal cord, facet joints, upper cervical nerves, atlanto-axial vertebrae, jaw, and related tissues, including those of the stylomandibular ligaments, offer further possibilities on headache and pain mechanisms. Also, ischemic disturbances of the brainstem and vestibular system, perhaps secondary to vertebral artery spasm, are likewise possible. A more complete discussion of cervical injury is found in Chapter 19.

Recently, Young and Packard (in *Headache,* Goadsby and Silberstein, 1997) summarized the similarity between proposed neurochemical changes in migraine and those in experimental brain injury. These include increased extracellular potassium and intracellular sodium, calcium, and chloride; excessive release of excitatory amino acids; alterations in serotonin function; alterations in other neurotransmitters and endogenous opioids; declining magnesium levels; impaired glucose metabolism; abnormalities in nitric oxide formation and function; and, alteration in neuropeptides.

Finally, headache symptoms may also arise from increased intracranial pressure and disturbances of intracranial pressure dynamics, including intracranial hypertension and hypotension (to be discussed).

III. Predispositional Conditions and Risk Factors

> *"It's not so much what happens to the head,*
> *but whose head it happens to."*
> —*(Modified from Symonds, 1937)*

It is likely that age, gender, and various genetic predispositional factors significantly influence the outcome of head injury. Women more than men seem predisposed (Jensen, 1990). Increasing age lessens recovery (Bohnen, 1992; Cartlidge, 1989), but age itself may not produce a greater vulnerability to the condition. Rotational factors seem to play a role, suggesting that if an individual is rotated prior to impact, or if the head is other than in a straightforward position, the condition is more likely to develop. Unpreparedness for the attack and rear-end collisions have been suggested as risk factors but are not proven.

The severity of injury does not correlate well with the severity of PTS. In fact, an inverse relationship between severity of injury and severity of post-traumatic headache has been suggested (Yamaguchi, 1992). Although pretraumatic migraine was not a risk for developing post-traumatic headache following cerebral concussion, in one study (Jensen, 1990) many authorities believe that a pre-existent headache condition may be provoked or aggravated by the trauma. In a study by Radanov (1995), pretraumatic headache was considered a significant risk factor for developing post-traumatic headache. Moreover, pre-existing psychological and behavioral illness may influence the development and course of PTS. Those with a significant history of pre-existing psychopathology or "unstable personalities" had more significant PTS (Ross, 1944). The available studies suggest that pre-existing psychopathology may influence the description of symptoms rather than subsequent disability, though general consensus does not exist (Young, 1997) and the studies have methodologic problems.

Thus, the issue of predispositional risk remains uncertain. Though it cannot be established with certainty, it seems reasonable to suggest that certain neurobiological and neuropsychiatric predispositional factors may explain why some patients subjected to mild to moderate head injury experience one or more of the sequelae, while others do not. Despite this "logic," the studies to date do not establish that this is so. It is interesting to note that children under the age of 15 may not be as likely to develop chronic symptoms.

IV. Key Clinical Features

Both immediately apparent symptoms and delayed phenomena (perhaps not initially recognized or evident) may occur. The delayed symptoms might result from a requisite interval between trauma and pathophysiological sequelae. This delay is seen in other neurological circumstances, such as *delayed post-traumatic epilepsy, delayed post-anoxic encephalopathy,* etc. Centralization and neurodegenerative changes (as discussed previously) might occur long after peripheral injury and may explain the delayed appearance or recognition of symptoms. Delay may also reflect the fact that deficits may not become apparent until convalescence progresses and normal function and high-level cognitive demands are present.

A. Pain and Headache

Headache, neck, and shoulder pain are usually present within the first 24–48 hours, although days or weeks may pass before onset. Neuralgic-like syndromes of the frontal or occipital regions may not appear for months or longer. The pattern of pain may change and the intensity may fluctuate over months and years.

Several pain patterns are noted:

1. Generalized, bilateral, persistent mild to moderate headache, similar to daily chronic or tension-type headache;
2. Neuralgic-like pain in occipitocervical or frontal regions (see Chapter 16);

3. Periodic, throbbing migraine or migraine-like attacks, sometimes accompanied by scintillating scotoma and other migrainous features, including nausea, light sensitivity, etc. May be occipital in location;

4. A cluster headache-like syndrome;

5. Suboccipital and cervical pain, with and without movement, perhaps from injury to suboccipital muscles, upper cervical vertebrae, zygapophyseal (facet) joints, etc. (see Chapter 19);

6. Cervical radiculopathy secondary to root injury;

7. Myofascial-like pain with "trigger points" in the occipital, cervical, shoulder (trapezius, supraspinatus), and paraspinal regions;

8. A low-pressure headache syndrome (with postural aggravation), possibly related to spontaneous dural tear (see Chapter 17);

9. Headache associated with increased intracranial pressure (intracranial hypertension) (Silberstein, 1990), perhaps the result of an alteration of cerebrospinal fluid (CSF) regulation, production, or drainage (see Chapter 18);

10. A brachial plexus-like syndrome (EMG rarely confirmatory) with features of positional arm and shoulder pain and headache aggravation following shoulder and arm exertion (Montalbetti, 1995);

11. Temporomandibular (TM) joint/myofascial syndrome, including injury to the joint itself, styloid process (fracture), styloid ligament, etc.; and

12. A hemicrania continua-like syndrome (see Chapter 15).

The majority of patients experience features of one or more of these patterns. Referred phenomena from suboccipital regions to frontal, vertex, or orbital regions have been documented and may account for the frequency of complex pain patterns (see Chapter 19).

B. Neurocognitive Impairment

Impaired memory, minor to major cognitive deficits, and reduced concentration are present in a significant number of patients with *PTS*. Key features include the inability to process information normally (or at a fast rate) and memory impairment. Recently, Keidel (1992) reporting on repeated neuropsychological tests in 30 patients with PTS after whiplash, demonstrated a hierarchy of functional recovery that occurred over a period greater than 12 weeks, even after apparently mild injury. Late neurobehavioral symptoms following mild head injury were reported by Bohnen (1995).

C. Neuropsychiatric and Behavioral Phenomena

Several neuropsychiatric symptoms are noted after mild to moderate head injury and are often present in PTS. Among these are:

1. Personality change;
2. Depression, with and without anxiety;
3. Irritability, with anger outbursts and emotional intolerance;
4. Loss of sense of humor;
5. Reduced motivation and social interaction;
6. Generalized lethargy (mental and physical);
7. Rage attacks;
8. Hypomania;
9. Hyperkinesis, mood changes, impaired attention, and enuresis (common in children); and
10. Post-traumatic stress disorder (PTSD).

Patients with PTS may fulfill criteria for PTSD. In a study by Chibnall (1994), the diagnosis was established in nearly 30% of a sample of patients with chronic post-traumatic headache. All were injured in motor vehicle accidents. Comparisons between the PTSD and non-PTSD groups demonstrated that depression and suppressed anger were significantly higher in those with PTSD. Also, they were more likely to have a history of pre-traumatic headache. Other variables were not different between the groups. Wallace (1997) noted amelioration of psychological disturbances in patients with these symptoms and neck pain when pain control was established.

D. Vertigo and Dizziness

Frank vertigo, as well as vague, nonspecific dizziness, are common. Positional vertigo may be present in up to 80% of patients reporting dizziness. It is worsened by movement of the head or a rapid change in body position. Imbalance or unsteadiness is a common complaint.

E. Sleep Disturbance

Sleep disturbances, including insomnia, frequent nocturnal awakening, and daytime sleepiness, are common. Patients report nonrestorative sleep and hypersomnolence, while polysomnographic studies demonstrate increased fragmentation of nocturnal sleep (Prigatano, 1982).

F. Spells

A variety of seizure-like events are reported in patients with PTS. These include:

1. True syncope (occurs rarely);
2. True epilepsy (occurs rarely); and

3. A variety of nonspecific periodic, paroxysmal events (pseudoseizures?), including:
   a. Staring spells
   b. Nonvestibular dizziness
   c. Sudden loss of memory (amnesia or confusion)
   d. Narcolepsy/cataplexy-like spells (Lankford, 1994)
   e. Episodic disorientation and fugue-like states.

The term "pseudoseizure" does not imply the absence of physiological legitimacy. Though the term is broad and may embody nonorganic circumstances, it is used here to include what appears to be physiological, bona fide cerebral events that do not fit existing epilepsy criteria.

G. Family Dysfunction

The family also generally suffers as a result of the trauma. Role reversal (dependency by a previously independent family member), loss of insurance and support, loss of consortium, rejection, disbelief, and anger toward the injured person are common, and contribute to the deterioration of quality and stability of life. These may be more common when there has been a loss of consciousness as a result of the injury (Lake, 1995).

H. Other Reported Symptoms/Signs

Other nonspecific symptoms reported in PTS include:

1. Weight loss or gain;
2. Changes in appetite;
3. Increased thirst;
4. Alcohol intolerance;
5. Menstrual irregularities, including amenorrhea;
6. Sexual dysfunction; loss or increase of libido;
7. A variety of "soft" neurological findings on examination; and
8. Others.

Traumatic disruption to the area of the hypothalamus and pituitary/adrenal axis may contribute to many of these complaints, but this remains speculative.

V. Specific Diagnostic Testing

There are no specific post-traumatic headache or PTS studies, and the diagnosis remains a clinical one. While modern neuroimaging studies and functional imaging, such as SPECT, demonstrate gross structural abnormalities and blood flow and metabolic disturbances, none thus far serves to diagnose these conditions.

A. Neurocognitive

The most reliable studies at this time involve neurocognitive evaluation, which often demonstrates impaired neurocognitive function. No other practical, widely available study so consistently demonstrates a basis for many of the features in this condition. (See Young, 1997, for current references on neurocognitive testing.) It is possible that the most sensitive tests for revealing cerebral dysfunction are those that evaluate the function of the greatest number of cortical and subcortical areas simultaneously (Gentilini, 1989).

B. Other Recommended Studies and Evaluations, When Appropriate

1. Electroencephalography (altered in 10–30% of patients but nonspecific in form and recommended primarily for the assessment of "spells" or frank seizures);
2. MRI/CT scan of head and neck (while clearly able to demonstrate "structural changes," they do not diagnose PTS or post-traumatic headache, and most published studies were done on patients with moderate to severe head injury);
3. Special sleep studies, which may demonstrate pattern abnormalities of sleep staging;
4. Dental/jaw evaluation;
5. Otolaryngological and vestibular evaluation including electronystagmography and other vestibular testing;
6. Lumbar puncture (LP) (to assess low or high pressure syndromes);
7. Diagnostic neuroblockade (vertebral [facet joint], supraorbital, paravertebral and suboccipital regions) (unfortunately, response to blockade is not a specific diagnostic marker in all cases); and
8. Positron emission tomography (PET) testing; not yet of practical value but has demonstrated changes that could explain post-traumatic behavioral disturbances (Starkstein, 1990). The test offers promise for future clinical substantiation of this condition.

Increasing refinement of neurophysiological methods for evaluating the brain and its function undoubtedly makes it likely that in the next several years more definitive observations regarding PTS and post-traumatic headache will occur. Methods such as advanced electroencephalography, polysomnography, advanced cerebral tomography, functional MRI, SPECT, and PET scanning will, in all likelihood, be more useful in the future than they are right now. Currently, the most reliable practical test for assessing the disturbances associated with PTS is sophisticated neurocognitive testing. Also, flow-sensitive MRI and cine-phase MRI may assist in detecting CSF leakage and abnormalities of flow dynamics in the cervical occipital region, respectively (see Chapter 3). Standard computed tomography (CT) and MR scanning currently assist in ruling out other pathology that, by exclusion, assist in establishing the diagnosis of PTS or post-traumatic headache.

C. Establishing the Diagnosis

The principal means of establishing the diagnosis of PTS is to rule out other sequelae to trauma, or the coincidental existence of other pathology. The key clinical elements to establish the diagnosis are:

1. The convincing presence of symptoms that are consistent with the key features of the syndrome;
2. A comprehensive history of the traumatic event and sequelae, which, *when compared with pretraumatic medical status, cognitive function, and job or school performance,* supports that a significant change in clinical status and cognitive function has occurred within a compatible temporal relationship to the injury;
3. The careful exclusion of other physiological, psychological, or organic disorders that might mimic or coexist with the symptoms of *PTS* and might arise from trauma. These include:
   a. Subdural/epidural hematoma
   b. CSF hypotension (CSF leak syndromes)/CSF hypertension
   c. Cerebral vein thrombosis/cavernous sinus thrombosis, fistula, aneurysm
   d. Cerebral hemorrhage
   e. True seizures
   f. Post-traumatic hydrocephalus
   g. Vertebral (facet joint)/cervical root/cervical nerve/suboccipital injury
   h. TM disorders, styloid ligament or process, facial injury, etc.

VI. Principles of Treatment

Patients with PTS are generally seriously distressed and seriously misunderstood. Appropriate treatment requires an objective approach to the complaints. Most patients are neither embellishing nor malingering. An objective, unbiased (neutral) appraisal is essential. This requires a comprehensive data collection process and a detailed, well-designed diagnostic evaluation.

VII. Specific Treatment Approaches

A comprehensive, interdisciplinary approach to treatment is generally required.

A. Headache and General Pain

1. Patients should be treated in the manner described in other sections of this book for various headache patterns, including migraine, daily chronic headache, or related headaches;
2. Cervical and shoulder syndromes and/or neuralgic-like syndromes may benefit from:
   a. Trigger point injection
   b. Various nerve and joint blocking procedures (including facet joint blockade, C2–C3 nerve blockade, etc.) (see Chapter 19)
   c. Epidural blockade, when appropriate
   d. Physical medicine therapies, including transneural stimulation (TNS), physical therapy, exercise, etc.
   e. Pharmacotherapy, using antidepressants, antineuralgic agents, muscle relaxants, neuroleptics, and nonsteroidal anti-inflammatory drugs
3. Biofeedback and relaxation therapy, other behavioral and cognitive interventions; and
4. Specific treatment for jaw or neck injury.

At times, patients require simultaneous therapies that provide intervention, both centrally and peripherally, as well as psychologically.

B. Spells

If true seizure activity is present, appropriate anticonvulsant therapy is indicated. Many patients do not benefit from standard anticonvulsant treatment but, anecdotally, may benefit from "stimulant-type" medication. Fluoxetine and other "activating" antidepressants, methylphenidate, and pemoline have been of anecdotal benefit in the treatment of both nonepileptic spells and neurocognitive dysfunction. Stimulant medication may be of particular value for daytime somnolence and narcolepsy-like syndromes. When true seizure-like activity occurs, divalproex sodium may be helpful for both the seizure-like activity and headache.

C. Neurocognitive Dysfunction and Neuropsychiatric Symptoms

Individually designed cognitive retraining, counseling, and vocational rehabilitation is often beneficial in treating PTS symptoms. Formal traumatic brain injury (TBI) programs can be very useful for many of the patients with impairment, with or without continuing pain. Head injury support groups may also be of value. Stimulant treatment may enhance neurocognitive performance.

Use of neuroleptics, lithium antidepressants, and divalproex may help mood and labile behavioral disturbances.

D. Family Dysfunction

Family therapy and consultation with employer and school personnel are recommended when appropriate. Careful explanation of cause, mechanism, and prognosis is helpful to all involved, particularly the patient.

VIII. Outcomes

Prognostications on post-traumatic headache and syndrome are difficult. In a review of the literature by Young and Packard (1997), after 1 month, 31–90% of patients still had headache. At 2–3 months post-injury, 32–78% of patients still had headache. One year after injury, 8–35% of patients still had headache. Between 2 and 4 years after injury, as many as 20–24% of patients have persistent headache. Neurocognitive, dizziness, and mood symptoms may persist for years (Evans, 1994).

The assumption that protracted cases result primarily from litigation-related motives or other nonphysiological circumstances is not supported by data. On balance, the prevailing studies fail to link impairment to litigational issues (Leininger, 1990; Mendelson, 1982; Packard, 1992; Rimel, 1981). Moreover, most studies appear to support the view that enduring and persistent impairment and pain can occur even after minor injury.

IX. Conclusions

PTS may well reflect the convergence of simultaneous processes that explain the condition better than any one phenomenon alone. Initial injury to both central structures and peripheral soft tissues may directly relate to the acceleration/deceleration forces involved in the injury. Diffuse axonal injury, cytotoxic metabolic changes, blood flow disturbances, disturbances of neurotransmitter and receptor physiology, and others yet to be defined may explain the painful symptoms, neuropsychological disturbances, and alterations in mood, behavior, and attention. Changes arising from the central disturbances and neuroplastic phenomena that occur as a result of chronic pain or injury to peripheral tissues or to stress-related factors may also be important. Moreover, behavioral and mood disturbances may result from either the neurophysiological changes or from the life alterations that occur following injury and the compelling presence of intractable pain (Wallace, 1997).

In most instances, the absence of objective markers is explained by the absence of sufficient diagnostic sophistication, not the legitimacy of the complaints. Patients have experienced symptoms long before doctors have known how to diagnose or treat them, or even known that they exist at all.

Delayed sequelae are possible and familiar to many neurological conditions, including post-traumatic epilepsy. Early recognition of the impairment, followed by aggressive, comprehensive, well-designed intervention may help prevent physiological and emotional deterioration.

Key factors in determining prognosis are the attitude and skill of the physician in charge of care. Objectivity must be maintained, and direct physician involvement in the strategy and delivery of treatment is necessary. One cannot assume that all that is reported is valid; and, a healthy, scholarly cynicism is appropriate. However, it is equally important to recognize that a clinician's honored responsibility is to trust his/her patient *unless reason exists to alter that posture.* The manner in which symptoms are described or the inability to immediately explain them with a recognized physiological mechanism should not of themselves threaten a serious and neutral assessment of a patient's complaints. That the patient is *usually right* is a well-accepted adage and a trusted principle of most experienced clinicians. Symptoms may persist for years and even a lifetime, despite qualified and appropriate interventions.

In short, PTS, while clearly unexplainable in many ways, can no longer be arbitrarily denied its physiological legitimacy, particularly with such compelling clinical support to its existence. There is yet much more to learn than is already known. Subjectivity does not imply absence of legitimacy. The history of medicine is replete with examples of illnesses suffered long before they were formally discovered. Prejudice and cynicism must give way to at least reasoned neutrality and objectivity in the face of strong, albeit subjective, clinical evidence, and growing, yet preliminary, objectifying data.

References

Abdul-Dayem H, Masdeu J, O'Connell R, et al. Brain perfusion abnormalities following minor/moderate closed head injury: Comparison between early and late imaging in two groups of patients. *Eur J Nucl Med*, 21:750, 1994.

Alavi A, Fazekas T, Alves W, et al. Position emission tomography in the evaluation of head injury. *J Cereb Blood Flow Metab*, 7:646, 1987.

Balla J, Iansek R. Headaches arising from disorders of the cervical spine. (In) *Headache: Problems in Diagnosis and Management.* A Hopkins (Ed), Pg 241, London, WB Saunders, 1988.

Blumbergs PC, Scott G, Manavis J, et al. Staining of amyloid precursor protein to study axonal damage in mild head injury. *Lancet*, 344:1055, 1994.

Bogduk N. Headache and the neck. (In) *Headache.* PJ Goadsby, SD Silberstein (Eds). Pgs 369–381, Boston, Butterworth-Heinemeann, 1997.

Bohnen NI, Jolles J, Twijnstra A, et al. Late neurobehavioral symptoms after mild head injury. *Brain Injury,* 9:27–33, 1995.

Bohnen N, Weijnstra A, Jolles J. Post-traumatic and emotional symptoms in different subgroups of patients with mild head injury. *Brain Injury,* 6:481–487, 1992.

Carlsson GS, Svardsudd K, Wellin L. Long-term effects of head injury sustained during life in three male populations. *J Neurosurg,* 67:197–205, 1987.

Cartlidge NEF, Shaw DA. Epidemiology of whiplash. (In) *Head Injury.* London, Saunders, 1981.

Chipnall JT, Duckro BN. Post-traumatic stress disorder in chronic post-traumatic headache patients. *Headache,* 34:357–361, 1994.

Davies RA, Luxon LM. Dizziness following head injury: A neurootologic study. *J Neurol,* 242:222–230, 1995.

Dila C, Bouchard L, Myer E, et al. Microvascular response to minimal brain trauma. (In) *Head Injuries.* R McLaurin (Ed). New York, Grune & Stratton, 1976.

Dillon H, Leopold RL. Children and the post-concussion syndrome. *JAMA,* 175:86–92, 1961.

Eisenberg HM. CT and MRI findings in mild to moderate head injury. (In) *Mild Head Injury.* HS Levin, HM Eisenberg, Al Benton (Eds). Pg 133, New York, Oxford University Press, 1989.

Elson LM, Ward CC. Mechanisms and pathophysiology of mild head injury. *Semin Neurol,* 14:8–18, 1994.

Erb DE, Povlishock JT. Neuroplasticity following traumatic brain injury: A study of GABAergic terminal loss and recovery in the cat dorsal lateral vestibular nucleus. *Exp Brain Res,* 83:253, 1991.

Evans RW. The postconcussion syndrome: 130 years of controversy. *Semin Neurol,* 14:32–39, 1994.

Feinsod M, Hoyt WF, Wilson WG, et al. Visual evoked response: Use in neurological evaluation of post- traumatic subjective visual complaints. *Arch Ophthalmol,* 94:237–240, 1976.

Fisher CM. Whiplash amnesia. *Neurology,* 32:667–668, 1982.

Fujiwara S, Yanagida Y, Nishimura A, et al. Recent advances in the study on the mechanism of brain injury. *Nippon Hoigaku Zasshi,* 47:387–397, 1993.

Gennarelli TA. Cerebral concussion and diffuse brain injuries. (In) *Head Injury.* PR Cooper (Ed). Pgs 83–97, Baltimore, Williams & Wilkins, 1982.

Gennarelli TA. Mechanisms of brain injury. *J Emerg Med,* 11(suppl):5–11, 1993.

Gennarelli TA, Thibault LE, Adams JH, et al. Diffuse axonal injury and traumatic coma in the primate. (In) *Trauma of the Central Nervous System.* RG Dacey, et al. (Eds). Pg 169, New York, Raven, 1985.

Gentilini TM, Michelli P, Schoenhuber R. Assessment of attention in mild head injury. (In) *Mild Head Injury.* HS Levin, HM Eisenberg, Al Benton (Eds). Pg 163, New York, Oxford University Press, 1989.

Gilkey SJ, Ramadan NM, Aurora TK, et al. Cerebral blood flow in chronic post-traumatic headache. *Headache,* 37:583–587, 1997.

Gray BG, Ichise M, Chung D, et al. Technetium-99m-HMPAO SPECT in the evaluation of patents with a remote history of traumatic brain injury: A comparison with x-ray computed tomography. *J Nucl Med,* 33:52, 1992.

Gronwall D, Wrightson P. Delayed recovery of intellectual function after minor head injury. *Lancet,* 2:605–609, 1984.

Haas DC, Pineda GS, Lourie H. Juvenile head trauma syndromes and their relationship to migraine. *Arch Neurol,* 32:727–730, 1975.

Hickling EJ, Blanchard EB, Silverman DJ, et al. Motor vehicle accidents, headaches, and posttraumatic stress disorder: Assessment findings in a consecutive series. *Headache,* 32:147–151, 1992.

Jacome DE. Basilar artery migraine after uncomplicated whiplash injuries. *Headache,* 26:515–516, 1986.

Jakobsen J, Daadsgaard SE, Thomsen S, et al. Prediction of post-concussional sequelae by reaction time test. *Acta Neurol Scand,* 75:341–345, 1987.

Jensen OK, Nielsen FF. The influence of sex and posttraumatic headache on the incidence and severity of headache after head injury. *Cephalalgia,* 10:285–293, 1990.

Keidel M, Yaguez L, Wilhelm H, et al. Prospective follow-up of neuropsychological deficits after cervicocephalic acceleration trauma. *Neurologische Klonik and Poliklinik,* Universitat Essen. Nervenarzt, 63:731, 1992.

Keith WS. Whiplash injury of the second cervical ganglion and nerve. *Can J Neurol Sci,* 13:133–137, 1986.

Kelly R. The post-traumatic syndrome. *Proc Royal Soc Med,* 24:242–244, 1981.

Kelly R. Headache after cranial trauma. (In) *Headache: Problems in Diagnosis and Management,* A Hopkins (Ed). Pg 219, London, Saunders, 1988.

Kerr FWL. A mechanism to account for frontal headache in a case of posterior fossa tumors. *J Neurosurg,* 18:605–609, 1961.

Khurana RK, Nirankari VW. Bilateral sympathetic dysfunction in post-traumatic headache. *Headache,* 26:183–188, 1986.

Klonoff PS, Snow WE, Costa LD. Quality of life in patients 2–4 years after closed head injury. *Neurosurgery,* 19:735–743, 1986.

Lake AE, Branca B, Lutz T, et al. Comorbid symptoms in chronic posttraumatic headache. I: Comparison to intractable migraine. II: Relationship to severity of injury and litigation (abstract). *Headache,* 35:302, 1995.

Lankford DA, Wellman JJ, O'Hara C. Posttraumatic narcolepsy in mild to moderate closed head injury. *Sleep,* 17(8 suppl):S25–S28, 1994.

Leininger BE. Neuropsychological deficits in symptomatic minor head injury patients after concussion and mild concussion. *J Neurol Neurosurg Psychiatry,* 53:293–296, 1990.

Levin HS, Amparo E, Eisenberg HM, et al. Magnetic resonance imaging and computerized tomography in relation to the neurobehavioral sequelae of mild and moderate head injuries. *J Neurosurg,* 66:706–713, 1987.

Levin HS, Mendelsohn D, Lilly MA, et al. Magnetic resonance imaging in relation to functional outcome of pediatric closed head injury: A test of the Ommaya-Gennarelli model. *Neurosurgery,* 40:432–440, 1997.

Levin HS, Williams DH, Eisenberg HM, et al. Serial MRI and neurobehavioral findings after mild to moderate head injuries. *J Neurol Neurosurg Psychiatry,* 55:255–262, 1992.

MacFlynn G, Montgomery EA, Fenton GW, et al. Measurement of reaction time following minor head injury. *J Neurol Neurosurg Psychiatry,* 47:1326–1331, 1984.

Masdeu JC, Abdel-Dayhem H, VanHeertum RL. Head trauma: Use of SPECT. *J Neuroimaging,* 5(supp 1):S53–S57, 1995.

Masdeu JC, VanHeertum RL, Kleiman A, et al. Early single-photon emission computed tomography in mild head trauma. A controlled study. *General Neuroimaging,* 4:177–181, 1994.

Matthews WB. Footballer's migraine, *Br Med J,* 2:326–327, 1972.

McIntosh TK, Smith DH, Meaney DF, et al. Neuropathological sequelae of traumatic brain injury: Relationship to neurochemical and biochemical mechanisms. *Lab Invest,* 74:315–342, 1996.

McKinley WW, Brooks DN, Bond MR. Post-concussional symptoms, financial compensation, and outcome of severe blunt head injury. *J Neurol Neurosurg Psychiatry,* 46:1084–1091, 1983.

Medina JL. Efficacy of an individualized outpatient program in the treatment of chronic posttraumatic headache. *Headache,* 32:180–183, 1992.

Mendelson G. Not "cured by a verdict." *Med J Aust,* 2:132–134, 1982.

Merskey H, Woodforde JM. Psychiatric sequelae of minor head injury. *Brain,* 95:521–528, 1972.

Noseworthy JH, Miller J, Murray TJ, et al. Auditory brainstem responses in postconcussion syndrome. *Arch Neurol,* 389:275–278, 1981.

Ommaya AK, Faas F, Yarnell P. Whiplash injury and brain damage: An experimental study. *JAMA,* 204:275–289, 1968.

Oppenheimer DR. Microscopic lesions in the brain following head injury. *J Neurol Neurosurg Psychiatry,* 31:299–306, 1968.

Packard RC. Post-traumatic headache. Permanency and relationship to legal settlement. *Headache,* 32:496, 1992.

Packard RC, Ham LP. Pathogenesis of post-traumatic headache and migraine. A common headache pathway. *Headache,* 37:142–152, 1997.

Post RM, Silberstein SD. Shared mechanisms in affective illness, epilepsy, and migraine. *Neurology,* 44:37, 1994.

Povlishok JT, Becker DP, Cheng CLY, et al. Axonal changes in minor head injury. *J Neuropathol Exp Neurol,* 42:225–242, 1983.

Povlishock JT, Coburn TH. Morphopathologic change associated with mild head injury. (In) *Mild Head Injury.* HS Levin, HM Eisenberg, Al Benton (Eds). New York, Oxford University Press, 1989.

Prigatano GP, Stahl ML, Orr WC, et al. Sleep and dreaming disturbances in closed head injury patients. *J Neurol Neurosurg Psychiatry,* 45:78–80, 1982.

Radanov BP, Sturzenegger M, DiStefano G. Long-term outcome after whiplash injury: A 2-year follow-up considering features of injury mechanism and somatic, radiologic, and psychosocial findings. *Medicine,* 74:281–297, 1995.

Raskin NH. *Headache.* New York, Churchill-Livingstone, 1988.

Rimel RW, Giordani B, Barth JT, et al. Disability caused by minor head injury. *Neurosurgery,* 9:221–228, 1981.

Rizzo PA, Pierelli F, Pozzessere G, et al. Subjective post-traumatic syndrome: A comparison of visual and brainstem auditory evoked responses. *Neuropsychobiology,* 9:78–82, 1983.

Ross WD, McNaughton FL. Head injury: A study of patients with chronic posttraumatic complaints. *Arch Neurol Psychiatry,* 52:255, 1944.

Rowe JM, Carlson C. Brainstem auditory evoked potential in post-concussion dizziness. *Arch Neurol,* 37:679–683, 1980.

Sackallares JC, Giordani B, Berent S, et al. Patients with pseudoseizures: Intellectual and cognitive performance. *Neurology,* 35:116–119, 1985.

Servadei P, Vergoni G, Pasini A, et al. Diffuse axonal injury with brainstem localization: Report of a case in a mild head injured patient. *J Neurosurg Sci,* 38:129–130, 1994.

Smith RG, Cherry JE. Traumatic Eagle's syndrome: Report of a case and review of the literature. *J Oral Maxillofac Surg,* 46:606–609, 1988.

Starkstein SE, Mayberg HS, Bertwier ML, et al. Mania after brain injury: Neuroradiological and metabolic findings. *Ann Neurol,* 27:652–659, 1990.

Stuss DT, Ely P, Hugenholtz H, et al. Subtle neuropsychological deficits in patients with good recovery after closed head injury. *Neurosurgery,* 17:41–47, 1985.

Symonds CP. Mental disorder following head injury. *Proc Royal Soc Med,* 30:1081, 1937.

Tarsh MJ, Royston C. A follow-up study of accident neurosis. *Br J Psychiatry,* 146:18–25, 1985.

Toglia JU, Rosenberg PE, Ronis ML. Post-traumatic dizziness. *Arch Otolaryngol,* 92:485–492, 1970.

Torres F, Shapiro SK. Electroencephalograms and whiplash injury. *Arch Neurol,* 5:40–47, 1961.

Trimbell MR. *Post-traumatic Neurosis: From Railway Spine to the Whiplash.* New York, John Wiley and Sons, 1981.

Vijayan N, Dreyfus PM. Post-traumatic dysautonomic cephalgia. *Arch Neurol,* 32:649–652, 1975.

Wei EP, Dietrich WD, Polvichek JT, et al. Functional, morphological, and metabolic abnormalities of the cerebral microcirculation after concussive brain injury in cats. *Circ Res,* 46:37–47, 1980.

Weiss HD, Stern BJ, Goldberg J. Post-traumatic migraine: Chronic migraine precipitated by minor head or neck trauma. *Headache,* 31:451–456, 1991.

West M, LaBella FS, Havlicek V, et al. Cerebral concussion in rats rapidly induces hypothalamic-specific effects on opiate and cholinergic receptors. *Brain Res,* 25:271–277, 1981.

Winston KR. Whiplash and its relationship to migraine. *Headache,* 27:452–457, 1987.

Yamaguchi M. Incidence of headache and severity of head injury. *Headache,* 32:427–431, 1992.

Young WB, Packard RC. Post-traumatic headache and post-traumatic syndrome. (In) *Headache,* PJ Goadsby, SD Silberstein (Eds). Pgs 253–277, Boston, Butterworth-Heinemeann, 1997.

14

Carotodynia and Arterial Dissections (Carotid and Vertebral)

I. Introduction

Syndromes of carotodynia and cervicocephalic arterial dissections will be considered together, because both represent potential neck pain syndromes of vascular origin. Moreover, both conditions generally prompt similar evaluations and, at least in the carotid region, represent entities that are in the differential diagnosis of each other.

II. Carotodynia
A. Introduction

Carotodynia refers to pain arising from the region of the cervical carotid artery, frequently radiating to the jaw, face, ear, and head (including the periorbital region) on the ipsilateral side. Both acute and chronic forms exist. *Carotodynia* may be overlooked as a cause of recurring facial pain (see Chapter 16). Recently, Clark (1994) proposed that carotodynia be divided into three distinct classifications: migrainous, nonmigrainous (or classic), and arteriosclerotic. Treatment choices depend upon the classification.

B. Key Clinical Features
1. Acute carotodynia

The acute or subacute onset of pain (stabbing, throbbing, or dull) lasts days to weeks. The pain is typically unilateral but bilateral pain has been reported. In some instances, the syndrome may appear to be provoked by an upper respiratory infection. The artery is tender, and neck and head motion, swallowing, sneezing, yawning, and coughing aggravate the pain.

2. Chronic carotodynia

The chronic form of carotodynia is better known and was initially identified in patients with chronic facial pain. Most patients are women, and an association with migraine is noted. Some consider chronic carotodynia a form of facial migraine. The carotid artery is tender, and headache may or may not be an accompaniment. The pain is persistent and is usually located in the neck, jaw, and periorbital regions. Periorbital and maxillary pain are not uncommon. The pain is dull, with throbbing elements. Periodic exacerbation lasting up to hours is noted, as well as icepick-like jabs (see Chapter 15). Ten-

derness and prominent pulsations, along with soft tissue
swelling overlying the carotid artery on the ipsilateral side, are
characteristic.

C. Mechanism

The primary mechanism of carotodynia may be similar to migraine and in the end may represent a migraine variant (see Chapter 8). Moreover, studies demonstrate that electrical stimulation
of the carotid artery wall at its bifurcation can produce pain in a
variety of areas about the head and jaw. Denervation of the carotid
artery produces cessation of facial pain.

D. Diagnosis

1. The diagnosis is established by ruling out other painful disorders of the neck, including:

   a. Giant cell arteritis;
   b. Spontaneous carotid dissection;
   c. Carotid atherosclerosis/thrombosis;
   d. Thyroiditis;
   e. Ruptured cervical carotid artery aneurysm;
   f. Fibromuscular dysplasia;
   g. Cluster headache/migraine;
   h. Elongation/fracture of styloid process;
   i. Tumor;
   j. Temporomandibular dysfunction (TMD) (including TM
      joint dysfunction); and
   k. Otitis/mastoiditis.

2. Recommended diagnostic studies include:

   a. MRI of the neck (MR angiogram);
   b. CT scan/MRI of head;
   c. Ultrasound of carotid artery;
   d. Carotid arteriogram (rarely required); and
   e. Appropriate blood and metabolic studies.

E. Specifics of Treatment
1. The acute syndrome:
   a. Analgesics
   b. NSAIDs
   c. DHE or a triptan
   d. Prednisone or
   e. Triamcinolone
      Steroids should be administered for 7 days, followed by
      gradual reduction (see Tables 6.11, 6.12, Chapter 6)

2. The chronic syndrome is treated with one or more of the following:
  a. Indomethacin 25–50 mg t.i.d.
  b. Methysergide/methylergonovine
  c Propranolol
  d. Nortriptyline
  e. Other migraine or cluster headache treatment

III. Arterial Dissections
A. Introduction

Acute headache and neck ache in the presence of stroke-like neurological symptoms (though often delayed) are the primary features of spontaneous dissection of either the internal carotid artery (ICA) or vertebral artery (VA). Estimated annual incidence is 2.6/100,000 population for carotid dissection and about one-third of that for vertebral dissection. Overall incidence for dissection is about 4.5/100,000 population (Mokri, 1997). Predisposing factors include:

1. Migraine?;
2. Fibromuscular dysplasia;
3. Cystic medial necrosis;
4. Marfan's syndrome;
5. Arteritis;
6. Atherosclerosis;
7. Other congenital abnormalities of the arterial wall; and
8. Hypertension. ?

B. ICA Dissection
1. Clinical features
  a. Sudden or gradual onset of ipsilateral neck pain or hemicrania (retro-orbital, face, head, and neck)
  b. Acute ischemic neurological events (often delayed)

    1) Incomplete ipsilateral Horner's syndrome (oculosympathetic palsy)
    2) Focal transient ischemic attack (TIA) or ischemic stroke-like symptoms (from carotid or vertebral vascular systems)
    3) Carotid bruit
    4) Subarachnoid hemorrhage from a leaking dissection intracranially
    5) Less commonly, lower cranial nerve palsies

The syndrome may be monosymptomatic, hemilingual only, or oculomotor only. Headache is present in about one-half of cases and usually precedes other symptoms. The onset of pain is usually gradual, but a "thunderclap" presentation has been reported (Mokri, 1997). Neck pain is present in about one-fourth of patients. A past history of migraine is a questionable predisposing factor.

2. Mechanism

Apparent weakness of the arterial wall, resulting in separation of the internal elastic lamina from the medial layer, is a consistent finding. Extravasation of blood into the arterial wall produces hematoma, with occlusion of the lumen. Embolic phenomena are possible, and intracranial bleeding is also possible. Traumatic events, often trivial, may also induce the syndrome. These include coughing, straining, or various neck movements. Rapid hyperextension of the neck as in "bottoms up" actions has resulted in dissection. Recently, roller-coaster rides were reported to account for three cases of cervical dissection (two carotid, one vertebral) (Kettaneh, 1998). Other cases of cervical and neurological injury were reported after roller-coaster rides as well.

Intrinsic predispositions lower the threshold to spontaneous events and were listed previously.

3. Diagnosis

The diagnosis of ICA dissection requires ruling out other causes for neck and head pain accompanied by neurological symptoms (see page 233 in this Chapter). Most dissections occur in middle age or younger. Seventy percent of patients are younger than 45 years of age (Mokri, 1997).

Historically, the diagnostic procedure of choice has been arteriography. MRI of the soft tissues of the neck and/or MR angiography of the carotids now replace arteriography in all but a few cases. A well-performed Doppler ultrasound examination may also be helpful. A lumbar puncture (LP) to rule out subarachnoid hemorrhage is advisable when clinical circumstances warrant. *Because the acute neurological symptoms frequently prompt an aggressive pursuit of intracranial pathology, the vasculature in the neck is sometimes overlooked.*

4. Treatment

Most cases undergo clinical and angiographic recovery spontaneously. Recurrence is rare. Anticoagulation and surgical intervention can be considered on a case-by-case basis. Controlled trials comparing antiplatelet vs. anticoagulant treatment are underway for acute ICA dissection. Unless a contraindication exists (hemorrhage, severe hypertension, or massive infarction), some authorities administer anticoagulation (warfarin or Heparin if urgent) for 3 months, followed by antiplatelet therapy for 3 months. Imaging studies and CSF evaluation for hemorrhage is advisable before initiating treatment. Surgical intervention is required in some cases, particularly if subarachnoid hemorrhage due to intracranial leaking from dissection is identified.

C. Vertebral Artery Dissection

In most ways, VA dissections are similar to that occurring in the internal carotid system (see page 235 for mechanism). Headache and neck pain are the most common symptoms. The headache is usually posterior and may be followed, after a period of some delay, by stroke or TIA symptomatology in the vertebrobasilar system. Monosymptomatic presentation is possible, as with internal carotid dissection. Subarachnoid hemorrhage may rarely be a presenting feature. Vertigo, "upside down vision" (Charles, 1992), hemifacial spasm (Matsumoto, 1991), and other clinical patterns may occur, including left upper limb pain mimicking myocardial infarction with respiratory arrest (Roos, 1992). Transient amnesia has also occurred. According to Mokri (1997), the most common presentation is headache or neck pain followed by the lateral medullary syndrome (Wallenberg's syndrome). The presence of the lateral medullary syndrome, particularly when preceded by a headache or neck pain in a younger person, should suggest a VA dissection. Diagnostic and treatment considerations for internal carotid dissection generally apply to that associated with VA dissection. The rate of recovery is about the same in both conditions, with more than 85% of patients making a complete or good recovery, though the presence of subarachnoid hemorrhage imposes a more guarded prognosis.

References

Bank H. Idiopathic carotiditis. *Lancet,* 1:726, 1978.

Cannon CR. Carotodynia: An unusual pain in the neck. *Otolaryngol Head Neck Surg,* 110:387–390, 1994.

Caplan LR, Baquis GD, Pessin MS, et al. Dissection of the intracranial vertebral artery. *Neurology,* 38:868, 1988.

Charles N, Froment C, Rode G, et al. Vertigo and upside down vision due to an infarct in the territory of medial branch of the posterior inferior cerebellar artery caused by dissection of a vertebral artery. *J Neurol Neurosurg Psychiatry,* 53:188, 1992.

Clark HB, King DE. Carotodynia. *Am Fam Physician,* 50:987–990, 1994.

Cox LK, Bertorini T, Lassiter RE. Headaches due to spontaneous internal carotid artery dissection: Magnetic resonance imaging evaluation follow-up. *Headache,* 31:12–16, 1991.

Fisher CM. The headache and pain of spontaneous carotid dissection. *Headache,* 22:660–665, 1982.

Hart RG, Easton JD. Dissections of cervical and cerebral arteries. *Neurol Clin,* 1:155–182, 1983.

Hicks PA, Leavitt JA, Mokri B. Ophthalmic manifestations of vertebral artery dissection: Patients seen at the Mayo Clinic from 1976 to 1992. *Opthalmology,* 101:1786–1792, 1994.

Kettaneh A, Biousse V, Bousser MG. Neurological complications of roller-coaster rides (abstract). Presented to American Academy of Neurology, Minneapolis, April 1998.

Linden D, Steinke W, Schwartz A, et al. Spontaneous vertebral artery dissection initially mimicking myocardial infarction. *Stroke,* 23:1021–1023, 1992.

Matsumoto K, Toshikazu S, Hideyuki K. Hemifacial spasm caused by spontaneous dissecting aneurysm of the vertebral artery. *J Neurosurg,* 74:650–652, 1991.

Mehigan JT, Olcott C. Carotodynia associated with carotid arterial disease and stroke. *Am J Surg,* 142:210–211, 1981.

Mokri B. Traumatic and spontaneous extracranial internal carotid artery dissections. *J Neurol,* 237:356–361, 1990.

Mokri B. Headache and spontaneous carotid vertebral artery dissections. (In) *Headache.* PJ Goadsby, SD Silberstein (Eds). Pgs 327–253, Boston, Butterworth-Heinemeann, 1997.

Mokri B, Houser OW, Stanson AW. Multivessel cervicocephalic and visceral arterial dissections: Pathogenic role of primary arterial disease in cervicocephalic arterial dissections. *J Stroke Cerebrovasc Dis,* 1:117, 1991.

Mokri B, Schievink WI, Olsen KD, et al. Spontaneous dissection of the cervical internal carotid artery: Presentation with lower cranial nerve palsies. *Arch Otolaryngol Head Neck Surg,* 118:431–435, 1992.

Mokri B, Silbert PL, Schievink WI, et al. Cranial nerve palsy and spontaneous dissection of the extracranial internal carotid artery. *Neurology,* 46:356–357,1996.

Mokri B, Sundt TM, Houser OW, et al. Spontaneous dissection of the cervical internal artery. *Ann Neurol,* 19:126–138, 1986.

Orfei R, Meienberg O. Carotodynia: Report of eight cases and prospective evaluation of therapy. *J Neurol,* 230:65–72, 1983.

Raskin NH, Prusiner S. Carotodynia. *Neurology,* 27:43–46, 1977.

Rittenhouse EA, Radke HM, Sumner DS. Carotid artery aneurysm. *Arch Surg,* 105:786–789, 1972.

Roos KL, Harris T. Vertebral artery dissection manifested by respiratory arrest. *J Neuroimaging,* 2:161, 1992.

Rothrock JF, Lim V, Press G, et al. Serial magnetic resonance and carotid duplex examinations in the management of carotid dissection. *Neurology,* 38:686–692, 1989.

Schievink WI, Mokri B, Garrity JA, et al. Oculomotor nerve palsy since spontaneous dissections of the cervical internal carotid artery. *Neurology,* 43:1938–1941, 1993.

Schievink WI, Mokri B, O'Fallon WM. Recurrent spontaneous cervical artery dissection. *N Engl J Med,* 330:393–397, 1994.

Schievink WI, Mokri B, Piepgras DG. Spontaneous dissections of the cervicocephalic arteries in childhood and adolescence. *Neurology,* 44:1607–1612, 1994.

Silbert PL, Mokri B, Schievink WI. Headache and neck pain in spontaneous internal carotid and vertebral artery dissections. *Neurology,* 45:1517–1522, 1995.

15

Headaches Provoked by Exertional Factors and/or Responsive to Indomethacin

I. Introduction

Several headache entities share the features of being particularly or exclusively (diagnostically) responsive to indomethacin. Some of these disorders appear to be provoked by physical stimulation (exertion, cough, flexion/extension of the neck, etc.), may have a relationship to migraine, and some may respond to migraine therapy (see Chapters 6, 8, and 9).

The headaches provoked by exertion and those that are extraordinarily sensitive to indomethacin are considered in the same chapter because the literature has reflected a potential, if not confusing, relationship based on general or exclusive responsiveness to indomethacin. The reader is warned that a mechanistic, etiological, or therapeutic relationship may not exist. Moreover, in the case of exertional-related headache, serious cervical or intracranial pathology may mimic that which has been considered otherwise benign.

II. Specific Exertional Syndromes
A. Exertional Headache
1. Introduction

Exertional headache encompasses several distinct entities, including cough headache (also induced by Valsalva maneuver), effort migraine, and coital cephalgia. Effort or exertional migraine is sometimes considered as two separate conditions (effort migraine and benign exertional headache). In a recent paper by Pascual (1996), 72 patients were evaluated because of headaches precipitated by coughing (30), physical exercise (28), or sexual excitement (14). Of the 72 cases, 30 (42%) were associated with structural pathology, of which 17 were secondary to Chiari Type I malformation, and the others were associated with subarachnoid hemorrhage.

Pascual points out that while the precipitant was the same, clinical factors differed, such as age of onset, associated clinical manifestations, and response to pharmacological treatment. *Benign cough headache* and *benign exertional headache,* while sharing male predominance, were considered by the author as separate conditions. *Benign cough headache* began significantly later (43 years on average) than *benign exertional headache*. The author concluded that benign and symptomatic (associated with pathology) cough headache are different from both benign and symptomatic (associated with pathology) exertional and sexual headaches.

Clearly, when considering exertional headaches, the literature is confusing and the classification and terminology is in a state of transition. What the reader must consider, however, is that in all or most cases of exertional headache, the potential for organic pathology exists and must be considered and pursued responsibly.

Exertional headaches share provocation by various types of exertion, including but not limited to coughing, sneezing, straining, weight lifting, bending, stooping, and sexual activity. While generally benign, headaches related to these maneuvers must be considered potentially pathological until appropriate investigation has been undertaken and excludes pathology.

2. Key clinical features

The clinical features of exertional headache consist of a severe, usually bilateral, sudden-onset headache that occurs within moments following the exertional stimulus. In the case of cough headache, it subsides within seconds. In the case of benign exertional headache, or *effort migraine,* it lingers for 5–24 hours. In both instances, dull aching may persist for hours, but patients are generally pain-free between attacks. Patients may be prone to other chronic headaches.

The location of the headache is often diffuse but can be lateralized. Accompaniments are generally absent, but effort migraine has been associated with transient neurological events and nausea and vomiting. Males are more likely affected than females.

3. Diagnosis

a. Differential diagnosis

Structural/organic causes of headache must be ruled out, even though many, if not most, will be of benign origin. Among the possible causes are:

1) Intracranial/intraspinal mass lesions (particularly tumors, subdural hematomas, structural or obstructive abnormalities of posterior fossa or occipital/cervical junction, such as Arnold-Chiari Type I malformation);

2) A-V malformation;
3) Aneurysm;
4) Intracranial hypertension (obstructive, nonobstructive);
5) Intracranial hypotension (for postural, movement-induced pain);
6) Sinusitis (paranasal, sphenoid sinusitis, etc.);
7) Cerebral venous thrombosis; and
8) Cervical disc disease.

b. Testing

1) Computerized tomography (CT scan)/magnetic resonance imagining (MRI) of head and neck should be obtained. A CT scan with and without contrast is helpful, but an MRI more effectively evaluates the presence of structural abnormalities of the posterior fossa and occipitocervical junction. Magnetic resonance angiography (MRA) and/or venous phase MRI are useful. Cine phase-contrast MRI can assess posterior fossa/cervical cerebrospinal fluid (CSF) flow and detect obstructive disease, and is recommended for serious consideration of cervico-occipital obstruction (Pujol, 1995). Flow-sensitive MRI can detect CSF leak sources.

Arnold-Chiari Type I malformation was historically assessed by myelography, in which patients would be placed in the upright position on a tilt table, with gravitational influence on the downward excursion of the tonsils. Current testing with MRI is performed with patients in the supine position, thereby denying the gravitational influence and perhaps resulting in oversight of the condition.

2) MR angiogram and arteriography must be considered on a case-by-case basis to rule out aneurysm.
3) Lumbar puncture (LP) should be performed to rule out pressure disturbances and subarachnoid hemorrhage when exertional pain is severe and occurs suddenly. *The performance of LP must await the performance and results of a CT scan (with and without enhancement) or MRI.*

4. Principles of treatment

a. The provoking effort must be curtailed until a diagnosis is established;
b. Pharmacological measures are generally indicated in benign cases; and

c. Attacks that occur predictably and occasionally can be treated by therapies given just before exertion, or if they occur unpredictably and frequently, through preventive therapy.

5. Specifics of treatment

a. *Symptomatic pharmacotherapy* (for established benign conditions). Symptomatic treatment can be administered 1–2 hours *before* the anticipated exertional event. Medications that may be useful in this setting include:

1) Indomethacin 25–50 mg
2) Specific migraine treatments (DHE, sumatriptan, naratriptan, zolmitriptan, rizatriptan, etc.)
3) Isometheptene mucate (Midrin, etc.)
4) Propranolol (20–40 mg)
5) Analgesics

b. Preventive pharmacotherapy:

1) Indomethacin
2) β-adrenergic blocking agents
3) Methysergide/methylergonovine
4) Other migraine preventive agents

c. *Lumbar puncture.* LP, perhaps by altering CSF pressure and dynamics, may be effective in terminating recurring exertional headache patterns (personal communication, Raskin, 1996).

B. Coital Headache/Headaches Associated with Sexual Activity/Benign Sexual Headaches
1. Introduction

Headaches associated with sexual activity may be simply exertional in nature, as described earlier, or have a particular relationship to orgasm or sexual excitement. Headache may occur just prior to, at the time of, or just after orgasm. The headache is rarely of psychological origin, although anticipatory anxiety regarding sexual activity could be provocative. In many instances, the syndrome correlates poorly with the degree of physical exertion or sexual excitement. In some instances, however, it does. Headache also has been reported after masturbation. The headache usually ceases if sexual activity stops but may continue, once started, to a more complete migraine-like attack. As in other exertion-related headaches, men appear more vulnerable to the syndrome than women (4:1).

2. Key clinical features

Three patterns of coital headache occur.

a. *Sudden onset.* In 70% of cases, the headache begins just before, during, or just after orgasm. The headache is of severe intensity, usually frontal or occipital, and may be throbbing. Usually the headache builds over minutes, but explosive attacks are reported. The duration of pain is usually several hours, and a low-grade discomfort may persist. Accompaniments are rare, but confusion, palpitations, and vomiting have been reported. A family history of headaches has been reported in about 25% of patients.

b. *Subacute, crescendo headache.* The second pattern is present in about 25% of cases and usually has onset much earlier than orgasm. It often increases in intensity until the time of orgasm. It has a dull, aching quality and is frequently located in the occiput.

c. *Postural headache.* The third and least common form of coital headache is a postural headache that occurs in the suboccipital area and is markedly accentuated when the patient is upright. It is more frequently associated with nausea and vomiting than the other forms. Low CSF pressure has been confirmed in at least one instance. The syndrome may result from a tear in the dura caused by exertion, and clinically resembles a post-LP headache and other CSF hypotension syndromes (see Chapter 17).

3. Diagnosis

See page 239. Silbert (1989) reported a case of benign sexual headache and benign exertional headache that occurred sequentially in the same patient in which arteriography demonstrated multiple areas of cerebral arterial spasm. This supports the concept that benign sexual headache and benign exertional headache may have a similar pathophysiological origin.

4. Principles of treatment

See pages 240–241.

If low CSF pressure is suspected, assessment and treatment guidelines for low-pressure headache should be followed (see Chapters 3 and 17).

C. Non-Exertional Headache (responsive to indomethacin)

1. Hemicrania continua

a. Introduction

In 1984, Sjaastad and Spierings described an unusual headache syndrome that was distinctly and completely responsive to indomethacin. Its main features included a continuous unilateral headache that was moderate to severe in intensity. Frequently, patients experienced a jabbing, icepick-like phenomenon, provoked by exertion. Since first described, hemicrania continua has been recognized as occurring in two patterns, both characterized by persistent, unilateral headache of moderate severity. In the first pattern, the continuous form, headaches persist continuously without remission for years. In the remitting form, periods of headache are separated by an interim of pain-free periods. Patients may evolve from episodic (remitting) hemicranial pain with migrainous features to chronic continuous pain. Icepick components are present in almost half of cases (Raskin, 1988). Traumatic onset is reported.

b. Key clinical features

1) The key clinical features include:

    a. Unilateral headache/variable location (rarely alteration of laterality occurs);

    b. Persisting pattern of pain (in episodic form, remission occurs; in continuous form, it does not);

    c. Moderate to severe intensity;

    d. Rare attack-related autonomic features;

    e. Absence of reliable precipitating features;

    f. Generally responsive to indomethacin;

    g. Female to male ratio—5:1;

    h. Mean age of onset—35.2 (11–58 years);

    i. Mean duration of illness–10.5 years; and

    j. Head trauma in 22% of cases.

2) Other clinical features include:

    a. Nocturnal awakening;

    b. Photophobia; and

    c. Menstrual aggravation.

c. Diagnosis

1) See pages 239–240.

2) The response to indomethacin is generally diagnostic, though exceptions exist.

d. **Principles of treatment**

1) Treatment with indomethacin is usually effective.
2) See pages 240–241.

2. Chronic Paroxysmal Hemicrania (CPH)
a. Introduction

Many consider chronic paroxysmal hemicrania (CPH) a variant of cluster headache. CPH was first described by Sjaastad and Dale in 1974. The condition occurs primarily in women, and sometimes young girls, and the attacks, unlike cluster headaches, may be precipitated by flexion and occasionally by rotation of the neck. It rarely responds to medications that are effective for cluster headache. The originally described pattern was characterized by multiple, short-lived, unilateral attacks occurring daily and without remission. Subsequently, Kudrow et al. described an episodic form in which headache phases were separated by prolonged pain-free remissions. This form was referred to as episodic hemicrania (Kudrow, 1987). The pattern may evolve from intermittent to continuous (chronic). Though rare, there are more than 100 cases of CPH in the literature. The chronic form seems to be more common than the episodic form. Though initially thought to be more likely in younger people, the mean age of reported cases is 33 years, with a range of 6–81 years (Newman, 1997). A family history of a similar condition is not found, although migraine may occur in families.

b. Key clinical features

1) Pain is strictly unilateral and localized to the temporal, frontal, ocular, aural, or maxillary region. Occasionally occipital or nuchal pain is reported; shifting to the alternate side is sometimes noted.
2) A range of pain forms (throbbing, boring, stabbing, etc.) is possible, with moderate to severe intensity. Persisting pain between acute attacks is reported.
3) Attacks of pain last 2–25 minutes, averaging 10–15 minutes (range 2–120 minutes). (Cluster headache attacks have a mean duration of 45 minutes.)
4) Patients generally prefer quiet and rest; some patients pace, as in cluster headache.

5) Attack frequency may be up to 40 per day but average 10–20 attacks per day.
6) In the episodic form, the headache phase is 2 days to 4.5 months. Remission is 1–30 months.
7) Nocturnal awakening occurs.
8) Ipsilateral autonomic symptoms occur, similar to those in cluster headache:
   a. lacrimation/rhinorrhea/nasal congestion/conjunctival injection;
   b. forehead perspiration;
   c. mild miosis;
   d. eyelid edema;
   e. photophobia;
   f. nausea;
   g. bradycardia/tachycardia; and
   h. ptosis.
9) Headache can be provoked by movement in 10% of cases; pressure on cervical region may precipitate an attack
10) Provocation by alcohol is sometimes noted.
11) Patients will frequently resort to excessive aspirin or over-the-counter (OTC) ibuprofen to control pain, perhaps due to the similarity in effect of indomethacin.

c. **Establishing the diagnosis**

Cluster headache is the most important differential diagnostic possibility, although hemicrania continua, trigeminal neuralgia, and short-lasting, unilateral neuralgiform headache attacks (SUNCT) must be considered (see Chapter 12). Attacks of CPH, as in cluster headache, have been mimicked by intracranial disease of either a structural or infiltrative, infectious type, including aneurysm of ophthalmic artery, pituitary and other intracranial tumors, sphenoid sinusitis, etc. (See Chapter 12 for differential diagnosis of CPH and cluster headache.) Table 15.1, published with permission of Newman (1997), compares features of CPH with cluster headache, hemicrania continua, trigeminal neuralgia, and SUNCT syndrome.

The following diagnostic studies are recommended:

1. CT scan with and without contrast, or preferably an MRI;
2. LP in questionable cases to rule out infiltrative disease;
3. MR angiogram or arteriogram as necessary; and

TABLE 15.1.   DIFFERENTIAL DIAGNOSIS OF THE PAROXYSMAL HEMICRANIAS

	Paroxysmal hemicrania	Cluster	Hemicrania continua	Trigeminal neuralgia	SUNCT syndrome[a]
Sex (F:M)	2:1	1:6	2:1	2:1	1:10
Age of onset (years)	6–81	20–40	11–58	50–60	30–68
Pain quality	Stabbing, pulsatile, throbbing	Stabbing, boring	Baseline dull ache, superimposed throbbing/stabbing	Lancinating	Lancinating
Site of maximal pain	Orbit/temple	Orbit/temple	Orbit/temple	V1–V2	Periorbital
Attacks per day	1–40	0–8	Varies	Varies/hundreds	Varies
Durations of attacks	2–120 minutes (average 2–25)	15–180 minutes (average 20–45)	Continuous	Seconds	Seconds
Autonomic features	Yes	Yes	Yes (but less pronounced than cluster)	No	Yes
Alcohol trigger	Yes	Sometimes	Yes	No	No

[a] SUNCT = short-lasting, unilateral neuralgiform headache attacks with conjunctival injection and tearing.
Used with permission of the authors and publisher. Newman LC, Lipton RB. Paroxysmal hemicranias. (In) *Headache (Blue Books of Practical Neurology).*
PJ Goadsby, SD Silberstein (Eds). Pgs 243–250, Boston, Butterworth-Heinemann, 1997.

4. Evaluation of the eyes for pathology, including glaucoma, orbital pseudotumor, etc.

Indomethacin is generally reliable and effective, and can be used for diagnostic purposes. Pursuit of the neurological workup can sometimes await a trial of treatment, although pathological conditions can occasionally respond to the analgesic and the anti-inflammatory effects of indomethacin.

d. **Specifics of treatment**

1) Indomethacin, 25–50 mg t.i.d. (high dosing may occasionally be necessary).
2) Failure to respond to modest dosages of indomethacin should challenge the diagnosis. Long-term therapy may require gastrointestinal protection. Calcium blockers, steroids, and other NSAIDs, such as piroxicam, may be helpful.

References

Akpunonu BE, Ahrens J. Sexual headaches: Case report. Review and treatment with calcium blocker. *Headache,* 31:141–145, 1991.

Biousse V, Bousser MG. The myth of carotodynia. *Neurology,* 44:993–995, 1994.

Bordini C, Antonaci F, Stovner LJ, et al. Hemicrania continua: A clinical review. *Headache,* 31:20–26, 1991.

Braun A, Klawans HL. Headaches associated with exercise and sexual activity. (In) *Handbook of Clinical Neurology,* Vol. 48. FC Rose (Ed). Pgs 373–382, Amsterdam, Elsevier Science Publishers, 1986.

Calandre L, Hernandez S, Lopez-Valdes E, et al. Benign valsalva's maneuver-related headache: An MRI study of 6 cases. *Headache,* 36:251–253, 1996.

Ekbom K. Cough headache. (In) *Handbook of Clinical Neurology,* Vol. 48. FC Rose (Ed). Pgs 367–371, Amsterdam, Elsevier Science Publishers, 1986.

Hannerz J, Ericson K, Bergstrand G. Chronic paroxysmal hemicrania: Orbital phlebography and steroid treatment. *Cephalalgia,* 7:189–192, 1987.

Johns DR. Benign sexual headache within a family. *Arch Neurol,* 43:1158–1160, 1986.

Kudrow, L, Esperanca P, Vijayan N. Episodic paroxysmal hemicrania? *Cephalalgia,* 7:197–201, 1987.

Kuritzky A. Indomethacin-resistant hemicrania continua. *Cephalalgia,* 12:57–59, 1992.

Moncada E, Graff-Radford SB. Benign indomethacin-responsive headaches presenting in the orofacial region: 8 case reports. *J Orofac Pain,* 9:276–284, 1995.

Newman LC, Lipton RB. Paroxysmal hemicranias. (In) *Headache (Blue Books of Practical Neurology).* PJ Goadsby, SD Silberstein (Eds). Pgs 243–250, Boston, Butterworth-Heinemeann, 1997.

Newman LC, Lipton RB, Russell M, et al. Hemicrania continua: Attacks may alternate sides. *Headache,* 32:237–238, 1992.

Newman LC, Lipton RB, Solomon S. Episodic paroxysmal hemicrania: Three new cases and a review of the literature. *Headache,* 3:195, 1993.

Newman LC, Lipton RB, Solomon S. Hemicrania continua: Ten new cases and a review of the literature. *Neurology,* 44:2111, 1994.

Pascual J, Iglesias F, Oterino A, et al. Cough, exertional, and sexual headaches: An analysis of 72 benign and symptomatic cases. *Neurology,* 46:1520–1524, 1996.

Paulson GW, Klawans HL. Benign orgasmic cephalgia. *Headache,* 13:181–187, 1974.

Porter M, Jankovic J. Benign coital cephalgia: Differential diagnosis and treatment. *Arch Neurol,* 38:710–712, 1981.

Pujol J, Roig C, Capdevila A, et al. Motion of the cerebellar tonsils in Chiari Type I malformation by cine-phase-contrast MRI. *Neurology,* 45:1746–1753, 1995.

Raskin NH. *Headache.* New York, Churchill-Livingstone, 1988.

Rooke ED. Benign exertional headache. *Med Clin North Am,* 52:801–808, 1968.

Russel D. Chronic paroxysmal hemicrania: Severity, duration, and time of occurrence of attacks. *Cephalalgia,* 4:53–56, 1984.

Sans GH, Newman L, Lipton R. Cough, exertional, and other miscellaneous headaches. *Med Clin North Am,* 75:733–747, 1991.

Selwyn DL. A study of coital-related headaches in 32 patients. *Cephalalgia,* 5(supp 3):300–301, 1985.

Silbert PL, Hankey GJ, Prentice DA, et al. Angiographically demonstrated arterial spasm in the case of benign sexual headache and benign exertional headache. *Aust N Z J Med,* 19:466–468, 1989.

Sjaastad O. Chronic paroxysmal hemicrania. (In) *Handbook of Clinical Neurology,* Vol. 48. FC Rose (Ed). Pgs 375–266, Amsterdam, Elsevier Science Publishers, 1986.

Sjaastad O, Antonaci F. A piroxican derivative partly effective in chronic paroxysmal hemicrania and hemicrania continua. *Headache,* 35:549–550, 1995.

Sjaastad O, Dale I. Evidence for a new (?) treatable headache entity. *Headache,* 14:105–108, 1974.

Sjaastad O, Spierings ELH. "Hemicrania continua": Another headache absolutely responsive to indomethacin. *Cephalalgia,* 4:65–70, 1984.

Sjaastad O, Stovner LJ, Stolt-Nielsen A, et al. Case reports CPH and hemicrania continua: Requirements of high-dose indomethacin dosages. An ominous sign? *Headache,* 35:363, 1995.

Spierings ELH. Case report: Episodic paroxysmal hemicrania and chronic paroxysmal hemicrania. *Clin J Pain,* 8:44, 1992.

16

Facial Pain and the Neuralgias

I. Introduction

The diagnosis and treatment of facial pain represents an important challenge, albeit often a gratifying one, to the clinician. Facial pain has many causes (see Table 16.1 for a list of some of the differential possibilities). Historically, pain not clearly identifiable as one of the "typical" (well-delineated) neuralgic syndromes was assumed to be of psychological origin. Most authorities now, however, believe that many, if not most, facial pain disorders, even if accompanied by depression, arise primarily from physiological dysfunction or organic disease. Psychological issues may represent comorbid factors.

II. General Diagnostic Approach
A. Complete History

The history is the key component to a successful evaluation. Factors that must be delineated include:

- Nature of onset;
- Time of day of onset;
- Character of pain;
- Location;
- Relationship to dental or ear-nose-throat (ENT) procedures;
- Aggravating and alleviating influences;
- Pattern of pain (constant, periodic, etc.); and
- Other health factors, such as sinus infection, dental disease, chest symptoms including cough and neck disease, and gastrointestinal (GI) complaints.

Although the location of pain in itself cannot be used to assign origin (pain involving the fifth cranial nerve, other cranial nerves, and cervical spine may be referred to any other region about the head and neck), its location and the presence of tenderness may provide important clues. Pain arising intracranially can be referred extracranially. The reverse is also true. *Pain arising in the thorax or portions of the esophagus or gastrum, and innervated by the vagus nerve, can be referred to the ear and face.*

Provoking phenomena may suggest etiology. Pain following a dental procedure, aggravated by hot or cold substances in the mouth or from chewing, may suggest dental or jaw origin, whereas

TABLE 16.1.   **SELECTED CONDITIONS CAUSING FACE PAIN**

Neurologic
  A. Neuralgic syndromes (trigeminal, glossopharyngeal, etc.)
  B. Posterior fossa tumors/aneurysm compressing trigeminal nerves, nervous intermedius, glossopharyngeal or vagus nerves
  C. Infiltrative intracranial disease (lymphomatous, etc.)
  D. Occipital/cervical and posterior fossa conditions, including Arnold Chiari malformation, Type I, obstructive hydrocephalus
  E. Postendarterectomy syndrome
  F. Cerebrovascular ischemic disease (thalamic pain, ischemia, etc.)
  G. Carotid/vertebral artery dissection/aneurysm
  H. Trauma
  I. Neuritis (trigeminal, optic nerve, occulomotor nerve)
  J. Herpes zoster (acute and postherpetic syndromes, including encephalitis)
  K. See PRIMARY HEADACHE CONDITIONS
  L. Gradenigo syndrome (apical petrositis)
  M. Raeder paratrigeminal syndrome
  N. Anesthesia dolorosa
  O. Giant cell arteritis

Selected Headache Conditions
  A. Carotodynia
  B. Cluster headache
  C. Chronic paroxysmal hemicrania
  D. Migraine
  E. "Icepick" pain
  F. Exertional headache syndromes
  G. Others

Dental
  A. Tooth abscesses
  B. Cracked tooth syndrome
  C. Postextraction syndromes
    1. Phantom tooth pain
    2. Postsurgical neuroma
    3. Postsurgical microabscesses
    4. Others
  D. Phantom tooth pain

Otolaryngological
  A. Sinus disease (particularly sphenoid sinus, including infectious, infiltrative, tumor, etc.) (See Chapters 3 and 5 and Druce, 1991)
  B. Bone, jaw disease (infection, infiltrative, tumor, etc.)
  C. Nasopharyngeal disease, including carcinoma, peritonsillar abscesses
  D. Otalgic disease
    1. External otitis, otitis media
    2. Herpes zoster
    3. Acoustic neuroma
  E. Nasal septal disease, deviation

Jaw and Cranial Abnormalities
  A. Styloid process syndromes (elongation, fracture, etc.)
  B. Stylomandibular ligament syndrome
  C. Primary disorders of the jaw
  D. Myofascial syndromes

continued

TABLE 16.1. **SELECTED CONDITIONS CAUSING FACE PAIN**

E. Osteoarthritis of cranial bones
F. Trauma
G. Multiple myeloma
H. Paget's disease

Ocular
A. Refraction errors
B. Heterophoria, heterotropia (weakness of muscles of eye movement)
C. Glaucoma (acute)
D. Corneal and conjunctival disease
E. Ischemic ocular disorders
F. Optic neuritis (retrobulbar neuritis)
G. Herpes zoster ophthalmicus
H. Painful ophthalmoplegia (Tolosa-Hunt syndrome)

Neck Disease
A. Vertebral abnormalities (disc disease/C2–C3 nerves, facet joints, etc.)
B. Root syndromes
C. Osteomyelitis
D. Trauma/fracture
E. Neuralgia (occipital)
F. Tumors
G. Soft tissue disorders
H. Dissections syndromes

Others
A. Thoracic tumors (esophageal, pulmonary, and gastric disorders can refer pain to face—usually right ear region) via the auricular branch of the vagus nerve.
B. Giant cell arteritis

---

pain provoked by cold wind to the face suggests *trigeminal neuralgia.* Pain induced by swallowing or taste stimuli may result from *glossopharyngeal neuralgia, superior laryngeal neuralgia,* or *carotodynia.*

Pain aggravated by alcohol, exertion, sleep, or menses may suggest migraine or a variant, such as carotodynia. Pain provoked by sneezing, coughing, or exertion may suggest intracranial structural disease, including arteriovenous (A-V) malformation, aneurysm, posterior fossa structural disease, occipitocervical syndromes, increased intracranial pressure, or "exertional migraine."

Face pain, often neuralgic in origin, when associated with headache and sinus symptoms might suggest acute sphenoid sinusitis. Other symptomatology involving the cavernous sinus (it lies immediately lateral to the sphenoid sinus) must be considered.

B. Diagnostic Testing

The diagnostic evaluation must be comprehensive if the source of pain and the diagnosis are not clear. A careful evaluation of the cranium, cervical spine, cerebral spinal fluid (CSF), and of dental, nasal, eye, throat, sinus, and ear structures is necessary. A complete neurological examination is mandatory.

The following diagnostic tests are recommended selectively when the origin of symptoms is not evident (see also Chapters 3 and 5):

1. Metabolic/hematological evaluation:
   - CBC and differential;
   - ESR;
   - Endocrinological parameters (including thyroid and parathyroid measurements); and
   - General chemistry exam.
2. Standard x-ray examinations (becoming less practical, but still with some value);
3. Computed tomography (CT scan)/magnetic resonance imaging (MRI)/MR angiogram (MRA) evaluating head, jaw, neck (soft tissues and bone), and sphenoid sinus regions;*
4. A complete dental and jaw evaluation, including selective alveolar blocks to rule out localized dental pathology, such as alveolar microabscess, neuroma, etc.;
5. A complete otolaryngological and ophthalmological evaluation, including intraocular pressure testing for glaucoma and visualization of nasal, ear, and pharyngeal structures;
6. "Diagnostic blocks," including sphenopalatine, occipital nerve, facet joints, and regions of the upper cervical spine** (see Chapter 19); and
7. An evaluation of soft tissues of the neck, including the carotid artery and glands.

*Routine CT scans may not demonstrate the sphenoid sinus sufficiently. Special views of the sinuses are required to rule out sphenoid disease on CT scanning (see Chapters 3 and 5).

**Relief through blockade does not reliably diagnose or localize the pathology.

III. Clinical Syndromes
A. Trigeminal Neuralgia
1. Introduction

Trigeminal neuralgia is the most well delineated of the formal neuralgic syndromes. Onset of the disorder is usually later in life (6th and 7th decades) but can occur earlier. Onset may follow a dental procedure. *Multiple sclerosis* may be causative when present in the younger population. Cases of trigeminal neuralgia may occur simultaneously with cluster headache in a syndrome referred to as *cluster-tic syndrome*. This topic and a review are more fully considered in Chapter 12.

2. Key clinical features

Brief unilateral paroxysms of electric-like pain are the primary symptomatic feature. The lancinating pain is in the distribution of one or more divisions of the trigeminal nerve. Maximum intensity of pain lasts a second or slightly longer and occurs repetitively. A sustaining deep, dull ache is often present between acute paroxysms. The pain does not cross to the other side but may be bilateral in 3–5% of cases.

The attacks of pain are characteristically "triggered" by one or more often trivial physical maneuvers (i.e., brushing teeth, chewing, talking, cold wind to the face, etc.). A "trigger zone" in the relevant division of the fifth cranial nerve is characteristic, but not always present.

Physical and neurological examinations are usually normal. The presence of impaired sensation along the course of the fifth nerve is atypical and should suggest the possibility of structural, demyelinating, or compressive lesions involving the trigeminal nerve, including acute sphenoid sinusitis, among other possibilities.

Periodic remissions are common, but permanent spontaneous remissions are rare. The natural history is variable and unpredictable. A remission of 6 months or more occurs in over 50% of patients.

3. Mechanism

Current theory suggests focal demyelination of the trigeminal nerve, often from vascular compression just prior to entry into the pons (Janetta, 1976). Dental pathology appears capable of activating the syndrome. Multiple sclerosis can produce a pattern of pain often indistinguishable from trigeminal neuralgia and should be considered in younger patients. Intracranial tumors, aneurysms, sphenoid sinusitis, vertebrobasilar ectasia, and infiltrative disease have produced painful paroxysms, at times indistinguishable from that of trigeminal neuralgia. Recently, neurochemical changes were noted in both "peripheral" and "central" cases of trigeminal neuralgia (Strittmatter, 1997).

4. Diagnosis

The diagnosis is established by the characteristic clinical features and by ruling out other pathology. Pain in the distribution of the fifth cranial nerve in association with decreased facial sensation can be the result of trigeminal neuropathy, mandibular or cranial malignancy, and intracranial disease, including acute sphenoid sinusitis and vertebrobasilar ectasia, among other considerations. Contrast-enhanced MRI (and MRA) of the brainstem (high resolution) can provide accurate information on the anatomical location and course of vessels in the cerebral pontine angle.

5. **General treatment**

Patients are desperate and frightened. Some will not eat, drink, brush their teeth, or shave out of fear of activating pain. Aggressive treatment is indicated.

6. **Specific treatment**

   a. **Medical treatment**

   Medical treatment is successful in most patients. Among the agents likely to be useful are:

   1) Carbamazepine—400–1200 mg/day;
   2) Phenytoin—300–600 mg/day;
   3) Baclofen—40–80 mg/day;
   4) Divalproex sodium—500–2,000 mg/day;
   5) Gabapentin—up to 3,600 mg/day;
   6) Clonazepam—2–8 mg/day;
   7) Pimozide—4–12 mg/day; and
   8) IV phenytoin—250 mg over 5 minutes.

   Most agents are administered in divided dosages, with the dose increased slowly over several days or weeks to minimize adverse effects. Drug combinations may be needed. Baclofen, an often overlooked agent, can be effectively combined with carbamazepine, phenytoin, and gabapentin. Phenytoin and carbamazepine can be used together, as can other of the agents.

   b. **Surgical treatment**

   A variety of surgical procedures have been used for the treatment of trigeminal neuralgia. Vascular compression of the trigeminal root at the root entry zone is present in up to 80–90% of patients. This is the basis of the Janetta procedure (Janetta, 1985), in which compression of the trigeminal nerve root by the superior cerebellar artery is relieved via an occipital craniotomy. Permanent beneficial results are reported in over 80% of patients. A 1% surgical mortality is present, with serious morbidity in 7%. Recently, with longer follow-up, a better understanding of recurrence has emerged. In some cases, recurrence has resulted from severe adhesions caused by the Teflon padding. In other cases, recompression has been identified.

Other less invasive but frequently equally effective surgical procedures are available, including percutaneous glycerol injection, radiofrequency rhizotomy, gamma knife radiosurgery, and others for pharmacotherapeutically refractory patients (estimated to be up to 50% over time, according to some estimates). Various surgical options are available. At this time, it is difficult to distinguish among these, balancing morbidity factors and long-term outcome results. Recurrence of symptoms is common, and repeat surgical intervention is often required.

B. Glossopharyngeal Neuralgia (GN)

1. Introduction

Glossopharyngeal Neuralgia (GN) is less common than trigeminal neuralgia. The pain is in the distribution of the glossopharyngeal and vagus nerves.

2. Key clinical features

The primary symptoms of GN include paroxysmal, usually unilateral pain in and around the throat, jaw, ear, larynx, or tongue. Radiation from the oral pharynx to the ear is common. The sudden pain paroxysms along the course of the glossopharyngeal and vagal nerves, including auricular branches, last for about 1 minute. Deep, continuing pain may be present between paroxysms. Multiple attacks per day, up to 30–40, are common and may awaken patients from sleep.

Aggravation by coughing, swallowing, cold liquids, chewing, talking, and yawning is characteristic. Stimulation of the external auditory canal and postauricular area may also provoke pain. Neurological exam is normal, but sensory impairment of cranial nerves IX and X is occasionally present.

In approximately 2% of cases, syncope caused by bradycardia or asystole has been noted, and in some cases seizures, presumably from cerebral ischemia, have occurred. (Atropine prevents bradycardia and fainting, suggesting vagal afferent discharge is the mechanism of the syncope.)

3. Mechanism

The usual cause of GN is vascular compression (as in trigeminal neuralgia). Ectopic impulse formation peripherally is likely to result in disinhibition centrally (similar to that in trigeminal neuralgia).

4. Diagnosis

The diagnosis for GN is established by history, physical examination, and ruling out other disease. The following conditions are among those associated with GN-like symptoms:

a. Cerebellopontine angle tumor
b. Nasopharyngeal carcinoma
c. Carotid aneurysm
d. Peritonsillar abscess
e. Osteophytic stylohyoid ligament (lateral to
   glossopharyngeal nerve)
   In 90% of patients tested, local anesthetic to the region
   of the tonsil and pharynx terminates the pain paroxysms
   and confirms the diagnosis. MRI of the head and neck, as
   well as a careful otolaryngological evaluation, is necessary. Also, see II. A. and B.

5. Treatment
a. *Drug treatment*—same as trigeminal neuralgia
b. *Surgical treatment*—Surgical treatment involves
   intracranial sectioning of the GN nerve and the upper
   rootlets of the vagus at the jugular foramen.

C. Superior Laryngeal Neuralgia
1. Introduction
The superior laryngeal nerve, a branch of the vagus, innervates the cricothyroid muscle of the larynx, which stretches,
tenses, and adducts the vocal cord. Paralysis of the nerve
causes hoarseness and fatigued voice, with altered pitch. The
syndrome occurs mostly in middle-aged men and may also occur following endarterectomy.

2. Key clinical features
Periodic, unilateral submandibular pain radiating through
the ear, eye or shoulder, is characteristic and at times indistinguishable clinically from GN. Pain may last seconds to minutes and be provoked by swallowing, straining the voice, turning, coughing, sneezing, yawning, or blowing the nose. An
irresistible urge to swallow is noted. A trigger point is frequently present just superior and lateral to the thyroid carti-
lage.

3. Mechanism
The mechanism is uncertain, but presumably is related to
injury or compression of the nerve, as in trigeminal neuralgia.

4. Diagnosis
The diagnostic procedures for superior laryngeal neuralgia
are the same as for GN.

5. Treatment
The drug therapy is the same as that for trigeminal neuralgia. Superior laryngeal nerve blocking and neurectomy are
also available.

D. Sphenopalatine Neuralgia

This disorder is known by many names, including *Vidian neuralgia, greater superficial petrosal neuralgia, Sluder's neuralgia, pterygopalatine neuralgia,* and others. It may be related to what is now regarded as a recurrent form of carotodynia or cluster headache. Key clinical features include unilateral pain in the face, usually around the nasal area, typically lasting hours to days, attended by congestion and nasal secretion. It may follow ethmoid or other sinusitis.

E. Geniculate Neuralgia (Nervus Intermedius Neuralgia)

This syndrome is characterized by lancinating pain in the ear presumably resulting from an alteration in the sensory portion of the facial nerve, the *nervus intermedius.* The syndrome is not distinct from GN. Accompanying hemifacial spasm and ear pain are occasionally noted.

F. Occipital Neuralgia
1. Introduction

Confusion prevails regarding the concept of "cervicogenic" headache. Many authorities now accept a classification that distinguishes between headaches etiologically related to the cervical spine disorders from those in which occipital pain occurs as a result of some other dynamic, including that which may occur in migraine and cluster headache. *Occipital neuralgia* belongs to the group related to anatomical disturbances of the cervical spine region. This group includes occipital neuralgia, cervicogenic headache, auriculotemporal neuralgia, cervicalgia, and cervicobrachialgia. (A further discussion of cervicogenic headache can be found in Chapter 19.) The discussion here will focus on occipital neuralgia.

Occipital neuralgia is a neuralgic-like syndrome involving the greater occipital nerve (GON), a continuation of the dorsal ramus of C2. The GON enters the scalp between the sternocleidomastoid and trapezius muscles. Compression induces paraesthesia or dysesthesia.

The C2 nerve runs behind the lateral atlanto-axial joint and rests on its capsule. The characteristic headache can be caused by lesions affecting the C2 nerve, which includes a variety of conditions ranging from meningioma to anomalous vertebral arteries and venous abnormalities. The *third occipital headache,* a controversial syndrome, may be related to disturbances of the C2–3 zygapophyseal (facet) joint and may be common in patients with whiplash injury (see Chapters 13 and 19). These and other headaches arising in the cervical area must be distinguished from occipital neuralgia, and this distinction is highly arbitrary at this time.

Tenderness of this nerve in the occipital cervical region is frequently encountered in patients with headaches (migraine or cluster headache) and without direct apparent involvement of the nerve, except perhaps by referral. The occipital area, but not specifically the nerve, is the site of referral of pain from upper cervical spine and facet joint disturbances.

The majority of pain authorities believe that true occipital neuralgia is generally secondary to traumatic injury. The nerve may be injured in some cases of flexion extension injury (whiplash) and other closed head injury syndromes. *Postherpetic neuralgia* may also occur in this area and affect the nerve.

Occipital migraine and other causes of occipital pain (such as those arising from C2–C3 upper cervical regions) may be misdiagnosed as occipital neuralgia (see Chapter 19).

2. Key clinical features

The primary clinical features of occipital neuralgia include continuous or paroxysmal pain from the occipitocervical junction, radiating anteriorly, and reduced sensation and paresthesias or dysesthesias in the affected distribution of the nerve. The International Headache Society (IHS) defines occipital neuralgia as a "paroxysmal jabbing pain in the distribution of the greater or lesser occipital nerves, accompanied by diminished sensation or dysesthesia in the affected area." In contrast, the International Association for the Study of Pain (IASP) defines occipital neuralgia as "pain, usually deep and aching, in the distribution of the cervical dorsal root." Thus, the distinctions differ in that the IHS stipulates the presence of paroxysmal or jabbing pain, whereas IASP describes it as deep and aching, with only occasional stabbing characteristics. Moreover, IASP does not require relief by neuroblockade as a criterion, but IHS insists that temporary relief by anesthetic block is diagnostic. Local tenderness is common, but there is no evidence that the occipital pain is due to irritation of the GON. Also, compelling, consistent evidence of entrapment cannot be found. The response to neuroblockade is a nonspecific, nondiagnostic feature, since neuroblockade of that region is not restricted to the nerve; other tissues are anesthetized as well. Pain may be referred to ipsilateral frontal, vertex, and eye areas, as well as to the occipital and parietal regions of the scalp.

3. Mechanism

The mechanism of pain is likely secondary to traumatic, infectious (zoster), or chronic compressive disease (vascular, lymph node, etc.) of the greater or lesser occipital nerves. Neuroma development secondary to trauma is noted in some surgical specimens. A similar syndrome has been reported in temporal arteritis, perhaps related to inflammation of the accompanying occipital artery. Generally no pathology is found.

4. Diagnosis

The diagnosis should be considered when typical features are present and temporarily ameliorated by local blockade. However, as noted earlier, neuroblockade is a nonspecific intervention in this region, and the response does not indicate specific etiology. The syndrome of occipital neuralgia may be mimicked by cervicogenic pain arising from the trapezius muscle, referral from atlanto-occipital joint and upper cervical segments, zygapophyseal (facet joints), C2–C3 roots, C2 and C3 spinal nerves, and migraine or cluster headache (see Chapter 19).

As noted earlier, a blocking procedure in this area may relieve the pain of migraine, cluster headache, and other referred conditions and therefore should not in itself constitute confirmation of the diagnosis. Ocular pain may be relieved in some instances by suboccipital injection (Ellis, 1995), further confirming the rich referral phenomena seen in head and neck pain disorders.

A careful evaluation of the upper cervical spine and posterior fossa is mandatory. Myofascial syndromes should be considered when paraspinal muscle and trapezius tenderness is present. While superficial occipital blockade is nonspecific in its implications, x-ray guided deep neuroblockade procedures have emerged as important tools in the modern study of cervical headaches (see Chapter 19). The blocks may be able to distinguish between C2 or C3 spinal nerves, the C2–3 zygapophyseal joint, and the lateral atlanto-occipital joint. Despite increasing sophistication, however, this area of diagnosis and treatment remains highly controversial and confusing.

5. General treatment

Despite its nonspecificity, repetitive nerve blocking is nonetheless helpful in many instances. A series of superficial nerve blocks may be appropriate over a course of weeks and months. Carbamazepine and other "antineuralgic" agents, as well as indomethacin, have been found to be useful. Neurolysis, neurectomy, and radiofrequency procedures may be of benefit in selected cases; however, neurectomy is regarded as a very last resort (if not contraindicated) since recurrence and neuropathic pain sequelae (deafferentation, anesthesia dolorosa) are noted. Invasive procedures remain controversial but are effective in some instances.

G. Atypical Facial Pain (AFP)/Facial Pain of Uncertain Etiology

1. Introduction

The term *atypical facial pain* (AFP) generally reflects the presence of continuous, deep, often burning pain in the absence of clear features defining the more delineated facial pain syndromes. The term *facial pain of unknown cause* may be more appropriate (Raskin, 1988). Despite assumptions regarding a psychiatric origin, the association with organic or physiological causes is likely, though not always identifiable.

2. Key clinical features

Continuous, unilateral (occasionally bilateral) pain or discomfort occurs in the distribution of the cheek, eyes, temples, gums, nose, or jaw. Women are more commonly affected than men. Depression with or without anxiety is a frequent accompaniment. Patients are often frightened, withdrawn, angry, and demoralized from pain as well as from rejection by health care professionals. They are vulnerable to a variety of inappropriate explanations and fad therapies.

3. Diagnosis

See pages 249–252.

The following conditions should be considered and excluded, if appropriate.

a. Maxillary and mandibular bone disease

Pain arising from occult, infected maxillary or mandibular bone cavities from previous tooth extractions is an often undetected cause of AFP. Oral surgical evaluation and blocking is required. Local selective alveolar blocks to the site of the tooth extraction are diagnostic. Curettage of the bone with antibiotic treatment is recommended when cavitous disease is noted.

b. Phantom tooth pain

Phantom tooth pain is a deafferentation disorder that results in pain in the region of previous tooth extractions. Studies by Sicuteri (1991) suggest a high correlation with a history of migraine or cluster headache. The condition responds to standard migraine or cluster headache treatment and perhaps to the neuralgic treatments as well.

c. Sphenoid sinusitis (see Chapters 3 and 5)

d. Post-traumatic facial pain

Trauma to the face often produces chronic facial pain, as can previous surgical trauma. The pain usually is self-limited, often subsiding 1–5 years after onset. The mechanism is presumed to be activation of central pain transmission pathways, but the exact mechanism is yet to be determined.

e. Hemicrania continua (see Chapter 15)

f. Anesthesia dolorosa

Painful anesthesia is a dysesthetic syndrome that arises from trauma to the trigeminal nerve or other cranial nerve often following surgical treatment for neuralgia. Its primary symptom is burning pain. The pain is difficult to treat and frequently requires aggressive pharmacological and nonpharmacological intervention. Depression is common. Anticonvulsant, antineuralgic therapies may be of benefit, as are antidepressants.

g. Thalamic pain

Thalamic pain may present as a unilateral facial pain with dysesthesia and usually follows ischemic lesions in the thalamus. Trunk and limb pain is usually present, as well. The pain is often of sudden onset and occurs most frequently in patients with ischemic disease or multiple sclerosis. Because the syndrome has been identified in patients with lesions in the brainstem, and without apparent involvement of the thalamus, the term central post-stroke pain (CPSP) may be more appropriate (Leijon, 1989).

h. Other causes

The role of psychiatric disease in AFP is a matter of controversy. Nondescript facial pain can be present and accompanied by significant depression and anxiety, which can also accompany all other forms of chronic pain. The coexistence of depression does not alone suggest a causal relationship and is better explained by the concept of comorbid disease or reactive presumption of phenomena. *The absence of identifiable, objective cause should not itself justify or constitute the presumption of psychogenic origin.* The absence of objective markers may be better explained by the failure of diagnostic science than the psychiatric profile of the patient. *Patients have had medical ailments long before doctors have identified causes or tests to diagnose them!*

4. Treatment

Initial treatment consists of employing varying combinations of the following medications:

a. Antidepressants;
b. Antineuralgic agents (anticonvulsants, baclofen, mexiletine, etc.);
c. Migraine drugs;
d. Cluster headache drugs;
e. Neuroleptics;
f. NSAIDs; and
g. Opioids.

Among the antidepressants, amitriptyline, nortriptyline, phenelzine, and desipramine are particularly valuable. Newer anticonvulsants, including gabapentin and lamotrigine, are possibly valuable by anecdotal report. Several personally treated refractory cases have responded well to chronic, long-acting opioids, without patterns of overuse or serious compromise. Resorting to opioids should be reserved for refractory cases in which serious concern for abuse is absent.

AFP generally requires pharmacotherapy. However, adjunctive and supportive psychological and behavioral therapy are often essential elements of successful treatment. Invasive treatments, including dental procedures, trigeminal blockade, and sphenopalatine blockade, must be considered in selected cases.

H. Postherpetic neuralgia (PHN)

1. Introduction

Postherpetic neuralgia (PHN) is a neuralgic syndrome resulting from a previous *acute herpes zoster* attack along a specific nerve distribution. It evolves several weeks to months after the acute attack and is more likely to occur in patients of advanced age.

The acute zoster episode is often preceded by a spectrum of sensory disturbances in the afflicted region, followed 4–5 days later by a vesicular eruption. The most typical areas of involvement in the head and neck are in the distribution of the ophthalmic division of the trigeminal nerve and the occipito-cervical junction. Most attacks are unilateral.

PHN follows the acute attack of herpes zoster by days or weeks and is more likely when the acute attack of zoster is more intense. It is also more common with increasing age, approaching a 50% incidence in the 7th decade and 75% after 70 years of age. It is as low as 5% in patients below the age of 40. Patients with myeloma have a higher rate of acute infection.

Antiviral agents, such as famciclovir at a dose of 500 mg three times a day, appear to reduce the duration of acute herpes zoster and perhaps reduce the duration of PHN when it develops, but does not reduce the risk of developing PHN (Tyring, 1995).

Overall, long-term prognosis is good for PHN, with spontaneous pain improvement in the majority of patients. Approximately 5% continue to have resistant pain.

2. Key clinical features

Following the acute vesicular eruption, pain may persist or return within weeks to months. Pain usually occurs in areas overlying abnormal skin, which is generally hypesthetic. Hyperesthesia or pain to light touch (allodynia) may also occur. The pain is usually superficial but may have a deep and burning quality. Repetitive stabs of pain and needle pricking sensations are common. Interruption of normal activities, including sleep, is typical. Light touch often provokes paroxysms of discomfort.

Ophthalmic herpes may follow involvement of cranial nerves III, IV, and VI. *Geniculate herpes* is associated with facial palsy (CN VII). Vesicles are apparent in the external auditory canal (Ramsay Hunt syndrome).

3. Mechanism

It is believed that the initial zoster infection produces inflammatory necrosis of the dorsal root ganglion that extends to the meninges and dorsal root entry zone of the involved segments. PHN probably reflects a deafferentation pain syndrome in which sensory nerve injury results in interruption of the involved neuron. The burning pain is often accompanied by increased sympathetic activity. Recently, there has been speculation that PHN may cause contralateral pain, a phenomenon perhaps explained by central changes occurring in the spinal cord and brainstem.

4. Treatment

a. Treatment for the pain of the *acute zoster* infection:

  1) oral steroids
  2) antiviral agents (acyclovir, famciclovir, vidarabine, and β-interferon)
  3) neuroblockade
  4) amitriptyline

In a recent report (Bowsher, 1997), it was suggested that low-dose amitriptyline, given in the acute phase of herpes zoster, reduced the prevalence of PHN and encouraged its use along with antiviral agents, particularly in the elderly who are at greater risk. As of now, there are no reliable methods to reduce the development of PHN following the acute infection, though the above recommendations may be promising.

b. Pharmacological treatment of PHN: The pharmacological treatment for PHN includes combinations of the following:

1) local application to the affected area of capsaicin cream (0.025% or 0.075%); alternatively, lidocaine or salicylate patches
2) amitriptyline up to 150 mg per day
3) gabapentin (recent preliminary reports suggest the possible value of gabapentin in the treatment of a variety of neuropathic painful disorders, including PHN)
4) divalproex or other antineuralgic agent (alone or in combination with amitriptyline)
5) perfenazine (or other neuroleptic), used in combination with amitriptyline
6) repetitive intravenous infusions of lidocaine/neuroblockade
7) opioid treament

c. Surgical treatment of PHN: Effective surgical therapy is not available for PHN that involves the facial regions, but dorsal root entry zone (DREZ) lesions have been effective for truncal pain; intraspinal stimulation or opioids may be useful.

I. Temporomandibular Joint Pain (TM Joint Pain)
1. Introduction

Temporomandibular dysfunction (TMD), which includes TM joint dysfunction, and related muscular symptoms (e.g., myofascial pain) are poorly defined and poorly delineated syndromes. According to most experienced headache authorities, TMD and related phenomena are overstated and exaggerated as causes of pain and are overtreated, in general. The clinical and basic science related to these disorders is seriously conflicting and rudimentary. Nonetheless, little doubt exists that major disturbances of bite and mandibular function with related muscular disturbances can contribute, if not cause, a variety of painful phenomena. Masticatory muscle spasm and fatigue can produce pain, as can major structural and inflammatory disturbances of the joint.

It is likely that disturbances of jaw and myofascial components aggravate preexisting or latent headache and face pain disorders, such as migraine, via central excitation. Thus, appropriate treatment of the peripheral (jaw and muscular) tissue may help reduce the activation, if not address the primary source of pain directly. Epidemiological and demographical data on the TM joint and related syndromes are in dispute.

2. Key clinical features

A wide range of painful, unilateral symptoms involving the jaw, face, ear, or preauricular area is noted, with radiation to temple, jaw, and neck. The pain is often deep, persistent, and worsened after clenching, chewing, or wide oral opening. Clicking or "locking" of the jaw is reported by some patients with actual joint abnormalities. Limitation of jaw motion with deviation on opening is common. Tenderness of the jaw, reduced range of motion, and pain with movement, together with crepitation, are usually present. In myofascial syndromes, muscle tenderness in temporalis and pterygoid muscles is often significant. True jaw dysfunction and/or myofascial symptoms may occur separately or concurrently.

3. Mechanism

The primary mechanism for myofascial pain, according to most reliable authorities, is muscle spasm involving the masticatory muscles leading to malocclusion, bruxism, or teeth clenching. Central mechanisms might well represent a primary process. The concept of condylar displacement is controversial and in dispute. The association with rheumatoid arthritis is uncertain. Post-traumatic injuries of the jaw or related soft tissues may be important and overlooked, including mandibular ligamentous or styloid process disruption (see Chapter 13). These may occur following flexion/extension injury to the neck. Notable exacerbation of preexisting jaw pathology also occurs occasionally as a result of otherwise apparently innocuous head and neck trauma. The finding that treatment of trapezius pain by trigger point injection resulted in reduction of pain and abnormal EMG activity in the masseter muscle reflects the complex central/peripheral mechanism for TMD pathogenesis and treatment (Carlson, 1993).

4. Diagnosis

See pages 249–252. Of special differential consideration are:

a. Neuralgic disorders
b. Post-traumatic syndromes, including fracture or elongation of the styloid process (Eagle's syndrome)
c. Stylomandibular ligamentous syndrome (Ernest syndrome)
d. Referred pain to the ear from vagus branches in the chest, esophagus, or gastrum
e. Jaw claudication from giant cell arteritis
f. Carotid/vertebral dissection
g. Referred pain from cervical or occipitocervical junction pathology
h. Acoustic neuroma

Careful physical examination of the jaw, intraoral, auditory, and muscular elements is necessary, as well as an evaluation of the chest (chest x-ray). Vagal branches in the chest, esophagus, and gastrum may be referred to the aural region. Physical examination generally reveals four primary findings in true TM joint dysfunction:

1. Pain;
2. Tenderness;
3. Clicking; and
4. Limitation of motion.

5. Treatment

a. *Conservative therapy* appears to be the most appropriate approach for both myofascial and joint disorders initially. It is effective in most cases. A serious effort at resting and relaxing the jaw and its musculature is mandatory. The methods include:

1) soft diet
2) behavioral/relaxation therapies/biofeedback
3) local heat
4) reduction of gross occlusal disturbances with a bite appliance
5) use of NSAIDs, tricyclic antidepressants, and other drugs useful in the treatment of facial pain
6) jaw exercises

Local injections may be helpful in selected cases. Reduction of pain and EMG activity in the masseter region has been demonstrated following trapezius trigger point injections (Carlson, 1993).

b. *Surgical procedures* should be avoided, except in extreme circumstances. The results have been inconsistent and can contribute to a worsening spiral of pain, inappropriate opioid use, and depression. Many of the patients personally evaluated who have had undesirable consequences from surgery appear to be patients with recognizable preexistent comorbid features, including major personality disorder, such as the borderline personality (see Chapter 20). Surgical risk must be seriously considered, particularly in this group.

6. Additional thoughts

A major dilemma in the treatment of TMD and related disorders is the possibility that a primary headache disorder, such as migraine or daily chronic headache, represents the fundamental underlying process. Clearly the interplay between occipital and anterior (trigeminal) pathways, with rich referral communication, contributes to this dilemma. Peripheral illness may activate and incite migraine and migraine-like disorders, but similarly, disturbances of the central mechanisms may produce peripheral phenomena, including pain enhancement, that appear muscular or myofascial in origin. Indeed, TMD and all facial pain disturbances should be considered in a perspective that addresses the full spectrum of other etiologies, including serious organic phenomena.

Moreover, the apparent though anecdotal observation that a high percentage of patients with complex TMD cases exhibit comorbid personality disturbances suggests an even greater challenge in diagnosing and treating these cases. Diagnosis and treatment should occur in the broad perspective of head and face pain syndromes, the predispositional factors that affect people with head and face pain syndromes, and a view that the jaw therapy of itself may be but a *component* rather than the focus of proper treatment. The prolonged use of opioid analgesics following surgical intervention may be a serious problem, as can the surgery itself. There is a place for opioids, but appropriate guidelines should be applied (see Chapter 6).

Behavioral and psychotherapeutic interventions may be critical in many cases. Addressing the psychological accompaniments that are often concurrent (comorbid, not necessarily causative) may be of equal, if not greater, importance than physical or medication treatment in some cases.

References

Arner S, Lindplom U, Meyerson BA, et al. Prolonged relief of neuralgia after regional anesthetic blocks: A call for further experimental and systematic clinical studies. *Pain*, 43:287–297, 1990.

Bindoff LA, Heseltine D. Unilateral face pain in patients with lung cancer. Referred pain via the vagus. *Lancet*, 1:812–815, 1988.

Bogduk N. Local anesthetic blocks of the second cervical ganglion: A technique with application in occipital headache. *Cephalalgia*, 1:41–50, 1981.

Bogduk N. Greater occipital neuralgia. (In) *Current Therapy in Neurological Surgery*. DM Long (Ed). Pgs 175–180, Toronto, BC Decker, 1985.

Bogduk N, Marsland A. On the concept of third occipital headache. *J Neurol Neurosurg Psychiatry*, 49:775–780, 1986.

Bovim G, Berg R, Dale LG. Cervicogenic headache: Anesthetic blockades of cervical nerves. (C2–C5) and facet joint (C2/C3). *Pain*, 49:315–320, 1992a.

Bovim G, Fredriksen TA, Stolt-Nielsen A, et al. Neurolysis of the greater occipital nerve in cervicogenic headache. A follow-up study. *Headache*, 32:175–179, 1992b.

Bruyn GW. Glossopharyngeal neuralgia. (In) *Handbook of Clinical Neurology*, Vol. 48. FC Rose (Ed). Pgs 459–473, Amsterdam, Elsevier Science Publishers, 1986.

Burchiel KJ, Clark EH, Haglund M, et al. Long-term efficacy of microvascular decompression of trigeminal neuralgia. *J Neurosurg*, 69:35–38, 1988.

Carlson CR, Okeson JP, Falace DA, et al. Reduction of pain and EMG activity in the masseter region by trapezius trigger point injection. *Pain*, 55:397–400, 1993.

Chawla JC, Falconer MA. Glossopharyngeal and vagal neuralgia. *Br Med J*, 3:529–531, 1967.

Cooper BC, Rabuzzi DD. Myofascial pain dysfunction syndrome: A clinical study of asymptomatic subjects. *Laryngoscope*, 94:68–75, 1984.

Court JE, Case CS. Treatment of tic douloureux with anticonvulsant (clonazepam). *J Neurol Neurosurg Psychiatry*, 39:297–299, 1976.

Denny-Brown D, Adams RD, Fitzgerald PJ. Pathologic features of herpes zoster: A note on "geniculate herpes." *Arch Neurol Psychiatry*, 51:216–231, 1944.

Druce HM, Slavin RG. Sinusitis: Critical need for further study. *J Allergy Clin Immunol*, 88:675–677, 1991.

Dwyer A, Aprill C, Bogduk N. Cervical zygapophyseal joint pain patterns I. A study in normal volunteers. *Spine*, 15:453–457, 1990.

Ekbom KA, Westerburg CE. Carbamazepine in glossopharyngeal neuralgia. *Arch Neurol*, 14:595–596, 1966.

Ellis BD, Kosmorsky GS. Referred ocular pain relief by suboccipital injection. *Headache*, 35:105–113, 1995.

Fromm GH, Terrence CF, Chattha AS. Baclofen in the treatment of trigeminal neuralgia: Double-blind study and long-term follow-up. *Ann Neurol*, 15:240–244, 1984.

Goadsby PJ, Zagami AS, Lambert GA. Neuroprocessing of craniovascular pain: A synthesis of the central structures involved in migraine. *Headache*, 31:365–371, 1991.

Graff-Radford SB. Oral mandibular disorders and headache: A critical appraisal. (In) *Neurologic Clinics*, NT Mathew (Ed). Pgs 929–943, Philadelphia, WB Saunders, November, 1990.

Graff-Radford SB, Reeves JL, Jagger B. Management of chronic head and neck pain: Effectiveness of altering factors perpetuating myofascial pain. *Headache*, 27:186–190, 1987.

Janetta PJ. Microsurgical management of trigeminal neuralgia. *Arch Neurol*, 42:800, 1985.

Kerr FWL. Central relationships of trigeminal and cervical primary afferents in the spinal cord and medulla. *Brain Res*, 43:561–572, 1972.

Kirsch E, Hausmann O, Kaim A, et al. Magnetic resonance imaging of vertebrobasilar ectasia in trigeminal neuralgia. *Acta Neurochir* (Wien), 138:1295–1298, 1996.

Kondziolka D, Flickinger JC, Lunsford LD, et al. Trigeminal neuralgia radiosurgery: University of Pittsburgh experience. *Stereotact Funct Neurosurg*, 66:343–348, 1996.

Kuroiwa T, Matsumoto S, Kato A, et al. MR imaging of idiopathic trigeminal neuralgia: Correlation with nonsurgical therapy. *Radiat Med*, 14:235–239,1996.

Lance JW, Anthony M. Neck-tongue syndrome on sudden turning of the head. *J Neurol Neurosurg Psychiatry*, 43:97–101, 1980.

Lechin F, Vanderdigs B, Lechin ME, et al. Pimozide therapy for trigeminal neuralgia. *Arch Neurol*, 9:960–964, 1989.

Leijon G, Boivia J, Johansson I. Central post-stroke pain: Neurological symptoms and pain characteristics. *Pain*, 36:13–25, 1989.

Liao JJ, Cheng WC, Chang CN, et al. Re-operation for recurring trigeminal neuralgia after microvascular decompression. *Surg Neurol*, 47:562–568, 1997.

Majoie CB, Hulsmans FJ, Verbeeten B Jr., et al. Trigeminal neuralgia: Comparison of two MR imaging techniques in the demonstration of neurovascular contact. *Radiology*, 204:455–460, 1997.

Margolis MT, Stein RL, Newton DH. Extracranial aneurysms of the internal carotid artery. *Neuroradiology*, 4:78–89, 1972.

Mehigan JT, Olcott C. Carotodynia associated with carotid arterial disease and stroke. *Am J Surg*, 142:210–211, 1981.

Montalbetti L, Ferrandi D, Pergami P, et al. Elongated styloid process and Eagle's syndrome. *Cephalalgia*, 15:80, 1995.

McNamara RM, O'Brien MC, David-Heiser S. Post-traumatic neck pain: A prospective and follow-up study. *Ann Emerg Med*, 17:906–911, 1988.

Oturai AD, Jensen K, Eriksen J, et al. Neurosurgery for trigeminal neuralgia: Comparison of alcohol block, neurectomy, and radiofrequency coagulation. *Clin J Pain*, 12:311–315, 1996.

Portenoy RK, Duma C, Foley KM. Acute herpetic and post-herpetic neuralgia: Clinical review and current management. *Ann Neurol*, 20:651–664, 1986.

Raskin NH, Prusiner S. Carotodynia. *Neurology*, 27:43–46, 1977.

Raskin NH, Schwartz RK. Icepick-like pain. *Neurology*, 30:203–205, 1980.

Rath SA, Klein HJ, Richter HP. Findings and long-term results of subsequent operations after failed microvascular decompression for trigeminal neuralgia. *Neurosurgery*, 39:933–938, 1996.

Ratner EJ, Langer B, Evins ML. Alveolar cavitational osteoporosis. *J Periodontol*, 57:593–603, 1986.

Ratner EJ, Person P, Kleinman DJ, et al. Jawbone cavities in trigeminal and atypical facial neuralgias. *Oral Surg*, 48:3–20, 1979.

Rittenhouse EA, Radke HM, Sumner DS. Carotid artery aneurysm. *Arch Surg*, 105:786–789, 1972.

Sessle BJ, Hu JW, Amano N, et al. Convergence of cutaneous, tooth pulp, visceral, neck, and muscle afferents onto nociceptive and non-nociceptive neurons in trigeminal subnucleus caudalis (medullary dorsal horn) and its implications for referred pain. *Pain,* 27:219–235, 1986.

Sicuteri F, Nicolodi M, Fusco BM, et al. Idiopathic headache as a possible risk factor for phantom tooth pain. *Headache,* 31:577–581, 1981.

Silberstein SD, Lipton RB, Saper JR, et al. Headache and facial pain: Part A. *Continuum,* 1:8, 1995.

Silberstein SD, Marcelis J. Headache associated with changes in intracranial pressure. *Headache,* 30:84–94, 1992.

Solomon S, Lipton RB. Facial pain. (In) *Neurologic Clinics.* NT Mathew (Ed). Pgs 913–928, Philadelphia, WB Saunders, November, 1990.

Strittmatter M, Grauer M, Eisenberg E, et al. Cerebrospinal fluid and neuropeptides in monoaminergic transmitters in patients with trigeminal neuralgia. *Headache,* 36:211–216, 1997.

Sweet WH. The treatment of trigeminal neuralgia. *N Engl J Med,* 316:692–693, 1987.

Swerdlow M. Anticonvulsant drugs and chronic pain. *Clin Neuropharmacol,* 7:51–82, 1984.

Tyring S, Barbarash RA, Nahlik JE, et al. Famciclovir for the treatment of acute herpes zoster: Effects on acute disease and post-herpetic neuralgia. *Ann Intern Med,* 123:89–96, 1995.

Wallin BJ, Westerberg CE, Sundlof G. Syncope induced by glossopharyngeal neuralgia: Sympathetic outflow to muscle. *Neurology,* 34:522–524, 1984.

Waltz TA, Dalessio DJ, Copeland B, et al. Percutaneous injection of glycerol for the treatment of trigeminal neuralgia. *Clin J Pain,* 5:195–198, 1989.

Watson CPN, Evans RJ. Post-herpetic neuralgia: A review. *Arch Neurol,* 43:836–840, 1986A.

Watson CPN, Evans RJ. Treatment of post-herpetic neuralgia. *Clin Neuropharmacol,* 9:533–541, 1986B.

Watson CPN, Evans RJ, Reed K, et al. Amitriptyline vs. placebo in post-herpetic neuralgic. *Neurology,* 32:671–673, 1982.

Yarri Y, Selzer ME, Pincus JH. Phenytoin: Mechanisms of anticonvulsant action. *Ann Neurol,* 20:171–184, 1986.

Young RF. Functional neurosurgery with the Leksell gamma knife. *Stereotact Funct Neurosurg,* 66:19–23, 1997.

17

CSF Hypotension
(Low-Pressure Headache)

I. Introduction

Headache almost invariably occurs when cerebrospinal fluid (CSF) pressure is low, usually under 90 mm of H_2O, although individual sensitivity varies. The production, absorption, and flow of CSF influence the pressure. Intracranial hypotension (ICH) can result from decreased production of CSF, increased absorption, or leakage. Although ICH occurs most commonly as a consequence of lumbar puncture (LP), many other causes, including spontaneous leakage (spontaneous intracranial hypotension [SIH]), must be considered. It is believed that headache results from traction on pain-sensitive intracranial and meningeal structures. Cranial nerves V, VI, IX, and X, as well as the upper three cervical nerves and bridging veins, are likely to be influenced by the "descent of the brain" or "ptotic brain," which can be seen on computed tomography (CT) and magnetic resonance imaging (MRI) (Benzon, 1996; Horton, 1994; Pannullo, 1993). Moreover, to compensate for the low pressure, secondary vasodilation of cerebral vessels may contribute to the throbbing component of the accompanying headache.

Recently, in a review of 26 patients with low-pressure headache unassociated with obvious leakage or trauma, Mokri (1997) demonstrated an opening pressure of 40 mm or less *in only half of the patients reviewed.* The remainder of patients had higher pressure, and occasionally had normal readings, even though they were symptomatic and had abnormal MRI findings. All patients in this study demonstrated gadolinium meningeal enhancement as a reason for referral.

II. Key Clinical Features

Headache is the most common symptom of CSF hypotension. According to the International Headache Society (IHS) classification, the characteristic low CSF headache occurs or worsens within 15 minutes of assuming the upright position and disappears or improves less than 30 minutes after resuming the recumbent position. More gradual worsening during the day and gradual improvement upon reclining is a phenomenon also seen, perhaps reflecting slower leakage patterns. The longer a patient is upright, the longer it takes the headache to subside after recumbency (Raskin, 1988). In prolonged chronic cases, the characteristic postural component may be minimal, and a more persistent pattern may occur, thus denying the clinician the clinical clue of the characteristic postural patterns. The headache may be frontal, occipital, or generalized. Frequently, nausea and vomiting, as well as dizziness, tinnitus, and other nonspecific symptoms, are present.

Characteristically, symptoms include:

1. Frontal headache that occurs or is accentuated within 15 minutes of assuming upright position and ameliorated within 15 minutes of recumbency;
2. Nausea and vomiting;
3. Dizziness, tinnitus, and anorexia;
4. Mild stiff neck;
5. Occasional bradycardia; and
6. Occasional cranial nerve palsy, particularly cranial nerve VI.

The headache itself can be gradual or sudden in onset and may be severe or mild, throbbing or dull. Head movement, coughing, straining, sneezing, or jugular compression may alter the headache. The anatomical connection between the subarachnoid space and the cochlea may provide the anatomical explanation for the development of labyrinthine hypotension and cochlear symptoms (Fishman, 1992).

III. Mechanism

The presumed mechanism of intracranial hypotension is varied. Two categories are noted: *spontaneous* intracranial hypotension (SIH), with no evidence of CSF leak or systemic illness, and *symptomatic intracranial hypotension,* which may be associated with demonstrable CSF leak. This classification is faulty, since traditional reliance on radioisotope techniques fails to reveal small leaks from such causes as ruptured spinal arachnoid cyst (Benzon, 1996; Rando, 1992; Weitz, 1996).

Classification may be further based on etiology, such as the following:

A. Lumbar Puncture (LP)

LP with persistent CSF leak (diagnostic myelography; spinal anesthesia; inadvertent puncture with epidural blockade; etc.).

B. Leakage (spontaneous or otherwise)

Leakage may arise from:

1. Spontaneous dural tear or rupture of spinal arachnoid cyst (Weitz, 1996);
2. Head/neck trauma/neck root evulsion;
3. Opening of cranial vault/spinal surgery/ventricular shunting; and
4. Exertion-induced tear (orgasmic headache). (See Chapter 15)

C. Decreased CSF Production or Volume

1. Dehydration;
2. Diabetic ketoacidosis;
3. Uremia;
4. Severe systemic infection/meningoencephalitis; and
5. Hyperpnea.

D. Systemic Hypotension
E. CSF Hyperabsorption ?
F. Arnold Chiari Malformation, Type I

Arnold Chiari malformation Type I has been associated with a low-pressure headache syndrome (see Khurana, 1991).

G. Excessive Drainage From Shunt Procedures

The most common complication of the LP is a headache, with incidence ranging from 10–30% and much higher in those with preexistent migraine. The incidence is greater in women than in men (2:1). Children younger than 13 and adults older than 60 are less likely to experience a post-LP headache. The volume of fluid removed at LP has not been shown to correlate with the headache. The headache may occur within minutes or days (up to 12), although usually within 12–24 hours following the LP. Most cases resolve spontaneously within 7 days. Despite attempts to prevent the post-LP headache, the only useful technique is to use a small gauge needle, though this is often impractical. Raskin (1988) suggests removing the needle while the patient is in the prone, rather than lateral cubitus position.

IV. Diagnosis
A. Characteristic Symptomatology

The diagnosis is suspected in the presence of characteristic symptomatology, particularly that of orthostatic headache or headache that worsens the longer a patient is upright, and begins to improve upon reclining.

B. Differential Diagnosis

Other headaches associated with postural or exertional aggravation, including the following, should be ruled out:

1. Intracranial tumors, including colloid cysts of the third ventricle, occipitocervical tumors, etc.;
2. Occipitocervical deformities (Arnold Chiari malformation, Type I, etc.);
3. Ventricular obstructive syndromes;
4. Exertional headache syndromes (see Chapter 15);
5. Cervical disc disease/spinal masses or obstruction;

6. Paranasal or sphenoid sinus disease;
7. Cerebral vein thrombosis;
8. Subdural hematoma; and
9. Others.

C. CT Scan and MRI

CT scan and MRI of head and neck are used to both rule out other intracranial and spinal diseases and confirm the presence of indirect indicators of low CSF pressure, such as "ptotic brain." "Slit-shaped" ventricles are thought to be due to secondary brain edema, perhaps a result of compensatory venous dilation. MRI studies enhanced with gadolinium may demonstrate diffuse meningeal enhancement (DME), first identified by Mokri (1993, 1997). DME is thought to be secondary to vascular dilatation, with venous engorgement reflected in greater concentration of gadolinium in the dural vasculature and interstitial fluid. Inflammatory changes may also occur. DME generally dissipates following resolution of the condition. Downward displacement of brain may be present and demonstrated on MRI findings which confirm the descent of the brainstem, flattening of the basis pontis, cerebellar tonsilar herniation, and bowing of the optic chiasm over the pituitary gland. Findings that mimic Arnold Chiari malformation Type I, which resolve with resolution of the headache, have been reported by Kasner (1969).

Recently Vakharia (1997) studied the efficacy of MRI in CSF leak syndromes, and demonstrated that MRI, using proton density (PD) and T2 weighted imaging, could identify the site of CSF leakage in the spinal canal, as well as the effect of blood patch tamponade. Pre-blood patch MRI showed extrathecal CSF and hemosiderosis, indicating the site of dural puncture in four of the five patients. Eljamel (1994) also showed that the MRI could localize the site of CSF fistulae. MRI cisternography identified the site of fistulae in each of the 11 patients. Levi (1995) showed the value of flow-sensitive MRI in the evaluation of CSF leaks which involved the skull base and temporal bone. Other authors have likewise added support to the growing utility of MRI in the evaluation of CSF leakage (Kabuto, 1996; Murata, 1995).

D. LP

Diagnosis is confirmed by LP demonstrating CSF pressure lower than 0–40mm CSF by manometric measurement, although patients may be symptomatic with less significant or even normal pressure readings (Mokri, 1997). LPs on patients with low pressure are often difficult because of the "dry tap" phenomenon that results from low pressure. Occasionally, the CSF pressure is negative (below that of atmospheric pressure), and a sucking noise may be heard when the stylet is removed from the LP needle (Lay, 1997). Mild pleocytosis may be present. Low CSF pressure readings, as measured by LP manometric evaluation, could result from an obstruction above the lumbar space entered or from obstruction intracranially. Failure of needle placement can result in inaccurate pressure readings.

Though not yet established with certainty, it is possible that an ostensibly normal CSF reading that drops significantly with a small amount of fluid withdrawal might indicate a low-pressure system. The authors have seen one such case of suspected CSF hypotension in which a normal reading (above 120 mm H_2O) dropped to 60 mm H_2O following withdrawal of 2 cc of fluid. Because a normal reading may reflect compensatory mechanisms, a small amount of fluid removal may prompt a precipitous drop in pressure.

E. Isotope Cisternography

Another diagnostic method is isotope cisternography with radioactive tracer to demonstrate:

1. Leakage (outside the normal confines of the subarachnoid space) from the cribriform plate or paranasal sinuses; and
2. Rapid transport and early visualization of kidneys and bladder.

F. CT Myelography

CT myelography is used to demonstrate the presence of a dural tear not otherwise apparent.

Currently, it appears that special MRI studies are surpassing other diagnostic techniques in localization of CSF leakage.

V. Treatment

The treatment is directed at supportive measures and at the cause, if identified.

A. General Symptomatic Treatment

1. Fluid replacement;
2. Bed rest;
3. Support hose;
4. Abdominal binder; and
5. Analgesics.

Use of the abdominal binder may be of some diagnostic value and can bring relief for periods of time. Increased fluid volume, raising of systemic blood pressure if the patient has systemic hypotension, increased salt intake, and administration of caffeine have all been recommended.

B. Specific Treatment

1. Treatment for a primary disorder (systemic hypotension, surgical treatment of dural tear, etc.)

2. Epidural blood patching

First introduced by Gormley in 1960, epidural blood patching has now become established as the treatment of choice for treating headaches following LP and for idiopathic cases. Some authors have even used the blood patch diagnostically. Fifteen to 20 ml of autologous blood is infused into the epidural space. A success rate approaches 97% in the treatment of spontaneous low-pressure headache, even of 2 years or longer duration. It is now believed that the value of the blood patch results from the tamponade effect that increases CSF pressure from the volume load against the dural sac. Vakharia (1997) demonstrated that the blood patch spread from its initial extradural site anteriorly up to 4.6 intervertebral spaces. This explains the observation that even when the cause of low pressure is not found or when a leak is not apparent, the epidural blood patch may nonetheless be effective. Compression of the dural sac seems to be the most likely therapeutic mechanism. Both lumbar and thoracic levels should be separately injected in refractory cases (Benzon, 1996). Insufficient volume (less than 15 cc) may be a cause for treatment failure.

3. Caffeine sodium benzoate infusion

Caffeine may increase CSF pressure.

a. 500 mg added to D–5 lactated Ringer's solution (500 ml–1,000 ml) and administered intravenously over several hours or longer; and

b. Careful monitoring for palpitations and other effects of caffeine is required. If a liter or more of fluid is given, monitor for fluid overload, electrolyte imbalance, etc.

4. Implementing continuous epidural saline infusion through a catheter is of temporary but significant benefit in some cases (Peterson, 1987).

5. In rare and refractory cases, CSF drainage has been used to close dural rents.

VI. Conclusion

Low CSF pressure is increasingly recognized as a cause of refractory headache. An LP and MRI are often necessary in pursuit of the diagnosis in patients with refractory headache, particularly those with postural components. Detailed history-taking may associate otherwise innocuous traumatic events, orgasmic episodes, or other benign activities (lifting, bending, turning, etc.) that may be related to the onset of the headache syndrome. Not all cases of bona fide CSF hypotension will be found to be associated with a cause or identified leakage.

Finally, while a low CSF pressure, as documented by LP, is the classic finding, a low reading may not be identifiable, even when symptoms of low pressure are present. Epidural blood patches may have a diagnostic value in such cases, though MR scanning of the cranium and spine and assessing for leakage may be useful prior to the blood patch. Therapeutically, epidural blood patches may be required more than once, at both the lumbar and thoracic levels, and infusion of 15–20 cc of blood per procedure is recommended.

References

Benzon HT, Nemickas R, Molloy RE, et al. Lumbar and thoracic epidural blood injections to treat spontaneous intracranial hypotension. *Anesthesiology,* 85: 920–922, 1996.

Eljamel MS, Pidgeon CN, Tolan J, et al. MRI cisternography in the localization of CSF fistulae. *Br J Neurosurg,* 8:433–437, 1994.

Fishman RA. *Cerebrospinal Fluid in Diseases of the Nervous System.* 2nd Edition. Philadelphia, WB Saunders, 1992.

Fishman RA, Dillon WP. Dural enhancement in cerebral displacement secondary to intracranial hypotension. *Neurology,* 43:609–611, 1993.

Friedman DI, Ingram P, Rogers MAM. Low tyramine diet in the treatment of idiopathic intracranial hypertension: A pilot study (abstract). To the American Academy of Neurology, 50th Annual Meeting. Minneapolis, April, 1998.

Hochman MS, Naidich TP, Kobetz SA, et al. Spontaneous intracranial hypotension with pachymeningeal enhancement on MRI. *Neurology,* 42:16–28, 1992.

Horton JC, Fishman RA. Neurovisual findings in the syndrome of spontaneous intracranial hypotension from dural cerebrospinal fluid leak. *Ophthalmology,* 101:244–251, 1994.

Kabuto M, Kabuto T, Kobayashi H, et al. MR imaging of cerebrospinal fluid rhinorrhea following the suboccipital approach to the cerebropontine angle and the internal auditory canal: Report of two cases. *Surg Neurol,* 45:336–340, 1996.

Kasner SE, Rosenfeld J, Farber RE. Spontaneous intracranial hypotension: Headache with a reversible Arnold Chiari malformation. *Headache,* 35:557–559, 1995.

Khurana RK. Headache spectrum and Arnold-Chiari malformation. *Headache,* 31:151–155, 1991.

Koller EA, Stadel BV, Malozowski SN. Papilledema in 15 renally compromised patients treated with growth hormone. *Pediatr Nephrol,* 11:451–454, 1997.

Lance JW, Branch GB. Persistent headache after lumbar puncture. *Lancet,* 343:414, 1994.

Lay CL, Campbell JK, Mokri B. Low cerebrospinal fluid pressure headache. (In) *Headache*. PJ Goadsby, SD Silverstein (Eds). Pgs 355–367, Boston, Butterworth-Heinemeann, 1997.

Levy LM, Gulya AJ, Davis SW, et al. Flow-sensitive magnetic resonance imaging in the evaluation of cerebral fluid leaks. *Am J Otol,* 16:591–596, 1995.

Malozowski S, Tanner LA, Wysowski DK, et al. Benign intracranial hypertension in children with growth hormone deficiency treated with growth hormone. *J Pediatr,* 126:996–999, 1995.

Marcelis J, Silberstein SD. Spontaneous low cerebral spinal fluid pressure headache. *Headache,* 30:192–196, 1990.

Marcelis J, Silberstein SD. Idiopathic intracranial hypertension without papilledema. *Arch Neurol,* 48:392–396, 1991.

Matthew RJ, Wilson WH. Caffeine-induced changes in cerebral circulation. *Stroke,* 16:814–817, 1985.

Mokri B, Krueger BR, Miller GM, et al. Meningeal gadolinium enhancement in low pressure headaches. *J Neuroimaging,* 3:11, 1993.

Mokri B, Piepgras DG, Miller GM. Syndrome of orthostatic headaches and diffuse pachymeningeal gadolinium enhancement. *Mayo Clin Proc,* 72:400–413, 1997.

Mokri B, Prisi JE, Scheithauer BW, et al. Meningeal biopsy in intracranial hypotension: Meningeal enhancement on MRI. *Neurology,* 45:1801–1807, 1995.

Murata Y, Yamada I, Isotani E, et al. MRI and spontaneous cerebrospinal fluid rhinorrhea. *Neuroradiology,* 37:453–455, 1995.

Panagopoulos G, Gotsi A, Piaditis G, et al. Treatment of benign intracranial hypertension with ostreotide (abstract). Presented to the American Academy of Neurology, 50th Annual Meeting. Minneapolis, April, 1998.

Pannullo S, Reich JB, Krol G, et al. MRI changes in intracranial hypotension. *Neurology,* 43:919, 1993.

Peterson RC, Freeman DP, Knox CA, et al. Successful treatment of spontaneous low cerebral fluid pressure. Headache (abstract). *Ann Neurol,* 22:148, 1987.

Rando TA, Fishman RA. Spontaneous intracranial hypotension: Report of two cases and review of the literature. *Neurology,* 42:481–487, 1992.

Schievink WI, Meyer FB, Atkinson JL. Spontaneous spinal cerebral fluid fluid leaks and intracranial hypotension. *J Neurosurg,* 84:598–605, 1996.

Sechzer PG, Abel L. Post-spinal anesthesia headache treated with caffeine: Evaluation with demand method. Part I. *Curr Ther Res,* 24:307–312, 1978.

Seebacher J, Ribeiro V, LeGuillou JL, et al. Epidural blood patch in the treatment of post-dural puncture headache: A double-blind study. *Headache,* 29:630–632, 1989.

Silberstein SD, Marcelis J. Headache associated with changes in intracranial pressure. *Headache,* 32:84–94, 1992.

Vakharia SB, Tomas PS, Rosenbaum AE, et al. Magnetic resonance imaging of cerebrospinal fluid leak and tamponade effect of blood patch in postdural puncture headache. *Anesth Analg,* 84:585–590, 1997.

Vilming ST, Titus F. Low cerebrospinal fluid pressure. (In) *The Headaches*. J Olesen, P Tfelt-Hansen, MA Welch (Eds). Pgs 687–695, New York, Raven, 1993.

Weitz SR, Drasner K. Spontaneous intracranial hypotension: A series. *Anaesthesia,* 85:923–925, 1996.

18

Idiopathic Intracranial Hypertension (Pseudotumor Cerebri, Benign Intracranial Hypertension)

I. Introduction

Idiopathic intracranial hypertension (IIH) is characterized by increased intracranial pressure of uncertain etiology. Although not always associated with a headache, this is the most consistent symptom. It may represent a new onset headache or a worsening of preexistent headaches. The condition occurs in the absence of intracranial structural lesions and primarily affects overweight women. In the general population, the overall incidence of the condition is 1 per 100,000, whereas the incidence within a population of obese women of childbearing age is 19 per 100,000. Women more than men (ratio of 8:1) suffer from the illness. The average age of onset is 29–30 years.

Interestingly, the cerebrospinal fluid (CSF) pressure does not directly correlate with the headache, since CSF pressure raised to many times normal levels (680–850 mm/H_2O) has been noted without accompanying head pain (Corbett, 1997).

II. Key Clinical Features
A. Primary Symptoms

The primary symptoms of IIH include:

1. Generalized, usually frontal headache, is most often accompanied by papilledema. The headache, which occurs in 75% of cases, may be unilateral or bioccipital. It is often associated with a postural component but is otherwise nonspecific in form. It may have migrainous or tension-type (migraine variant) features. Patients with daily chronic headache who fit the profile (obese women of childbearing age) may have increased pressure without papilledema (Mathew, 1996). The headache frequently persists even after pressure reduction occurs, particularly in long-standing cases. It may exacerbate a preexistent migraine disorder;
2. Nausea and vomiting;
3. Progressive visual loss if sustained, unrelieved papilledema occurs;
4. Occasional cranial nerve VI paresis (also rarely, cranial nerve VII paresis, facial pain, and hearing loss);

5. Dizziness and unsteadiness of gait, possibly related to postural hypotension;
6. Stiff neck;
7. Pulsatile tinnitus (may improve with ipsilateral, internal jugular vein compression and/or lumber puncture [LP]);
8. Cranial bruit that may be perceived by the patient or auscultated over the mastoid or temporalis, while mouth held open (due to major venous sinus turbulence); and
9. Somnolence, fever, and systemic symptoms in severe cases, and which should suggest venous sinus occlusion or other organic cause of increased pressure.

B. Clinical Findings

Major clinical findings include:

1. Papilledema (present in over 75% of patients);
2. Visual findings may include:
   - Enlargement of the physiological blind spot;
   - Persistent visual blurring and moderate to severe reduction in visual acuity;
   - Constriction of the visual fields; and
   - Inferonasal visual field defects.
3. Elevation of pressure over 200 (some authorities believe 250) mm of H_2O on manometric reading during LP; headache most often, but not always, improves following spinal tap, except in long-standing cases in which a persistent headache, usually refractory to standard treatment, continues.

CSF pressure fluctuates throughout the day. A one-time reading, high, normal, or low, does not necessarily accurately reflect the dynamic changes over a 24-hour period. More than one reading or CSF monitoring may be necessary.

III. Mechanism

Recent speculation suggests that the monoamine system may be relevant to the pathogenesis of the disorder (Friedman, 1998). This is based upon the observation that the production of CSF by the choroid plexus is regulated by monoamines. Increasing epinephrine or norepinephrine levels in animals is associated with a decrease of CSF production. Theoretically, increased CSF production could result from lowered monoamine levels or function.

Moreover, growth hormone or insulin-like growth factor 1 may cause the development of intracranial hypertension (Koller, 1997; Malozowski, 1993). Recently, Panagopoulos (1998) reported that treatment of intracranial hypertension with octreotide, a somatostatin analog, was highly effective in the treatment of 13 of 15 patients with benign intracranial hypertension, reducing both headache and papilledema.

It is believed that traction or stimulation is responsible for the headache, but this is not a certainty. The posterior fossa is innervated by the vagus and glossopharyngeal nerves, as well as the upper cervical nerves (C2 and C3). These project to neurons of the caudal trigeminal nucleus, and provide the basis for frontal headache. Moreover, the roof of the posterior fossa (the tentorium cerebelli) and the dural structures are pain sensitive and refer pain to the forehead ipsilaterally.

Despite the likelihood that the headache is due to traction or pressure on pain-sensitive structures (venous sinuses, arteries, and dura) and on pain-carrying cranial and cervical nerves, the cause of increased pressure often remains unknown. Some authorities suggest occult venous sinus occlusive disease or increased central venous pressure to be frequent, though undiagnosed, causes. Increased flow resistance in the arachnoid villi and/or increase in dural sinus pressure are recognized. Other changes may include cerebral vasomotor instability or a loss of cerebrovascular regulation (Raskin, 1988).

The original case of IIH was the result of lateral venous thrombosis, thus initially called *otitic hydrocephalus.*

IV. Diagnosis
A. Making the Diagnosis

The diagnosis is established by:

1. Ruling out other causes of increased intracranial pressure and papilledema:
   a. Obstructive hydrocephalus
   b. Cerebral edema
   c. Cerebral venous/sinus thrombosis
   d. Vasculitis
   e. Intracranial mass: tumor, AVM, subdural hematoma, etc.
   f. Infectious/infiltrative central nervous system (CNS) disease
   g. Spinal mass (may result in increased intracranial pressure, but low readings on LP below the mass)
   h. Others
2. Confirming elevation of CSF pressure by the performance of serial LP and manometric measurements after computed tomography (CT)/magnetic resonance imagining (MRI) has been performed to rule out mass that would contraindicate the performance of an LP.

B. Other Diagnostic Considerations

1. Most diagnostic tests are normal; delayed visual-evoked potential (VEP) latency of P–100 is present in some cases.
2. CT scan is generally normal, but slightly enlarged or diminished ventricles have been noted; venous phase MRI and MR angiogram (MRA) may reveal venous occlusive disease, if present.
3. Evidence of causative/associated conditions, including:
   a. Endocrine abnormalities
      1) Disturbances of cortisol secretions
      2) Hypoparathyroidism
      3) Other
   b. Hyper/hypovitaminosis, particularly hypervitaminosis A (Friedland, 1996)
   c. Antibiotic treatment
   d. Hematological abnormalities
   e. Toxic exposure
   f. Danazol (danocrine) therapy
   g. Anticardiolipin antibodies (Acl-Ab) (Leker and Steiner, 1998)

   Recently, Leker and Steiner (1998) have shown a possible association between Alc-Ab and intracranial hypertension in the absence of venous thrombosis. Intracranial hypertension may be a presenting feature of antiphospholipid syndrome.

V. Principles of Treatment
A. Treatment Objectives

1. Reducing increased intracranial pressure;
2. Reducing pressure on optic nerves; and
3. Treating headache.

B. Reduction of Pressure

Pressure is reduced by the following methods:

1. Acetazolamide (Diamox) at dosages of 500 mg b.i.d. and up to 2 g daily (side effects include nausea, depression, numbness and tingling, renal stones, and occasionally hepatic failure). Metabolic acidosis is expected;
2. Diuretics, primarily furosemide, at a dose of 40–160 mg per day with potassium supplementation;
3. Combinations of 1 and 2;
4. Steroids (used less now than in the past);

5. Repetitive LPs to maintain reduced pressure. Some patients will respond dramatically after one LP and require only occasional LPs. Repetitive LPs are not recommended for long-term treatment and may result in spinal epidermoid tumor, chronic back pain, and a low pressure headache syndrome; and

6. Two recent reports, via abstract, offer preliminary evidence of two new novel treatments: First, a low tyramine diet resulted in improvement in headache and perhaps CSF pressure in five patients with intracranial hypertension (Friedman, 1998). It is uncertain if the headache improvement was the result of the low tyramine diet or from lowering of the pressure. Second, administration of octreotide, a somatostatin analog, resulted in reduction in papilledema and headache in 13 of 15 patients with intracranial hypertension within days of administration (Panagopoulos, 1998).

C. Resistant Cases

For resistant cases of increased intracranial pressure, the following is suggested:

1. Optic nerve sheath fenestration (decompression) to improve and protect visual function and lower CSF pressure; and

2. Shunt procedures (shunting relieves pressure but may result in a low-pressure postural headache syndrome. Acquired disturbance of occipital-cervical anatomy may occur with lumboperitoneal shunting).

D. Headache Control:

1. Drugs used to control migraine and its variants;
2. Analgesics; and
3. See above.

VI. Special Considerations

1. Obesity in females is the most apparent predisposing factor.
2. The most common visual disturbance is transient visual obscuration (loss of vision usually lasting for a few seconds). Permanent visual impairment occurs with chronic papilledema.
3. Disc swelling is poorly correlated to increased intracranial pressure. Individual optic sheath anatomy influences the presence or absence of papilledema, and in chronic cases, optic cup gliosis occurs, thereby denying ophthalmoscopic visualization of evidence

of increased intracranial pressure. Regular ophthalmological evaluations and visual field examinations are required to document visual function.

4. Visual field testing may be the most important test for assessing visual impairment, although prolonged visual-evoked responses have been used by some authors.

5. If gliosis develops in the optic nerve, ophthalmoscopic visualization for papilledema is no longer reliable. Regular ophthalmological evaluations and visual field examinations are required to document visual function accurately.

6. Headache does not necessarily abate when pressure is reduced, particularly in prolonged chronic cases.

7. Because papilledema is not always present, reliance on LP and manometric readings is necessary in suspected cases.

8. Symptoms persist in 25% of cases, which become chronic and associated with asthenia, memory dysfunction, and/or persistent headache.

IIH is an important cause of headache. Mathew (1996) recently demonstrated that 12 of 85 patients with refractory transformed migraine had CSF pressures ranging from 230 to 450 mm of H_2O. Papilledema is not a reliable sign, and LP is warranted in cases of refractory headache. Treatments include occasional or periodic LPs, pharmacotherapy to reduce pressure and to treat the headache (including the use of migraine prophylaxis), and careful monitoring of visual systems. While shunting and fenestration are appropriate in selected cases, lumboperitoneal and ventricular shunting may be associated with other severe sequelae and headache events.

References

Benzon HT, Nemickas R, Molloy RE, et al. Lumbar and thoracic epidural blood injections to treat spontaneous intracranial hypotension. *Anesthesiology,* 85: 920–922, 1996.

Eljamel MS, Pidgeon CN, Tolan J, et al. MRI cisternography in the localization of CSF fistulae. *Br J Neurosurg,* 8:433–437, 1994.

Fishman RA. *Cerebrospinal Fluid in Diseases of the Nervous System.* 2nd Edition. Philadelphia, WB Saunders, 1992.

Fishman RA, Dillon WP. Dural enhancement in cerebral displacement secondary to intracranial hypotension. *Neurology,* 43:609–611, 1993.

Friedman DI, Ingram P, Rogers MAM. Low tyramine diet in the treatment of idiopathic intracranial hypertension: A pilot study (abstract). To the American Academy of Neurology, 50th Annual Meeting. Minneapolis, April, 1998.

Hochman MS, Naidich TP, Kobetz SA, et al. Spontaneous intracranial hypotension with pachymeningeal enhancement on MRI. *Neurology,* 42:16–28, 1992.

Horton JC, Fishman RA. Neurovisual findings in the syndrome of spontaneous intracranial hypotension from dural cerebrospinal fluid leak. *Ophthalmology,* 101:244–251, 1994.

Kabuto M, Kabuto T, Kobayashi H, et al. MR imaging of cerebrospinal fluid rhinorrhea following the suboccipital approach to the cerebropontine angle and the internal auditory canal: Report of two cases. *Surg Neurol,* 45:336–340, 1996.

Kasner SE, Rosenfeld J, Farber RE. Spontaneous intracranial hypotension: Headache with a reversible Arnold Chiari malformation. *Headache,* 35:557–559, 1995.

Khurana RK. Headache spectrum and Arnold-Chiari malformation. *Headache,* 31:151–155, 1991.

Koller EA, Stadel BV, Malozowski SN. Papilledema in 15 renally compromised patients treated with growth hormone. *Pediatr Nephrol,* 11:451–454, 1997.

Lance JW, Branch GB. Persistent headache after lumbar puncture. *Lancet,* 343:414, 1994.

Lay CL, Campbell JK, Mokri B. Low cerebrospinal fluid pressure headache. (In) *Headache.* PJ Goadsby, SD Silverstein (Eds). Pgs 355–367, Boston, Butterworth-Heinemeann, 1997.

Leker RR, Steiner J. Anticardial-lipid antibodies are frequently present in patients with intercranial hypertension. *Arch Neurol,* 55: R817–820, 1988

Levy LM, Gulya AJ, Davis SW, et al. Flow-sensitive magnetic resonance imaging in the evaluation of cerebral fluid leaks. *Am J Otol,* 16:591–596, 1995.

Malozowski S, Tanner LA, Wysowski DK, et al. Benign intracranial hypertension in children with growth hormone deficiency treated with growth hormone. *J Pediatr,* 126:996–999, 1995.

Marcelis J, Silberstein SD. Spontaneous low cerebral spinal fluid pressure headache. *Headache,* 30:192–196, 1990.

Marcelis J, Silberstein SD. Idiopathic intracranial hypertension without papilledema. *Arch Neurol,* 48:392–396, 1991.

Mathew NT, Ravishankar K, Sanin LC. Coexistence of migraine and idiopathic intracranial hypertension without papilledema. *Neurology,* 46:1226–30, 1996.

Mathew RJ, Wilson WH. Caffeine-induced changes in cerebral circulation. *Stroke,* 16:814–817, 1985.

Mokri B, Krueger BR, Miller GM, et al. Meningeal gadolinium enhancement in low pressure headaches. *J Neuroimaging,* 3:11, 1993.

Mokri B, Piepgras DG, Miller GM. Syndrome of orthostatic headaches and diffuse pachymeningeal gadolinium enhancement. *Mayo Clin Proc,* 72:400–413, 1997.

Mokri B, Prisi JE, Scheithauer BW, et al. Meningeal biopsy in intracranial hypotension: Meningeal enhancement on MRI. *Neurology,* 45:1801–1807, 1995.

Murata Y, Yamada I, Isotani E, et al. MRI and spontaneous cerebrospinal fluid rhinorrhea. *Neuroradiology,* 37:453–455, 1995.

Panagopoulos G, Gotsi A, Piaditis G, et al. Treatment of benign intracranial hypertension with ostreotide (abstract). Presented to the American Academy of Neurology, 50th Annual Meeting. Minneapolis, April, 1998,

Pannullo S, Reich JB, Krol G, et al. MRI changes in intracranial hypotension. *Neurology,* 43:919, 1993.

Peterson RC, Freeman DP, Knox CA, et al. Successful treatment of spontaneous low cerebral fluid pressure. Headache (abstract). *Ann Neurol,* 22:148, 1987.

Rando TA, Fishman RA. Spontaneous intracranial hypotension: Report of two cases and review of the literature. *Neurology,* 42:481–487, 1992.

Schievink WI, Meyer FB, Atkinson JL. Spontaneous spinal cerebral fluid fluid leaks and intracranial hypotension. *J Neurosurg,* 84:598–605, 1996.

Sechzer PG, Abel L. Post-spinal anesthesia headache treated with caffeine: Evaluation with demand method. Part I. *Curr Ther Res,* 24:307–312, 1978.

Seebacher J, Ribeiro V, LeGuillou JL, et al. Epidural blood patch in the treatment of post-dural puncture headache: A double-blind study. *Headache,* 29:630–632, 1989.

Silberstein SD, Marcelis J. Headache associated with changes in intracranial pressure. *Headache,* 32:84–94, 1992.

Vakharia SB, Tomas PS, Rosenbaum AE, et al. Magnetic resonance imaging of cerebrospinal fluid leak and tamponade effect of blood patch in postdural puncture headache. *Anesth Analg,* 84:585–590, 1997.

Vilming ST, Titus F. Low cerebrospinal fluid pressure. (In) *The Headaches.* J Olesen, P Tfelt-Hansen, MA Welch (Eds). Pgs 687–695, New York, Raven, 1993.

Weitz SR, Drasner K. Spontaneous intracranial hypotension: A series. *Anaesthesia,* 85:923–925, 1996.

19

The Neck and Headache: Cervical Headache, Cervicogenic Headache, and Others

"A headache is surely more than just a pain in the neck; but it is that too!"
—Saper, 1993

I. Introduction

Controversy and confusion surround the role of the cervical spine and the development of headache. Classification and semantic differences contribute to the confusion. The scope of this book does not allow a detailed review of this controversy. Instead, an overview of cause and treatment considerations will be offered.

Based upon current data, it is likely that pain arising or felt in the neck rarely represents a distinctive clinical entity. There is no single cause of "cervical headache." Muscles, joints, nerves, components of the upper cervical spine, and migraine and cluster headache symptoms might all represent causes of pain felt in or arising in the neck. Moreover, the clinical examination and history are not generally capable of reliably distinguishing between these entities. In fact, it may be that contemporary investigators, reporting on various forms and syndromes of cervical headache, may be confronting variants of the same phenomenon (Bogduk, 1997), differing primarily in the source or origin of pain and the manner in which investigation has been undertaken.

Clearly, there are but a few headache disorders that *do not* occasionally, if not more frequently, include accompanying neck pain. Conversely, most neck pain disorders with identifiable pathology are associated with elements of headache, some of which occur in the orbital, temporal, and frontal regions.

The following cervical entities and syndromes are believed currently to represent primary disorders of the neck which can produce both headache and neck ache:

- Cervicogenic headache;
- C2 neuralgia;
- Neck-tongue syndrome;
- Third occipital headache;
- Atlantoaxial joint pain; and
- Occipital neuralgia.

II. Anatomy, Physiology, and Possible Mechanisms

(For pain pathways of head and neck, see Chapter 4.)

The trigeminal cervical nucleus (gray matter composed of the pars caudalis of the spinal nucleus of the trigeminal nerve and the gray matter of the upper cervical spinal cord segments) is the anatomical structure critical to the concept of cervical headache and head/neck referral patterns. Afferents from the trigeminal nerve and from the first three cervical spinal nerves relay through the trigeminal cervical nucleus. Overlapping and convergence form second-order neurons, the basis for referred pain (Bogduk, 1997). Cervical pain can be perceived in the territory of the trigeminal nerve, particularly the first division. In fact, pain of cervical origin is, perhaps frequently, referred to orbital and frontal regions. The "red ear syndrome" is a painful, burning red ear which is associated with the third cervical root, temporomandibular joint dysfunction or thalamic syndrome (Lance, 1996). The condition may occur without structural origin. It might reflect the angry back-firing C-nociceptive (ABC) syndrome. Antidromic release of vasoactive peptides may cause the ear symptoms.

Possible anatomical sources of headache within the cervical spine include the following:

1. The joints and ligaments of the median atlantoaxial joint, the atlanto-occipital joint, and the lateral atlantoaxial joints;
2. C2–3 zygapophyseal joint (facet joint)/nerves;
3. Suboccipital and upper posterior neck muscles;
4. Upper paravertebral muscles;
5. Spinal dura matter;
6. The vertebral artery;
7. C2–3 intervertebral disc; and
8. Trapezius and sternocleidomastoid muscles.

Figure 19.1 shows a map of the distribution of pain from zygapophyseal joints at segments C2–C3 to C6–C7, as reported by Dwyer and associates (1990).

III. Clinical Conditions

Many clinical conditions can cause headache and neck pain. These include:

A. Migraine

B. Cluster headache

C. Anomalies of the Craniocervical Junction

1. Basilar invagination;
2. Arnold Chiari malformation, Type I;
3. Congenital atlantoaxial dislocation;

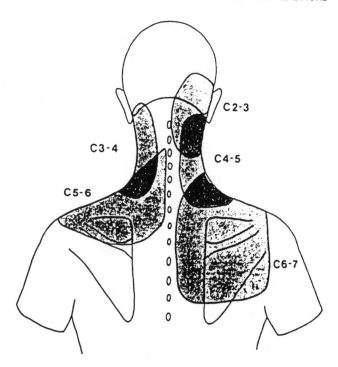

Figure 19.1. A composite map of the results in all volunteers depicting the putative characteristic distribution of pain from zygapophyseal joints at segments C2–3 to C6–7. (From Dwyer A, Aprill C, Bogduk N. Cervical zygapophyseal joint patterns I: A study in normal volunteers. *Spine* 15:453–457, 1990.)

    4. Dandy-Walker syndrome;
    5. Occipitalization of the axis; and
    6. Others.

D. Craniocervical Junction Disease

    1. Tumor;
    2. Neurofibroma;
    3. Infection;
    4. Paget's disease; and
    5. Others.

E. Arthritis/Ankylosing Spondylitis
F. Cervical Disc or Root Disease
G. Trauma
H. Others

IV. Specific Cervical Headache Syndromes

The following syndromes, several of which are the center of controversy, represent the key entities within this category.

A. Cervicogenic Headache.

First proposed by Sjaastad (1983), cervicogenic headache is a headache syndrome in which unilateral pain is provoked by neck movements or by pressure over areas of the neck. Reduced range of motion of the neck and neck pain are common. The headache is characterized by:

1. Continuing pain;
2. Varying duration;
3. Nonthrobbing discomfort from the neck; and
4. Spread to the oculofrontal regions.

The pain may be accompanied by photophobia, phonophobia, nausea, vomiting, dizziness, difficulty swallowing, and blurred vision. Diagnostically, blockade of cervical structures or cervical nerves relieves the headache, but this is not always the case and is thus not an essential diagnostic criterion.

B. C2 Neuralgia

C2 neuralgia is characterized by intermittent, lancinating pain in the occipital area, often associated with lacrimation and conjunctival injection. Dull occipital pain, as well as dull temporal, frontal, and orbital pain, are noted. A "cutting or tearing" sensation in the occipital region is frequently reported. The attacks are episodic and vary from a few per week to 5 per day, followed by a pain-free interval of days, weeks, or months. Approximately 75% of patients experience the autonomic disturbances. Also noted are blurred vision, rhinorrhea, and dizziness. Frequently, hypesthesia in the territory of the trigeminal and cervical nerves is present.

C2 neuralgia has been characterized as a "cluster-like" occipital headache. Pain relief generally follows local anesthetic blockade of the suspected nerve root, typically the C2 spinal nerve, performed with radiographic control. It does not respond to pharmacotherapy (Bogduk, 1997); however, surgery that frees entrapped nerves has been reported as effective. A dense venous network has been found around the C2 roots and identified in 50% of cadavers. However, surgical removal of venous anomalies in symptomatic patients does not reliably relieve the pain. Resection or thermal coagulation of the nerve apparently is more likely to bring relief (Jansen, 1989).

Anatomically, the C2 nerve travels behind the lateral atlantoaxial joint, in close proximity to its capsule. Diseases of the joint (inflammation, fibrosis, etc.) and entrapment are suspected as a cause of the syndrome.

C. Neck-Tongue Syndrome

This rare disorder is characterized clinically by the development of acute, unilateral, occipital pain provoked by sudden movement of the head (usually rotation). A sensation of numbness occurs in the ipsilateral half of the tongue. Currently, it is believed that subluxation of a lateral atlantoaxial joint causes the syndrome. Since proprioceptive afferents from the tongue pass into the C2 ventral ramus, it is believed that impingement or stretching of the C2 ventral ramus by the subluxated articular process results in tongue numbness. The condition is associated with disorders of the neck, which include rheumatoid arthritis and congenital joint laxity. A soft cervical collar may provide appropriate treatment, whereas in other cases, fusion or resection of C2 is required.

D. Third Occipital Headache (The Headache of Whiplash?)

Third occipital headache involves the C2–3 zygapophyseal (facet) joint. Entrapment or trauma to the third occipital nerve by osteophytes of C2–3 or traumatic arthritis of C2–3 appear to be fundamental to this syndrome. Bogduk (1988), using radiographically-controlled neuroblockade, demonstrated a number of patients whose headache could be relieved by anesthetizing either the C2–3 joint or the third occipital nerve. Although disputed, it now appears that this syndrome may be common in whiplash patients and is estimated to account for 58% of patients whose major complaint after whiplash is headache (Lord, 1994). The condition is diagnosed by radiographically-controlled blockade of the third occipital nerve and joint. Percutaneous thermal coagulation of the nerve has been tried, but the results are variable (Lord, 1995). In subsequent work, Lord, Bogduk, and others further established that cervical zygapophyseal joint pain is common among patients with chronic neck pain after whiplash. During a follow-up study, these same authors showed that in patients with chronic cervical zygapophyseal joint pain, confirmed with double-blind, placebo-controlled local anesthesia, a percutaneous radiofrequency neurotomy with multiple lesions of target nerves provided lasting relief.

E. Occipital Neuralgia

A detailed discussion of occipital neuralgia is found in Chapter 16. There is similarity between the lancinating form of occipital neuralgia and that described as a C2 neuralgia (Bogduk, 1997). Dorsal rhizotomy at C1–3 or C1–4 offers relief for up to 5 years, but recurrences are common. Partial posterior rhizotomy also provides relief to some patients but recurrence is likewise a problem and neuropathic sequelae are reported. Neurectomy is no longer advisable.

V. Overview of Cervical Syndromes

A variety of other pain patterns could arise from cervical disorders. Neuralgic syndromes, muscular and myofascial phenomena, and referred pain may all present as neck pain. Occipital pain may arise as a component of migraine and cluster headache.

VI. The Diagnosis

The diagnosis of cervical headache is complex. Clearly, computed tomography (CT) and magnetic resonance imaging (MRI) are important to rule out identifiable pathology. Electromyographic studies are generally not reliable in the high cervical region. Furthermore, since physical examination and clinical features do not distinguish these entities from each other, the use of diagnostic blocks has emerged as an important tool (Bogduk, 1997), although specificity and diagnostic certainty are lacking, according to some authorities. These blocks must be performed under radiographic control and by those experienced in the procedure. Technical limitations are present.

VII. Treatment

The treatment of neck pain with or without headache must take into account the general broad categories of illness described above, as well as the overall approach to treating head pain. Specific pathological disorders of the neck must be addressed appropriately. The following therapeutic methods are available:

1. Pharmacotherapy, using drugs generally effective for migraine, neuralgic syndromes, etc.;
2. Trigger point and neuroblockade (zygapophyseal/facet joint, and occipital nerve blocking);
3. Treating specific organic conditions, if identified;
4. Conservative physical medicine measures, including physical therapy, transneural stimulation (TNS), traction (can aggravate some cases of headache and neck pain), and biofeedback; and
5. Surgery and radiofrequency procedures.

VIII. Suggested Criteria for Suboccipital Blocking Procedures

1. The presence of persistent neck pain following appropriate conservative therapy;

2. The onset of pain following neck or head injury;
3. The identified or suspected presence of cervico-occipital pathology;
4. Provocation of headache by neck movement; and
5. The clear presence of localized pain foci in the occipitocervical junction.

IX. Special Considerations

Much more must be understood before a definitive relationship between cervical pathology and persistent headache can be defined fully and gain the consensus of most authorities. Persistent, nociceptive, afferent input to the nucleus caudalis, perhaps from as low as C5–6, could play a primary role in the development of headache. Similarly, intracranial irritation of dural veins and sinuses produces changes in the nucleus caudalis that might reflect pain perceived in the neck (Goadsby, 1991). Supraspinal, vascular, and other input to the system may be important. *Post-traumatic migraine* (Russell, 1996) following neck injury in patients not previously experiencing headache supports the possibility that injuries or disturbances of the neck region may result in "new onset" migraine. That superficial blockade in the occipitocervical junction brings temporary or even more permanent relief in some patients continues to defy simple explanation. Clearly, a constellation of central and peripheral phenomena, including changes in central modulation as a result of chronic peripheral pain, might contribute individually or concurrently to this confusing set of circumstances.

References

Aprill C, Dwyer A, Bogduk N. Cervical zygapophyseal joint pain patterns II: A clinical evaluation. *Spine*, 15:458–461, 1990.

Arner S, Lindbolm U, Meyerson BA, et al. Prolonged relief of neuralgia after regional anesthetic blocks: A call for further experimental and systemic clinical studies. *Pain*, 43:287–297, 1990.

Bogduk N. Local anesthetic blocks of the second cervical ganglion: Technique with application in occipital headache. *Cephalalgia*, 1:41–50, 1981.

Bogduk N. The clinical anatomy of the cervical dorsal rami. *Spine*, 7:319–330, 1982.

Bogduk N, Marsland A. The cervical zygapophyseal joints as a source of neck pain. *Spine*, 13:610–617, 1988.

Bogduk N. Headache and the neck. (In) *Headache*. PJ Goadsby, SD Silberstein (Eds). Pgs 369–381, Boston, Butterworth-Heinemeann, 1997.

Bovim G, Berg R, Dale LG. Cervicogenic headache: Anesthetic blockades of cervical nerves (C2–C5) and facet joint (C2/C3). *Pain*, 49:315–320, 1992a.

Bovim G, Fredriksen TA, Stolt-Nielsen A, et al. Neurolysis of the greater occipital nerve in cervicogenic headache: A follow-up study. *Headache*, 32:175–179, 1992b.

Busch E, Wilson PR. Atlanto-occipital and atlanto-axial injections in the treatment of headache and neck pain. *Reg Anesth*, 14 (supp 2):45, 1989.

Dwyer A, Aprill C, Bogduk N. Cervical zygapophyseal joint patterns I: A study in normal volunteers. *Spine*, 15:453–457, 1990.

Ehni G, Benner B. Occipital neuralgia in C1–C2 arthrosis syndrome. *J Neurosurg,* 61:961–965, 1984.

Gawel MJ, Rothbart PJ. Occipital nerve block in the management of headache and cervical pain. *Cephalalgia,* 12:9–13, 1992.

Goadsby PJ, Zagami AS. Stimulation of the superior sagittal sinus increases metabolic activity and blood flow in certain regions of the brainstem and upper cervical spinal cord of the cat. *Brain,* 114:1001–1011, 1991.

Gore DR, Sepic FB, Gardner GM, et al. Neck pain: A long-term follow-up of 205 patients. *Spine,* 12:1–5, 1987.

Graff-Radford SB, Reeves JL, Jaeger B. Management of chronic head and neck pain: Effectiveness of altering factors perpetuating myofascial pain. *Headache,* 27:186–190, 1987.

Jansen J, Bardosi A, Hildebrandt J, et al. Cervicogenic, hemicranial attacks associated with vascular irritation or compression of the cervical nerve root C2: Clinical manifestations and morphological findings. *Pain,* 39:203, 1989.

Keith WS. "Whiplash" injury of the second cervical ganglion and nerve. *Can J Neurol Sci,* 13:133–137, 1986.

Kerr FWL. A mechanism to account for frontal headache in cases of posterior fossa tumors. *J Neurosurg,* 18:605–609, 1961.

Kerr FWL. Central relationships of trigeminal and cervical primary afferents in the cord and medulla. *Brain Res,* 43:561–572, 1972.

Lamer TJ. Ear pain due to cervical spine arthritis: Treatment with cervical facet injection. *Headache,* 31:682–683, 1991.

Lance, JW. The red ear syndrome. *Neurology,* 47:617–620, 1996.

LaRocca H. Cervical sprain syndrome: Diagnosis, treatment, and long-term outcome. (In) *The Adult Spine: Principles and Practices.* JW Frymoyer (Ed). Pg 1051, New York, Raven Press, 1991.

Lord S, Barnsley L, Bogduk N. Percutaneous radiofrequency neurotomy in the treatment of cervical zygapophyseal joint pain: A caution. *Neurosurgery,* 36:732–739, 1995.

Lord S, Barnsley L, Bogduk N. The utility of comparative local anesthetic blocks vs. placebo-controlled blocks for the diagnosis of cervical zygapophyseal joint pain. *Clin J Pain,* 11:208, 1995.

Lord S, Barnsley L, Wallis BJ, et al. Third occipital headache: A prevalence study. *J Neurol Neurosurg, Neuropsych,* 57:1187–1190, 1994.

Lord S, Barnsley L, Wallis BJ, et al. Chronic cervical zygapophyseal joint pain after whiplash: A placebo-controlled prevalence study. *Spine,* 12:1737–1744, 1996.

McNamera RM, O'Brien MC, Davidheizer S. Post-traumatic neck pain: A prospective and follow-up study. *Ann Emerg Med,* 17:906–911, 1988.

Olesen J. Clinical and pathophysiological observations in migraine and tension-type headache explained by integration of vascular, supraspinal, and myofascial input. *Pain,* 46:125–132, 1991.

Russell MB, Olesen J. Migraine associated with head trauma. *Eur J Neurol,* 3:424–428, 1996.

Russell MD, Rasmussen BK, Fenger K, et al. Migraine without aura and migraine with aura are distinct clinical entities: A study of 484 male and female migraineurs from the general population. *Cephalalgia,* 16:239–245, 1996.

Sjaastad O, Fredriksen TA, Pfaffenrath V. Cervicogenic headache: Diagnostic criteria. *Headache,* 30:725, 1990.

Sjaastad O, Saunte C, Hovdahl H, et al. "Cervicogenic" headache: An hypothesis. *Cephalalgia,* 3:249, 1983.

Travell JG, Dimons DJ. Posterior cervical muscles: Semispinalis capitis, semispinalis cervices, and multifidi: "Pain in the neck." (In) *Myofascial Pain and Dysfunction: The Trigger Point Manual.* JG Travell, DG Simons (Eds). Pg 305, Baltimore, Williams & Wilkins, 1983.

Winston KR. Whiplash and its relationship to migraine. *Headache,* 27:452–467, 1987.

20

Borderline Personality Disorder

I. Introduction

The treatment of headache is frequently confounded by the presence of psychological comorbidities, including personality disorders. Among the personality disorders, the one that presents the most challenging dilemmas during the treatment of headache is the Borderline Personality Disorder (BPD). Though not necessarily recognizing it as such, many physicians who share their anecdotes about impossible and angry patients are describing patients with BPD. This chapter will review BPD and recommend a variety of management approaches that might aid in the treatment of patients with BPD who suffer from headache and related painful phenomena.

A personality disorder (PD) is an *enduring pattern of inner experience and behavior that deviates significantly from the expectations of an individual's culture and peer group, is pervasive and inflexible, and has an onset in adolescence or early adulthood.* It is generally stable over time but can be exacerbated and intensified by life stressors. It leads to distress and impairment.

There are ten specific PDs (see Table 20.1). Please refer to the Diagnostic and Statistical Manual of Mental Disorders-Revised (DSM IV-R) for detailed descriptions. The Personality Disorders are referred to as "Axis II" diagnoses, which include personality disorders and mental retardation. Axis I disorders are generally those of the major psychiatric conditions, such as major depression, psychosis, etc. *The presence of an Axis II disorder, particularly BPD, in a patient with headache reliably converts even the most straight-forward borderline case to a supreme clinical "challenge."*

II. General Clinical Features of Personality Disorders

In general, PD traits represent continuing and enduring patterns of interpreting, perceiving, thinking about, and relating to one's environment, as well as oneself. They are exhibited in a broad spectrum of social and personal contexts. When a personality trait becomes inflexible, disruptive, and causes functional impairment, it then constitutes a more formal definition of PD. The diagnosis of a PD requires an assessment of an individual's long-term patterns of functioning, although certain traits of behavior may prompt suspicion of its presence. A single interview rarely is sufficient to confirm the diagnosis. Certain personality features may be sufficiently subtle

TABLE 20.1. **SPECIFIC PERSONALITY DISORDERS**

- Paranoid P.D.
- Schizoid P.D.
- Schizotypal P.D.
- Antisocial P.D.
- Borderline P.D.
- Histrionic P.D.
- Narcissistic P.D.
- Avoidant P.D.
- Dependent P.D.
- Obsessive-Compulsive P.D.
- P.D., Not Otherwise Specified

so as not be readily evident. Moreover, in some disorders, such as BPD, inaccurate, deceptive, or even delusional interpretations of events can be misleading. *A proper diagnosis requires collateral information from others.* Finally, some behavioral patterns may result from crisis situations and do not span a broad enough period to fulfill diagnostic criteria.

Borderline and histrionic, as well as dependent PD, occur more frequently, if not dominantly, in women. The course of the illness is such that recognition is often possible in adolescence or early adulthood, but the pattern, by definition, is persistent and reflects the way a person thinks, feels, and behaves through a good part of his life. Some of the PD, including borderline, may "burn out" and become somewhat less evident after the age of 50.

III. Clinical Features of Borderline Personality Disorder (BPD)

Patients with BPD are frequently characterized as angry, impulsive, and unpredictable individuals. Their behavior frequently makes other people feel "on edge," and they may often display a hurtful, sullen, or distressed appearance. They are frequently described by others as nasty and obstinate, often volatile. They may be manipulative and unpredictable. Events are frequently exaggerated and distorted, and intense expectations are on others with respect to support and caring. Patients are prone to punish people by silence or by other behaviors, and are frequently offended by trivial disappointments, disagreements, or setbacks. They are frequently impatient and irritable unless things go according to their expectations and demands.

BPD individuals often feel unappreciated, cheated, or discontent. They often believe that they are misunderstood. Terms such as obstructive, pessimistic, and immature are frequently applied to them, and they blame others for the distress or disruption that their behavior causes.

Many, but not all, BPD patients are unable to achieve the social status they seek, and this may reflect either rejection or other obstacles that result from their behavior and erratic personal nature. They often have repeated failures, including educational efforts and marriages, and complicate their own lives and those around them by their behavior.

BPD patients may have stress-provoked transient psychotic events. Some are paranoid in nature and can be prolonged.

Failed relationships, hormonal changes, and other factors that often alter stability can cause an escalation. A loss of boundary-setting influences, through divorce, death, rejection, or other, can be provocative and cause decompensation.

IV. Specific Diagnostic Criteria for BPD

The following are criteria of BPD. Five are necessary to establish the diagnosis.

1. Frantic efforts to avoid abandonment;
2. Unstable and intense interpersonal relationships that may vary between extremes of idealization and devaluation;
3. "Identity disturbance"—markedly and persistently unstable self-image or sense of self;
4. Impulsivity, which can be self-damaging (spending, sex, substance abuse, reckless driving, binge eating);
5. Recurrent suicidal or self-destructive threats or self-mutilating behavior (weight loss, overuse of medications, or frank efforts at attention-getting through risk behaviors);
6. Affective instability due to reactivity of mood, e.g., intense, episodic dysphoria and/or irritability, or anxiety, usually lasting a few hours or rarely more than a few days;
7. Chronic feelings of emptiness;
8. Inappropriate, intense anger or difficulty controlling anger (frequent displays of temper, constant anger, recurrent physical fights); and
9. Transient stress-related paranoid ideation or severe dissociated symptoms ("You are out to hurt me; you don't want to help me anymore," etc.).

V. Etiology of BPD

The etiology of BPD is uncertain. Biological origins are possible, and genetic implications are suspected. From a psychological point of view, childhood neglect, emotional trauma, and abuse (often sexual) are considered potential origins and are frequently found in the history of those with BPD. The accuracy of "abuse" reports has been questioned, since individuals with BPD either intentionally or otherwise misinterpret or distort the events and relationships of their lives.

VI. Prevalence

BPD is found in 2% of the general population. Ten percent of patients in an outpatient mental health clinic suffer from BPD. BPD is five times more common in first-degree biological relatives of those with BPD. There is an increased risk for substance-related disorders and antisocial disorders.

VII. Comorbidity: Migraine and BPD

Hegarty (1993) evaluated 112 sequential patients (24 male, 88 female) who had been diagnosed with BPD and were attending outpatient and emergency psychiatric departments in a metropolitan hospital center. The overall prevalence of severe headache was 60.4% in those with BPD, clearly substantially higher than in the general population, and was associated with high prevalence in both men (24%) and women (50%). Accompanying symptoms included suicide attempts (20% males, 63% females), violent outbursts, and substance abuse. In women more than men, a history of impulse control was noted. The author emphasized that depression, suicidality, impulsivity, violence, and migraine all have been associated with central biochemical disturbance, particularly serotoninergic disregulation. Perhaps serotoninergic and other biochemical mechanisms are common to BPD and certain headache disorders.

VIII. Behaviors that Affect (Sabotage) or Influence Headache Treatment

The patient with BPD is frequently an individual who early in the course of headache treatment will give signs of the disturbance and will come to the attention of the alert physician or staff as a result of these behaviors. These include:

1. The malevolent "hug sign" (coined by Robert Hamel, P.A.-C, 1993). It includes inappropriate physical and/or emotional "hugging." Patients will demonstrate early in the relationship overly familiar physical and verbal behavior and a tendency to prematurely glorify with praise (often followed by sharp criticism when disappointed). Frequently encountered statements may include, "You are the first physician who has ever taken my symptoms seriously"; "I know you will make me better"; "You are the best physician I've ever seen." Bringing gifts and food to staff is often characteristic following the first visit.

2. Pushing limits, unsatisfiable neediness, inappropriate requests for medications or other special favors;

3. Irritability or anger with the physician or staff (often expressed through others) when demands are not met;

4. A recurring pattern of chaos, distress, or unexplained clinical phenomena, such as unusual and extreme side effects, disruptive behavior, manipulative behaviors, etc.;

5. Severe reactions to any distancing, limit-setting, or reduction in medications;

6. Behaviors which serve to "split" physician from other physicians, staff members from each other, or in other ways to interfere with orderliness in the day-to-day patient-doctor relationship;

7. Persistent efforts to acquire more medication than prescribed, excessive usage, and the use of devious means to obtain prescriptions;

8. Perceiving events of care in an "all or nothing" fashion (reflects the extreme idealization and devaluation pattern). The care is seen as all good or all bad, a physician's statement of encouragement is seen as a *promise* to help, or a physician's limit setting is perceived as an accusation, as in "You called me a drug addict."; and

9. Failure to take responsibility for behaviors. This manifests in the "blame game," whereby others are blamed for the plight of the patient, without a willingness to accept responsibility for one's own behavior.

These behaviors and others make it very difficult to treat the headaches of patients with BPD. Patients may exhibit *cephalgiaphobia,* a term we believe was first used by Harvey Featherstone, M.D., and which reflects anxiety over painful events, which prompts excessive and obsessive drug-taking behavior and ultimately medication overuse. Simple drug overuse patterns, as well as frank addictive disease, are both encountered in patients with headache and BPD, and attempts to set limits often result in sharp, confrontational interactions.

The use of opioids in patients with BPD and headache is likely to fail and result in serious overuse patterns, if not an intensification of disrupted behaviors. Hospitalization is generally disorderly and can result in confrontational behavior and interaction, splitting of staff and other patients, and frequently, though not always, an unsuccessful stay.

It may be that the pressure of pain provides a means to control relationships and avoid "abandonment". Relief of pain may threaten stability and the means with which to control others.

IX. Treatment Approaches for BPD
A. Primary Treatments

The most useful treatment for BPD appears to be a combination of psychotherapy and pharmacotherapy. One of the more popular behavioral therapies is referred to as dialectical behavioral therapy (DBT), as popularized by Linehan (1991). This therapy contains elements of behavioral, cognitive, and supportive psychotherapy. Therapy is often conducted weekly, in both individual and group sessions. Other forms of psychotherapy are also employed.

Pharmacological treatments are of potential value. No treatment is universally effective, but most psychiatrists administer some medication to control symptoms. Anecdotal personal experience (JRS, BH) demonstrates that neuroleptics (risperidone and olanzapine) may be of considerable value in some patients. Dosages should generally be kept low and are useful for impulse control, psychotic-type symptoms, depression, and anxiety. Headache benefit is possible.

Tricyclic antidepressants may be of value in patients with depression but may also increase anger and lessen impulse control. MAO inhibitors may be useful in some patients.

Open-label trials of fluoxetine, as well as sertraline, have unproven efficacy in reducing self-injury, suicidality, affective instability, rage, impulsivity, psychosis, and obsessionality. No single SSRI has emerged as the treatment of choice, and individuals failing one may respond to another.

The anticonvulsants are sometimes effective in managing anger and impulse control. Divalproex and carbamazepine are both noted to be of potential benefit. Divalproex has established headache control benefits as well, and may thus be of particular value.

Anxiolytics, and perhaps opioids and alchohol, may increase behavioral discontrol and generally should be avoided.

Medications are frequently abused. Since dependency on drugs is a significant risk, long-term maintenance therapy has not been shown to be of particular benefit, but short-term adjunctive use of medication may be important in the management of patients with BPD.

B. Other Therapeutic Recommendations

A key factor in approaching a patient with BPD and headache is the *setting of firm limits and expectations regarding behavior and treatment*. Precise limits must be established and boundaries defined. Specific goals must be identified. Inappropriate behaviors must be confronted, and there must be an insistence upon psychological/psychiatric treatment. The following guidelines are recommended as soon as the diagnosis is suspected:

- Identify potential problems early;
- Establish early and clear limit setting and boundary definitions regarding treatment, drug use, and behavior;
- Establish the principle that the problems are not "someone

else's" fault, and that the patient must accept his/her role in his/her own distress and therapy (internal locus of control);

- Focus on specific goals for treatment;
- Confront behavior problems with firmness, candor, and consistency;
- Identify splitting behaviors and don't become a "victim"; don't enable the patient or "buy into" the trap;
- Insist as a condition of care that coordinated psychological/psychiatric treatment be undertaken;
- Discontinue treatment when appropriate; and
- Establish a treatment contract.

X. A Treatment Contract

Once a BPD patient has been diagnosed or strongly suspected as having BPD, a treatment contract is essential. Elements of a treatment contract include the following:

1. Emphasize patient responsibility for compliance (not staff's responsibility)
   - Agreement to comply
   - Acceptance of drug and dose limitations
   - Agreement to psychiatric referral
2. Agreement upon goals of treatment and time limitations for outpatient visits, hospitalization, etc.
3. Agreement to tolerate some level of pain until best treatments can be found
4. Identification of expectations for pain control
   - Complete pain relief is not possible
   - Some pain will have to be tolerated
   - Medications must be used according to established limits
5. Specify unacceptable disruptive behavior and consequences*
   - No intense anger expressions or outbursts
   - No profanity
   - No throwing objects
   - No self-harm
   - No destruction of property
   - No medication excesses or limit violations
6. Specify means of informing staff of suicidal feelings
7. Identify consequences for noncompliance or failure to keep contract
   - Transfer to other physician, psychiatrist
   - Discontinuance of care

8. Frequent visits may help to control behavior and lessen anxiety.

   * A recently hospitalized headache patient proudly proclaimed that she had "trashed" the last hospital she was in, as well as loudly cursed the staff. As part of her pre-admission contract, she specifically agreed not to do any trashing, verbally or physically. She did not, and the hospital stay was orderly.

   Do not acquiesce or enable a patient by accepting or tolerating manipulation, anger, or any other unacceptable behavior.

   Finally, a suggested statement to patients who are angry and disruptive: "I know that anger is a problem for you. Your anger is also a problem for me and my staff. Anger cannot be tolerated when it is as inappropriate as is yours. Anger is also important in headache provocation. You must address your anger and control it as part of your treatment. It is your responsibility. If it is not controlled, we will no longer care for you."

   Special thanks to Alvin E. Lake III, Ph.D. for sharing his material, experience, and advice, and to Robert Hamel, P.A.-C for his astute clinical observations.

References

Allen DM. Techniques for reducing therapy: Interfering behavior in patients with borderline personality disorder. Similarities in four diverse treatment paradigms. *J Psychother Pract Res,* 6:25–35, 1997.

Beck AT, Freeman A, et al. *Cognitive Therapy of Personality Disorders.* New York, Guilford Press, 1990.

Clarkin JF, Marziali E, Nunroe-Blum H. *Borderline Personality Disorder: Clinical and Empirical Perspectives.* New York, Guilford Press, 1992.

Hegarty AM. The prevalence of migraine in borderline personality disorder (abstract). *Headache,* 33:291, 1993.

Kutcher S, Papathe O, Dorou G, et al. The successful pharmacological treatment of adolescents and young adults with borderline personality disorder: A preliminary open trial of flupenthixol. *J Psychiatry Neurosci,* 20:113–118, 1995.

Lake AE III. Behavioral assessment considerations in the management of headache. *Headache,* 21:170–178, 1981.

Linehan MM. *Cognitive-Behavioral Treatment of Borderline Personality Disorder.* New York, Guilford Press, 1993.

Linehan MM, Oldham JM, Silk KR. Dx: Personality Disorder . . . Now What? *Patient Care,* pp. 75–84, 1995.

Markovitz PJ, Wagner SC, Venlafaxin E. In the treatment of borderline personality disorder. *Psychopharmacol Bull,* 31:773–777, 1995.

Primavera JP III, Kaiser RS. The relationship between locus of control, amount of preadmission analgesic/ergot use, and length of stay for patients admitted for inpatient treatment of chronic headache. *Headache,* 34:204–208, 1994.

Salzman C, Wolfson AN, Schatzberg A, et al. The effect of fluoxetine on anger in symptomatic volunteers with borderline personality disorder. *J Clin Psychopharmacol,* 15:23–29, 1995.

Silk KR, Eisner W, Allport C, et al. Focused time-limited inpatient treatment of borderline personality disorder. *J Pers Disord,* 8:268–278, 1994.

Stein DG, Simeon D, Frenkel M. An open trial of valproate in borderline personality disorder. *J Clin Psychiatry,* 56:506–510, 1995.

Wilcox JA. Divalproex sodium as a treatment for borderline personality disorder. *Ann Clin Psychiatry,* 7:33–37, 1995.

Zanarini MC, Williams AA, Lewis RE, et al. Reported pathological childhood experiences associated with the development of borderline personality disorder. *Am J Psychiatry,* 154:1101–1106, 1997.

21

When All Else Fails: What to Do and When to Refer

Note to readers: This chapter consolidates thoughts contained elsewhere in the text and should be used in conjunction with Chapters 3 and 5 (diagnostic evaluation and differential diagnosis) as well as treatment chapters, including Chapters 6, 8, 9, 11, 12, and others that deal with specific entities.

The physician frequently encounters patients with headache who do not respond to what appear to be appropriately administered standard interventions. The patient reports persisting or recurring pain despite even aggressive efforts. Standard diagnostic tests provide little in the way of relevant information or data with which to alter the diagnosis or provide an alternative treatment or identified etiology. Often the patient's desperation and demeanor leave little doubt as to the legitimacy of the reported pain. He/she seeks over and again the means to achieve effective treatment and pain relief.

I. Reasons Why Headache Patients Do Not Get Better (modified from Buchholz, 1996)

- Wrong diagnosis;
- "Rebound" or excessive medication usage, toxicity, etc.;
- Failure of patient to avoid "triggers" and activators;
- Medication selection not proper or dosages not adequate;
- Comorbid conditions have not been addressed; the presence of Borderline Personality Disorder or other personality disorder;
- Goals and outcome expectations are unreliable;
- "Hidden agenda";
- Physiological mechanisms or factors not yet understood and/or effectively treated with current interventions; and
- Others.

The following represents an approach to such patients.

II. More History

Among the most valuable adages in clinical neurology is, "When all else fails, take more history." This exhortation has appeared and reappeared over and again during medical training, because it recognizes that more clinical information may ultimately lead to better diagnosis and ultimately to effective treatment.

The following considerations are **among** the most important:

A History of Trauma

Is there a traumatic history? Frequently overlooked in the standard history is a mild to moderate closed head injury or cervical injury, which can cause headache or render an individual more likely to be refractory to standard headache treatments. Such a history will also explain other coexisting phenomena or findings that may accompany mild closed head injury, including the presence of occipitocervical local pain (which might respond to blocking procedures, including facet joint and cervical nerve blockade), depression, sleep disturbance, and others. The "red ear syndrome," for example, may indicate a 3rd cervical root syndrome (see Chapter 19, Lance, 1996).

B. Relieving/Aggravating Factors

A clue to the diagnosis and often to a different approach to treatment can sometimes be found by a careful pursuit of relieving and aggravating factors that might go beyond those that would be otherwise asked in a standard historical review. Among these include any postural components (pain differences when lying down and standing up) and provocation from straining or movement of the head and neck. Positional lightheadedness, neck pain, and provocation by flexion or extension of the neck are among the important factors in such a review. Consideration should also be given to "low-pressure" headache patterns from previous lumbar puncture (LP) or epidural block, spontaneous cerebrospinal fluid (CSF) leakage, etc.

C. General Medical Symptoms

Any recent general medical or neurological symptom or change in medicines used for unrelated reasons is important, with a particular emphasis on headache-provoking treatments. Headache associated illnesses, infection, or hormonal disturbances are likewise important.

D. Reconsideration of Onset

Also helpful can be a reconsideration of onset. What were the events and details at onset; and how rapidly did the headache begin? New onset headache and sudden, rapid acceleration of the headache are important. Consider sphenoid sinusitis among important new onset disorders.

E. Environmental Causes

Exposure to fumes, toxins, or other environmental elements can be headache provoking. Specific inquiry into carbon monoxide exposure is prudent. Obtain a smoking history, including frequency and quantity.

F. Dental History

The presence or absence of recent symptoms or intervention of a dental nature should be explored. Root canals, tooth extractions, or bite disturbances may provoke or be associated with the development of an intractable headache, including migraine.

G. Dermatological Concerns

The recent development of a skin rash (as in Lyme disease) or vesicles (as in herpes zoster) or other dermatological problem that might indicate the presence or absence of systemic or localized disease related to headache need to be investigated.

H. Ocular History

The presence of ocular disturbances, such as increased intraocular pressure, or localized infection, tearing, or related disturbances must be considered.

I. Otological Problems

Otological problems, such as nasal blockage, drainage, pressure, or other features, should be pursued (consider nasopharyngeal carcinoma, which can present with headache).

J. Medication Review

A review of all medications, over-the-counter (OTC) and prescribed, is a worthwhile undertaking. Give special consideration to caffeine usage, OTC medication and "health food" supplements (including vitamins), and other drugs which individually or collectively (toxic influence) can produce headache symptoms. The SSRIs may be useful for headache in some patients, but they are well known to produce pain and aggravate headache in others. Aspartame and monosodium glutamate (MSG) produce headache in some people.

In addition, establish true pattern of usage of previous medications that have "failed":

- Were these medicines provided at a time when the patient was "rebounding" and thus of less value?
- Were dosages taken to the appropriate level to provide therapeutic impact?
- Were they used in combination appropriately to provide an added measure of intervention in patients with refractory symptoms?
- What was the duration of usage?

K. Life Style

The patient's work hours, sleep/wakefulness cycles, the presence of sleep apnea, etc. should be considered.

These and many variables must be considered and reconsidered in patients with intractable conditions. Although many of these questions might have been asked initially, a reconsideration of these and other standard and more subtle nuances is essential and may lead to greater understanding of patients with headache.

III. Head/Neck and Neurological Evaluation

Very little can substitute for a careful neurological examination, with attention to those parts that are particularly important in headache provocation, such as eyes, ears, neck, and other trigeminal regions. Special attention should be paid to:

- Movement of the neck;
- The presence of occipitocervical pain on palpation and movement;
- The presence of submandibular pain (indicating styloid process factors, lymph nodes, carotid artery disturbances or masses);
- Disc margin clarity, visual function, and eye movement;
- Oral cavity health or pain sources;
- Facial sensation; and
- Others.

The clinician should obtain appropriate consultations from:

- Mental health professionals;
- Ear-nose-throat, ophthalmological, and dental consultants; and
- Endocrinological/gynecological consultants when appropriate and suggested by the nature of the patient's headache pattern.

IV. Illnesses to be Considered or Reconsidered That Can "Mimic" or Aggravate/Activate Benign Headache Syndromes (also see Chapters 3, 5, 16, 19, and others)

1. Low/high CSF pressure syndromes (increased intracranial pressure [ICP] or low pressure syndromes, such as idiopathic intracranial hypertension or hypotension [spontaneous or provoked "leak" syndromes])
2. Acute or chronic sphenoid sinusitis;
3. Infections—Lyme disease, HIV, encephalitis, fungal meningitis, etc.;
4. Carotid or vertebral artery dissection/cerebrovascular disease;
5. Cerebral vein or sinus thrombosis;
6. Occipital/cervical disease, including Arnold Chiari Malformation Type I, upper cervical and facet joint, root, or nerve (neuralgic) syndromes;
7. Hormonal disturbances/endocrinological disease (e.g., estrogen

factors, recent treatment with progesterone, thyroid disease, prolactin elevation, etc.);

8. Metabolic disturbances (including hepatitis, renal disease, B_{12} deficiency, anemia, toxins, hyponatremia, carbon monoxide elevation, vitamin A or D toxicity, etc.);
9. Overuse of medications (rebound or toxic drug overuse syndromes);
10. Otolaryngological disease, including acute or chronic sphenoid sinusitis (or other sinus disease) and nasopharyngeal disturbances, including tumor (may require ENT visualization/assessment);
11. Disorders along the course of the trigeminal nerve, including dental and oral disease, and jaw pathology;
12. Glaucoma and other ocular diseases; and
13. Vasculitis/rheumatic/connective tissue disorders.

V. Additional Diagnostic Tests (see Chapter 3 and others)

Experience demonstrates that initial testing may provide normal results, but repeat study will occasionally demonstrate pathology that was either not initially evident. In the presence of intractable symptoms of pain, responsible repeat testing and additional testing are sometimes justified.

- LP to assess the presence of inflammatory or infectious changes or alteration of CSF pressure;
- Cisternography, computed tomography (CT) myelogram, or flow-sensitive magnetic resonance imaging (MRI) if CSF leak is suspected;
- Repeat MRI and CT scanning with special attention to the posterior fossa and occipitocervical junction, nasopharyngeal regions, and sphenoid sinus. (Standard CT scanning may not provide adequate views of the sphenoid, and radiological attention should be focused, and sinus views ordered, when evaluating patients with suspected sphenoid disease.);
- Otolaryngological, ophthalmological, and dental consultation if appropriate; and
- MRI/MR angiogram (MRA) of the carotid or vertebral arteries or venous studies for cerebrovenous thrombosis.

More extensive studies, including arteriography, are rarely justified but should be considered in individuals when the symptoms of headache or pain are accompanied by factors which would otherwise be considered not identifiable **except** by arteriographic procedures.

VI. Treatments of Intractable Headaches see Chapter 8 and 9)

The treatments considered in Chapters 6, 8, 9, 11, 12, and others will not be repeated here. The reader is referred to these and other chapters for review of treatment.

VII. Consider Referral to a Tertiary Facility for Inpatient Management and Comprehensive Programming (see Chapters 2, 9, and 11)

The use of tertiary systems for the care of intractable headache patients remains ill-defined and arbitrary, but outcome studies suggest benefit (see Chapter 2). Criteria that might be used to make such a referral would include:

1. Patients with intractable severe pain who fail to respond to standard treatments;
2. Patients unable to refrain from the excessive use of treatments that might contribute to the persisting pain (rebounding, etc.);
3. Patients with medical illnesses that confound and/or complicate the treatment of pain;
4. Patients in whom behavioral and psychological factors are interwoven and enmeshed with the headache disorder, such that outpatient treatment is not likely to produce effective control;
5. Patients requiring a combination of detoxification, headache interruption, and the development of a preventive program such that outpatient treatment is unlikely to provide an adequate pace or the appropriate intensity of treatment to achieve maximal results;
6. When the severity of pain and the patient's desperation require the most aggressive and speedy pain control available;
7. Cases of headache that require comprehensive team-oriented, coordinated, interdisciplinary intervention; and
8. Persistent headache that requires advanced diagnostic and treatment services not found in primary or secondary levels of care.

References

Baumgartner CP, Wesseley P, Bingol C, et al. Long-term prognosis of analgesic withdrawal in patients with drug-induced headache. *Headache,* 29:510–514, 1989.

Belegrade MJ, Ling LJ, Schleevogt MB, et al. Comparison of single dose meperidine, butorphanol, and dihydroergotamine in treatment of vascular headache. *Neurology,* 39:590–592, 1989.

Bell R, Montoya D, Shuaib A, et al. A comparative trial of three agents in the treatment of acute migraine headache. *Ann Emerg Med,* 19:1079–1082, 1990.

Buchholz D. Personal Communication, 1996.

Busson EG, et al. Short-lasting unilateral neuralgiform headache attacks with tearing and conjunctival injection: The first "symptomatic" case? *Cephalalgia,* 11:123–127, 1991.

Callaham M, Raskin NH. A controlled study of dihydroergotamine in the treatment of acute migraine headache. *Headache,* 26:168–171, 1986.

Diener HC, Dichgans J, Scholz E, et al. Analgesic-induced chronic headache: Long-term results of withdrawal therapy. *J Neurol,* 236:9–14, 1989.

Edmeads J. Emergency management of headache. *Headache,* 28:675–9, 1988.

Fusco BM, Marabine S, Maggi CA, et al. Preventive effective repeated nasal applications of capsaicin in cluster headache. *Pain,* 59:321–325, 1994.

Gaukroger PB, Brownridge R. Epidural blood patch in treatment of chronic headache. *Can J Anaesth,* 35:322–323, 1988.

Gordon RE, Moser FG, Pressman BD, et al. Resolution of pachymeningeal enhancement following dural puncture and blood patch. *Neuroradiology,* 37: 557–558, 1995.

Jones J, Sklar D, Dogherty J, et al. Randomized double-blind trial of intravenous prochlorperazine for the treatment of acute headache. *JAMA,* 261:1174–1176, 1989.

Lance JW, Branch GB. Persistent headaches after lumbar puncture (letter). *Lancet* 343:414, 1994.

Mathew NT. Advances in cluster headache. *Neurol Clin,* 8:867–890, 1990.

Mathew NT, Hurt W. Percutaneous radiofrequency trigeminal gangliorhizolysis in intractable cluster headache. *Headache,* 28:328–231, 1988.

Neuman M, Demarez JP, Harmer JR, et al. Prevention of migraine attacks through use of dihydroergotamine. *Int J Clin Pharmacol Res,* 6:11–13, 1986.

Pareja, et al. SUNCT syndrome: Repetitive and overlapping attacks. *Headache,* 34:114–116, 1994.

Rapoport AM, Silberstein SD. Emergency treatment of headache. SD Silberstein (Ed). *Neurology,* Supp 2, March, 1992.

Rapoport A, Weeks R, Sheftell F, et al. Analgesic rebound headache: Theoretical and practical implications. *Cephalalgia,* 5(supp 3):448–450, 1985.

Raskin NH. Repetitive intravenous dihydroergotamine as therapy for intractable migraine. *Neurology,* 36:995–997, 1986.

Sable SG, Ramadan NM. Meningeal enhancement in low CSF pressure headache: An MRI study. *Cephalalgia,* 11:275–276, 1991.

Saper JR. Diagnosis and symptomatic treatment of migraine. *Headache,* 37 (Suppl 1):S1–S14, 1997.

Saper JR, Jones JM. Ergotamine tartrate dependency: Features and possible mechanisms. *Clin Neuropharmacol,* 9:244–256, 1986.

Silberstein SD, Schulman EA, Hopkins MM. Repetitive intravenous DHE in the treatment of refractory headache. *Headache,* 30:334–339, 1990.

Silberstein SD, Silberstein JR. Analgesic/ergotamine rebound headache: Prognosis following detoxification and treatment with repetitive IV DHE. *Headache,* 32:352, 1992.

Sjaastad O, Saunter C, Salveen R, et al. Short-lasting unilateral neuralgiform headache with conjunctival injection and tearing and rhinorrhea. *Cephalalgia,* 9:147–156, 1989.

Tahu JM, Tew JM. Long-term results of radiofrequency rhizotomy in the treatment of cluster headache. *Headache,* 35:193–196, 1995.

Index